ON THE THEORY AND PRACTICAL APPLICATION OF CHANNELS AND COLLATERALS

Guan Zun hui

Translated and edited by Andrew McPherson

BALBOA.PRESS

A DIVISION OF HAY HOUSE

Balboa Press books may be ordered through booksellers or by contacting:

Balboa Press
A Division of Hay House
1663 Liberty Drive
Bloomington, IN 47403
www.balboapress.com.au
AU TFN: 1 800 844 925 (Toll Free inside Australia)
AU Local: (02) 8310 7086 (+61 2 8310 7086 from outside Australia)

ISBN: 978-1-5043-1882-2 (sc)
ISBN: 978-1-5043-1883-9 (e)

Print information available on the last page.

Balboa Press rev. date: 08/13/2024

FOREWORD

I have translated and edited this document in order that people have a better understanding of acupuncture, and also TCM theory, as practised in China today. Where-as most of the current literature is found in publications from the 1970's and early 80's in China, there is little from the last decade or two. While, this book was, in fact, written and published originally in the mid - 1980's in China, I have found that much of what is written here is still not known or understood in the West. Although, primarily an epidemiological work, I have tested everything Professor Guan says in his book. I believe this dispenses with the need for any highly questionable conclusions or theories made by some members of the acupuncture community in modern times because of the lack of more advanced material like what is presented now. In fact, much of the material here is backed with many many quotes from the classics.

This, then is my translation of Professor Guan Zun hui's book and while, in many cases, I have had to virtually invent words to describe what Professor Guan means, I believe it to be a good translation of the original. Ever since my days at university, I have been warned against too literal a translation or too broad. Much of what language Professor Guan uses will have to be excused as the Chinese government way of saying things, at the time, or enthusiasm as a result of reading so much Chinese literature. With this in mind, this book will provide many hours of informative reading.

Andrew McPherson.

Channels and collaterals (jing-luo) theory is the basic theory of Chinese medicine. It makes up the complete Chinese medicine theory system which includes ying yang, wu zang, zang xiang, ying wei and qi xue etc. Channels and collaterals theory is the main theoretical basis that Chinese medicine demonstrates and analyses, physiologically and pathologically, and is used for diagnosis and treatment. Channels and collaterals theory, not only is the theoretical nucleus of acupuncture study, it also has general guidance meaning for each Department of Chinese medicine in the clinical situation.

The purpose of writing this book is to systematically introduce the theory of channels and collaterals, and to demonstrate the control function of channels and collaterals theory in the Chinese medicine treatment system. Hopefully it will represent the leading functions and important meaning of channels and collaterals theory in the identification pattern of illnesses for treatment, via the description of the Chinese application of channels and collaterals theory and illness case example analysis.

This book is divided into first and second sections, and appendices. The first section describes channels and collaterals theory. The demonstration part of this section describes in total the concept of channels and collaterals, the clinical value of channels and collaterals theory, and the formation and development of channels and collaterals theory. Each demonstrative part completely describes the 12 channels illness conditions, the eight extra ordinary channels, the jing bie luo mai, the jing jin theory and the pi bu theory. The second section demonstrates the guidance meaning of channels and collaterals. In the clinical application aspects of acupuncture combination points, needling insertion hand techniques, channels and collaterals treatment methods, and medicines formulae etc. are all shown to represent needling function and treatment in accordance with channels and collaterals in Chinese medicine theory. In the Chinese medicine aspect, "li, fa, fang, yao" ("theory, technique, formulae, medicine"), is used to look at specific illness case examples from different angles, the appendix chooses to edit three papers to reinforce the book's contents and represents the old doctors academic views - it has a deep relationship with his book's contents.

This book uses my father Guan Zun zai's past doctors lecture notes as the basis of this version and also combines much personal study, understanding, and clinical experience. It was revised three times, and ultimately produced in this book form. In the autumn of 1978, after the first manuscript was finished, my father during his last few days read it completely and revised and corrected it. After making the necessary changes and correction to the manuscript, it was received and given a lot of useful suggestions by Kunming city's Yan and hospital professors, Zhang Pei ling Kunming medical colleges affiliated first hospital professor Yang Bo ren, Yunnan Chinese medicine College Associate Professor Xu Zhi jian. I appreciate all their help during the course of this work.

Because of the author's limited academic level, this book's contents must have a lot of omissions and possible mistakes, I ask any experts in the area of acupuncture not to withhold their criticism so as to be able to continue to revise and improve upon Chinese medicine.

<u>Guan Zun hui</u>

CONTENTS

APPENDIX

PART 1
··
THE THEORY OF JING LUO

CHAPTER 1

A General Introduction to Jing Luo Theory

Jing luo theory is an important part of the theoretical system of Chinese medicine. It has a close relationship with zang-xiang theory; they combine, supplement, and prove each other, reflecting as a whole the basic point of view of Chinese medicine concerning human physiology and pathology. Together, they become the core of Chinese medicine's theoretical system.

In Chinese medicine's theoretical system, jing luo theory is an academic theory and developed very early. It has decisive significance in the formation of the basic points of view in Chinese medicine. These basic points of view—such as the organic concept of the human body and viewing its various parts as forming an organic whole, dynamic and balanced—are the most fundamental theoretical documents for dialectical analysis and treatment. They are also the starting points for any traditional Chinese medicine (TCM) theory discussion. After long-term medical practice and repeated verifications, it has been without a doubt proven that jing luo theory not only has very high research values in academic theory but also has a popular directing significance in therapeutic practice in various clinical areas in Chinese medicine. So to study the theory of jing luo comprehensively and to combine it with clinical practice, it is not only necessary to carry on and practice the heritage of Chinese medicine, it also has an important current and long-term historical significance.

Section 1
The Concept of Jing Luo

The Meaning of Jing Luo

Jing luo is the general name of *jing mai* and *luo mai*, but they do have different meanings. "Jing" has the meaning of "path." For example, a path is the key road of the jing luo system. "Luo" means "network." In terms of network, it is thin and smaller than the jing mai and distributes all over the body. It is a branch of the jing luo system.

Jing and luo combine into a whole circulation system, reaction system, and regulating system, connecting upwards and downwards, inside and outside. It includes the four limbs and one hundred bones; that is, all limbs and most of the bones in a human adult).

Qi and blood circulate endlessly through the jing luo, nourishing organs and muscles, smoothing skin, and helping vessels and bones to accomplish their functions of metabolising and adapting the body to its external environment.

The Contents of the Jing Luo System

The contents of the jing luo system can be divided into jing luo parts and related parts. The jing luo parts are divided into jing mai and luo mai. With regard to jing mai, the twelve jing mai are the main body of the whole jing luo system (including jing mai and luo mai), so people also later called this the twelve zheng jing (real meridians). The branches separating off the joining to the twelve real meridians are called jing *bie* (jing sub-route).

Besides the twelve jing mai, eight special jing mai are not connected to the organs and have no connection between the external and internal. These are called the *qi ing ba mai* (eight extraordinary meridians). Their main function is to regulate the *mai* qi (channel qi) regarding the overflow and storage of the zheng jing.

In connection with the luo mai, the fifteen luo make up the main body of the luo mai system and are often called the fifteen bie luo (sub-route luo). The mai, which are hence derived, are diagonally distributed from the fifteen bie luo; normally, all are called mai luo.

The thin, small branch mai derived from the luo mai are called sun luo (grandson luo). The luo mai distributed on the body surface are called *fu* luo (floating luo).

The related parts of the jing luo system can be divided into the internal and external parts. On the inside, the jing luo go deep into the *ti qiang* (body cavity/chamber) and belong to the *wu zang liu fu* (five solid and six hollow organs). The relationship between jing luo and the organs is close; they cannot be separated. Jing qi originates from the qi of the organs, so the strength and weakness of the organs' qi determines the deficiency and excesses of the jing qi.

The externally related part of the mai luo penetrates and preserves the tissues of the body's exterior. The relationship between the jing luo and the outer body is mainly reflected in the twelve jing jin (jing tendons) and the twelve *pi* luo (skin positions).

The system located at the *jing rou* (tendons and flesh) and joints within which the qi of the twelve jing clumps, gathers, or disperses (i.e., luos) is called jing-jin. Those positions, administered by the twelve jing, are called the twelve pi *bu*.

The jing luo system is the path through which blood and qi is circulated and distributed via the jing luo and the jing mai. Inside the body, it is connected to each related organ. Outside the body, it is connected to the jing rou and the skin. The interior and exterior are connected and cross-linked, and these closely relate to human organs and limbs to form an inseparable unit. The context of the jing luo system is summarised in table 1.

Jing Luo System	**Jing Luo Parts**	**Jing Mai**	12 Channels:	Internal belong zang fu; external follows the joints. Circulating between the muscles is the qi blood stagnant circulate path. Note point treatment flow.
			12 Jing Bie:	Bie travelling its true channel; 12 channels combine, with branch channels coming out. Internal parts heavy travelled, with points becoming "liu he."
			Extraordinary 8 Channels:	Bie path, extraordinary cycling channel branches but at true channels, increase balance joints qi and blood. Opposite 12 channels elements combined.
		Luo Mai	Bie Luo:	Controls big luo. Inside are the 12 unblocked interior and external channels and qi and blood. Combines with ren, du, spleen big luo to become the "is luo." Used to balance the whole body's luo mai.
			Floating Luo:	Floating and often seen. Branches go horizontally. Moistens and softens body exterior's muscles and skin.
			Sun Luo:	Luo mai branches and thin small ones. Luo's bie.
	Line Parts	**Internally Belongs**	5 Zang:	Liver, heart, spleen, lungs, kidneys, and pericardium becomes 6 zang. Becomes jing mai (and parts, luo mai) on the same line.
			6 Fu:	Gallbladder, small intestines, stomach, large intestines, bladder; triple heater becomes 6 fu.
		External Line	12 Jing Jin:	External body external, enters zang fu, becomes 12 jing qi. Accumulation spreads luo at jin muscles and joints systems. Points become "4 jie," heavy and adds 3 yin channels; 3 yang channels become mechanised system.
			12 Skin Parts:	Jing luo at outer body helps protective qi. External evil and inverse zang fu jing luo brings illness.

Table 1.

3

The Concept of Jing Qi, with the Meaning of Jing Shui

Jing luo (channels and collaterals) are the pathways through which qi and blood of the human body circulate. Jing qi circulates non-stop through the entire human body to push blood to circulate, thereby maintaining life activity in the body.

What is jing qi? How does jing qi drive circulation of qi and blood? These are the first questions discussed in the jing luo study.

To clear up the concept of jing qi, it is necessary to briefly review the concepts of qi, blood, *wei* qi, ying qi, zong qi, yuan qi, zheng qi, and so on.

Qi: In Chinese medicine, the general concept of qi has two aspects to its meaning. The first relates to the fundamental materials to maintaining life activity, such as breathing, and the jing qi of water and grains transformed from the spleen. The second relates to the real qi—jing qi, zang fu qi (viscera and bowel qi), and so on power that drives the functioning of human organs and tissues.

Blood: Blood circulating in the mai (vessels) carries the jing qi, nourishes the whole body, helps circulate and improve the flow of red blood cells, and is the main substance in maintaining human life. The formation of blood comes mainly through the following sources.

The spleen and stomach are the biochemical origins of blood. "*Zhong jiao shou*" qi (the central heater receives/accepts the qi), receives the juices ("*qu zhi bian hua er chi*"), and transforms them into the red *shi weixu*. This is called blood.

Ying qi goes to the vessels and transforms and produces blood. "*Ying qi zhe, mi qi jin ye, zhu zhi yu mai hua yi wei xu*" (Ying qi secretes its fluid, injects it into the vessels, and then transforms it into blood.

Jing and blood can be transformed into each other. The kidney is used mainly for storing jing semen essence and controls the production of marrow in the bones. Jing and marrow can be transformed into blood. Therefore, there are theories of "*xue zhi yuan tou zai shen*" (the origin of blood is from the kidney) and "*jing xue tong yuan*" (jing and blood are of the same origin).

Qi and blood are dependent on each other. They produce each other and are inseparable. Blood relies on the driving force of qi, and qi relies on the transformation of the blood. "*Qi wei xue zhi shuai, xue wei qi zhi mu, qi xing. Ze xue xing, qi zhi ze xue yu*" (Qi is the leader of blood, blood is the mother of qi, if qi circulates, blood circulates too. If qi is stagnant, then blood is also stagnant). Of the two, one is yin and the other is yang. They are closely related.

Ying qi: It is jing qi that works in the mai. Produced by water and grain and originating from the spleen and stomach, it comes out of the middle heater. It transforms and produces blood to tone the whole body. So the "Ling shu-xie ke"

4

chapter said, *"ying qi zhe, mi qi jin ye, zhu zhi yu mai, hua yi wei xue, yi rong si mo, nei zhu wu zang liu fu"* (Ying qi secretes its body fluid and injects it into the mai and transforms it into blood to tonify the whole body and eventually puts it into all the five visera and six bowels").

Wei qi - produced from water and grain, originates from the spleen and stomach, coming out from the upper heater, it is strong, quick, smooth, promoting in nature and is good at "walking around" and penetrating and is not controlled by the mai (vessels). It stays in the mang mo (mang diaphragm) and disperses into the chest and abdomen to warmly preserve all the organs; externally it circulates in the space between the muscles and the skin to moisten and warmly preserve muscle and skin *"Ling shu ben zang"* chapter said "wei qi zhe, suo yi wen fen rou, chong pi fu, fei cou li, si kai he zhe ye" the wei qi it can warm the flesh, preserve the skin and the pores and deals with their opening and closing.") This is a brief generalisation of the functions of the wei qi.

Zong qi - the ying qi and the wei qi produced from water and grain combining with the qi from nature, and accumulating in the chest is called the "zong qi". It is also "hou tian zhi qi" ("the qi afterbirth"). Its functions are: zou xi dao yi si hu xi; guan xin mai yi xing xue qi. (It travels in the tracks to control the breath, spreads into the heart vessel to circulate the blood and qi). So the strength of the sound of breathing and the circulation of qi and blood both are related to zong qi.

Zhen qi - the qi born with at birth (yuan qi) and the qi born after birth (the jingqi of nature and water and grain), both combine together and form zhen qi. So the *Ling shu-ci jie zhen* <u>xie</u>) chapter said "Zhong qi zhe, suo shou yu tian, yu gu qi bin ge chong shen ye" ("Zhen qi received from heaven and combined with grain qi and tonifies the body").

The relation of the above each qi is summarised in Table 2:

Before heaven Qi – Yuan qi (Yuan Yang's Qi), Also "in between kidney's moving qi", belongs to kidney (ming men), at dan tian lower qi hai

True Qi	After Heaven's Qi - Zong Qi	Food enters stomach, spleen channel transforms circulating qi transforms and creates blood nutrition for the whole body	Yang Qi	
				Stores in chest upper Qi Hai
		Circulates externally in the mai, softens nourishes and warms the skin and hair	Wei Qi	
		Lungs breathing enters "self jing qi" (same as empty qi")		

Table 2

Because the mature connection and mature combination help the qi born with birth and the qi born after birth, they all travel in the jing mai to supply nutrients to the whole body and preserve life. So, the qi which travels in the jing mai - jing qi is zhen qi in reality. The *Su wen - li he zhen xie lun* said clearly "zhen qi zhe jing qi ye". So it can be seen, the so-called "jing qi" is the spirit transformed from water and grain, inhaled air and the jing qi stored in the kidney, display that function in general. Summarising the discussion above, the jing qi in jing luo theory includes ying qi, wei qi, zong qi and yuan qi. Ying qi and wei qi circulates in the whole body, zong qi is the driving force, yuan qi is the basis of the activities of jing luo functions. They closely work together and cannot be separated from each other. The meaning of jing qi is summarised in Table 3.

True Qi Channel Qi	At tian		Before Heaven's Qi – Yuan Qi – Jing Luo Function	
			Big Qi	
	And Grain Qi Combined	Zong Qi	– Unblocks heart qi, up and out at lungs – nutrition and protection circulates	Channel Qi Transports and circulates
		Ying Qi	– water grains' jing qi, transforms blood fluids – circulates in the vessels	
		Wei Qi	– water grains' fierce qi, illnesses smooth unblocks – circulates outside the vessels	

Table 3

According to the theory of jing luo, jing luo is internally belonging to zang fu and spreads externally to the limbs and forms a complete jing luo system. The jing qi circulates and spreads over the whole body without stopping. It also has other more specialised names according to its position and physiological functions which are summarised in Table 4.

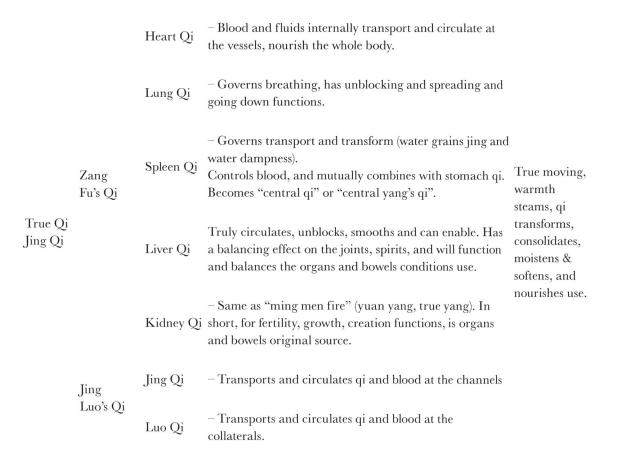

True Qi Jing Qi	Zang Fu's Qi	Heart Qi	– Blood and fluids internally transport and circulate at the vessels, nourish the whole body.	True moving, warmth steams, qi transforms, consolidates, moistens & softens, and nourishes use.
		Lung Qi	– Governs breathing, has unblocking and spreading and going down functions.	
		Spleen Qi	– Governs transport and transform (water grains jing and water dampness). Controls blood, and mutually combines with stomach qi. Becomes "central qi" or "central yang's qi".	
		Liver Qi	Truly circulates, unblocks, smooths and can enable. Has a balancing effect on the joints, spirits, and will function and balances the organs and bowels conditions use.	
		Kidney Qi	– Same as "ming men fire" (yuan yang, true yang). In short, for fertility, growth, creation functions, is organs and bowels original source.	
	Jing Luo's Qi	Jing Qi	– Transports and circulates qi and blood at the channels	
		Luo Qi	– Transports and circulates qi and blood at the collaterals.	

Table 4

"Jing shui" according to the records in the book *Ling shu - jing shui* has the names of qing shui, wei shu, hai shui, hu shui, ru shui, mian shui, huai shui, luo shui jiang, he shui, ji shu, zhang shui, et cetera. 12 big waters. It was the author of the Nei jing, who use them to stimulate the 12 jing of the human body according to a map. The main idea was to use the origins and the flowing area crossings and the separation of the 12 rivers to show the circulation of qi and blood in the 12 jing (channels) and indicate the effects of the flow and presentation of the 12 jing as a circulating and non-stopping system. As for the human body itself, it means the jing luo of the human body is related to the external nature. The *jing shu* chapter mainly discussed the functional cooperation between the 12 jing and the 12 shui with a separate discussion on the most appropriate needling depth and time for the yin and yang jing of the hands and feet, and the importance of applying acupuncture flexibly according to the different cases; it also discussed the consequences of overdosage and inadequate dosage.

In jing luo theory, jing shui and jing qi are different and this should be given due attention.

The definition of jing luo theory

Jing luo theory is the study of physiology, pathological changes and the relationship to the corresponding viscera and bowels of the human jing luo system. It is an important part of Chinese medicine theory system. It is a summary of the experience of the Chinese people after thousands of years of fighting disease.

Jing luo theory is the summary of the objective principles of the human anatomy, physiology and pathology by ancient doctors.

Jing luo theory is the theory set up after a long term medical practice. According to the effects of point treatment the summarising of pathological reaction, and the deducing of the functions of the pathological activity, we can see that from perceptual knowledge it has been taken into rational knowledge.

Jing luo theory shows the point of view of the whole body in Chinese medicine and emphasises that the human body is a united organism consisting of a jing luo system.

Jing luo theory is a body connection theory which discusses the principles of the systematic life activities, and studies the functional relationship and functional influence between the human zang fu, organs and tissues.

Section 2
The clinical value of Jing Luo theory

The function of jing luo and clinical meaning

The Jing luo have a qi and blood circulating, as well as health preserving function. Qi and blood is the energy and basis for human life activities. The *Mai jing-er shi er nan* said, "qi zhu he zhi, xue zhu ru zhi." This means qi is the energy for the functional activities, blood is the source for maintaining and preserving, but qi and blood must be spread through jing luo to ensure the normal physiological functions of tissues and organs. So the *Ling Shu-ben zang* chapter said "Jing mai zhi, sou yi xing xue qi er ying yin yang ru un gu, li guan jie zhe ye." This points out that the jing mai are the pathways of qi and blood circulation, the jing luo vertically and horizontally distribute inside the body and the skin to preserve the whole body and play an important role in maintaining the normal human body functional activities.

The jing luo have the function of reflecting abnormal changes in the human body.

When the human body is invaded by various kinds of disease factors and the normal functions of the organs are interrupted and one starts to have a disease, because the jing luo have special relationships with each individual part, so various kinds of abnormal changes such as pressing pain points and energy points can be detected from the jing luo connected position on the body surface by observation and pressing, etc. methods; alternatively there may be observable changes in the body such as those relating to the nodes under the skin, or papules or red lines or changes in the skin colour along the jing luo or overgrowth of hair. These can provide reference for the diagnosis of disease. There has been a relatively large development in the application of jing luo reactions in diagnosis and treatment, such as changes in the skin electro-resistance measurement of the twelve jing yuan (original) points or the measurement of the twelve jing jing (well) points, tolerance to temperature, which can facilitate disease diagnosis. At the same time, it has been expanded beyond specific shu points (such as yuan points, jing - well points, cleft points, mu points, back shu points, etc) Such as "Lan wei xue", "Kui yang bei xue" ("ulcer back point"), Kui yang di xue ("ulcer bone point"), "Guan xin xue ("Coronary heart point"), Dan nang xue ("Gall bladder point") etc. These body surface reactions can not only be used for reference in disease diagnosis, they can also be used as points of acupuncture treatment. It has been said, "Ren you bing tong, ji jin nie qi shang, ruo li dang chu, bu wen kong xue, ji be bian kuai huo tong" (if someone has pain and you press down the pain area, if it is correct to do not bother with points, the pain can be resolved.") The ancient documents recorded the "yi tong wei shu" and later the so-called "ah shi xue", "tian ying xue" while even later the so-called pressing pain points, sensitive points are all based on this principle.

In addition, in Zang-fu theory it is said that the heart opens its orifice at the tongue, the lung at the nose, the spleen at the mouth, the liver at the eyes, and the kidney at the ears, it is also showing in this way the jing luo connections.

The jing luo reflect the abnormal changes in the body as another kind of symptom indication of the whole body, i.e. the jing luo classification of symptoms. It was earliest recorded in the *Nei-Jing* the 12 jing symptoms (i.e. whenever a jing luo and the related organ are in disease it will have different whole-body symptoms). The later medical doctors developed the 12 jing symptoms into Zang fu theory, iu jing (6 jing) theory and wei qi ying xue theories, etc, and provided the basis for dialectical treatment of Chinese medicine.

The jing luo has conductive functions re disease evil invasion and acupuncture stimulus.

The jing luo have conductive effects on the invasion of disease evils, when the skin meets the invasion of disease evils, the evils can be transmitted through the jing luo into the internal organs by way of connection between the organs with the jing luo. Disease evils can be transmitted from one organ to another which is called "the transfer of disease evils", in brief chuan (passed on to the jing) jing.

The Su wen miu ci lun said, "Fu xie zhi ke yu xing, bi xian she yu pi mao, liu er bu qu, ru she yu, jun mai, liu er bu qu, ru she yu luo mai, liu er bu qu, ru she jing mai luo, nei lin wu zang, san wu chang wei" (must first stay in the skin and hair and stay there, then it invades the deep sun mai and stays there, then invades the luo mai and stays there, then invades the jing mai which connects with the five zang, then it disperses into the intestines and stomach"). This is the general concept of the conduction (transduction) of disease evils by the jing luo by the ancient medical doctors and it is in accordance with objective reality to a certain extent. The later medical doctors on the basis of summarising clinical experience made more clear statements and developments, such as the transmission of disease evil as in the symptom groups of liu jing theory of *Shang han lun*, and the transmission and transformation of wei qi ying, xue in "Wen Bing" theory; all used the conductive functions of jing luo as their theoretical basis. When this theory is used in the dialectic treatment of Chinese medicine, it cannot only give us conclusions on the development and transformation of disease, it can also provide corresponding treatment measures with a certain value in disease prevention.

Acupuncture treatment and some other modern treatment methods such as dian zhen (electric acupuncture) and shui zhen (liquid acupuncture) use physical and chemical factors to treat certain positions of the body surface and achieve the aims of disease treatment, they are all based on the principle of conduction function of the jing luo. The qi of jing luo of the human body starts from the shu points on the body. The *Ling shu-jiu zhen shi er yuan* said, "Jie zhi jiao, san bai liu shi wu hui, suo yan jie (shu xue) zhe, shen qi suo you xing chu ru ye". (The crossing of the jie has 365 points, so-called jie (shu points) other places where the spirit qi ("Shen qi" passes') so the key point of acupuncture is to regulate qi, as it is said "ci zhi yao, qi z her you xiao, ci zhi er qi bu zhi, wu wen qi shu" ("the important point of acupuncture is to have the qi come then it is effective, if the qi doesn't come with acupuncture then it is useless"), to regulate the qi is to regulate qi and blood caused by the transduction of jing luo. When the jing luo or the functions of internal organs are out of regulation, by the stimulus of acupuncture of certain points of the body surface, the jing luo can transport treatment stimulus to the related positions and organs. Along with the regulatory functions of human qi mechanisms, it can make qi and blood circulation become fluent, and ying and wei harmonious and hence provide a cure for disease.

The relationship between acupuncture treatment and jing luo conduction is shown in detail by the selection of points along the route of jing luo circulation ie.

treatments such as he gu point (L 14) for the treatment of toothache, nei guan point (P6) for stomach and abdomen pain, zu san li (ST 36) for stomach and intestinal diseases, etc., all have quite good clinical results which are closely related to the transduction function of the jing luo. The transduction function of jing luo is also shown by the sour and fullness feeling which disperses along the circulation line of jing luo. When the patients receive acupuncture, individual patients can even feel the effect of reaching the disease area directly. There are some cases where after acupuncture there are extended lines of abnormal colour on the patient's skin with distribution basically the same as the distribution of jing luo. According to clinical experience, proper acupuncture hand techniques and proper stimulation strength are important factors to the achievement of acupuncture treatment results but the keynote point of treatment is the location of acupuncture reaction - this is also an indication of the transduction function of the jing luo. As it is said in *Biao you fu* (written by a famous acupuncturist Dou Han qing in the Jin Yuan Dynasty), "qi zhi zhi ye, ru yu tun gou er zhi chen fu; qi wei zhi ye, ru xian chu you tang zhi shen sui. Qi su zhi er su xiao, qi chi zhi er bu zhi." ("when the qi comes, it is like a fish which bites on the hook, when the qi still hasn't come, it is very very quiet. When the qi comes quickly it has results quickly, if the qi comes late then it has no effects"). So it can be seen that the transductive effect of the jing luo is the main internal reason for this and that the applied stimulating environment conditions become effective via the internal connections of jing luo.

The jing lou present the principles of special connections of the internal human body.

The jing luo, in addition to their common definitions of a mixture of common connections within the human body and the point of view of integrity, also emphasised the principles of special connections within the human body particularly in three aspects: (1) special connections on the skin and body surface indicating their special connections to each certain position in the upper and lower, left and right, front and back, true centre and side parts (2) The special connections of the internal human zang fu indicating the special influences between some internal organs and other internal organs, (3) the special connections between the body surface and the zang fu indicating the internal and external united relationship between certain positions and the skin, and different organs inside the body, the special connection principles can be used in diagnosis re the abnormal reactions in a position far from the disease area, or other special symptoms, to deduce an organ in the state of disease. The commonly used colour observation, touching of the body surface as well as the moderately developed "jing xue ce ding" and ear needlepoint detection etc. in

Chinese medicine are all the detailed applications of jing luo theory in diagnosis. The application of jing luo treatment is even wider, for example the 15 kinds of associated point methods commonly used in acupuncture is the detailed application of the special connection theory of jing luo. The ba gang theory, zang fu theory, liu jing theory, wei qi ying xue theory, etc. in Chinese internal medicine have an inseparable relationship with jing luo theory in their formation and development. The diagnosis of children's diseases puts important emphasis on wang zhen (visual diagnosis) however wang mian se (checking face colour), shen miao qiao (examining children's orifices), kan zhi wen (checking the finger prints) etc. in visual diagnosis have their theoretical basis in jing luo theory, especially fingerprint examination which is the development of jing luo se zhen (colour diagnosis) in jing luo theory. Jing luo theory is particularly important in women's diseases, jing dai chan (periods, leucorrhoea, fertility; reproduction etc.) women's diseases are closely related to the chong ren dai and heart, liver, spleen and kidney. Every generation of medical doctors pay attention to jing luo theory to direct their diagnosis and treatment of women's diseases.

The human eyes are the place where the jing qi of the five organs and six bowels intersect and where the circulation of the jing qi instantly relies on the jing mai and hence all the mai belong to the eyes and it can be seen that the relationship between the eyes and jing luo theory are very important. Therefore in the treatment of eye diseases, to distinguish the jing of the eye diseases and the qi jing (usually the yin and yang two qiao) is a very important consideration.

The wu lun ba kuo theory is another method based on jing luo theory (the whole eye is divided into five parts called the five wheels in association with the five organs. Again the whole eye is divided into eight parts called the ba kuo in association with the six bowels and the heart and mingmen. The theory of the "wu lun" is originally from wu xing lun, the theory of ba kuo is originally from the distribution of the ba gua. The interpretation of eye disease in relation to yin yang wu xing, jing luo zang fu demonstrates the principles of the connection between zang fu and the connection of the twelve jing).

In addition, in the areas of external woundage, massage, qi gong etc. jing luo theory has certain directing meanings and has inseparable connections.

Summarising the above, the jing luo system is closely related to the tissues and organs of the whole body and also possesses the function of transporting qi and blood, reflecting changes and conducting stimulus etc. jing luo theory states and discusses the special connection principles inside the human body. So jing luo does not only have an important function in physiological and pathological changes, it also has directing meaning and very high practical clinical value in disease diagnosis and various clinical treatments.

The position of jing luo theory in Chinese medicine.

The *Ling shu - jing bie* chapter says, "fu shi er jing mai zhe, ren zhi suo yi sheng, bing zhi sou yi cheng ren zhi suo yi zhi, bing zhi sou yi xue, qi, zhi suo shi, gong zhi sou zhi ye" (the twelve jing mai is where a human is born, diseases formed, a patient is treated, a disease starts, learning begins, work stops.") Ming dynasty Dr Zhang Jie bin explained, "the Jing mai are the branches and leaves of the zang fu, the zang fu is the root of the jing mai, if the principle of 12 meridians is clear, then you understand yin and yang, exterior and interior, qi and blood, deficiency and excess, i.e. obeyance and disobeyance of the principles can be examined, the safety and the danger of evil and good can be told, and the birth of normal people, the formation of disease, the treatment of patients, the start of disease can be seen to emanate from here. So, beginner should start from here, while good doctors also stop here." So it can be seen that even though jing luo theory is only one part of the Chinese medicine theoretical system, its connections and influences penetrate yin yang, wu xing, zang fu, qi and blood, exterior and interior deficiency and excess, evil and true (zheng) safety and danger, etc., physiological and pathological process. So the *Ling shu jing mai* chapter pointed out even more strenuously that "jing mai zhe, suo yi neng jue si sheng, chu bai bing, tiao xin shi, bu ke bu tong." (the jing mai determine death and survival, are able to treat various kinds of disease and regulate deficiency and excess, this must be understood.")

From all statements it is not difficult to see the important academic position held by jing luo theory in Chinese medicine and hence later doctors paid much attention to the theory and application of jing lou theory. For example Ming dynasty Ma yuan said in the *Ling Shu zhu zheng fa wei*, "shi er jing mai … shi xue zhe xi yi zhi di yi yao yi, bu su jiu xin shou wan ye, hou shi neng yan, bu shi er jing luo, kai kou dong shou bian cuo, er yu ci meng ran, xi zai" ("The 12 jing mai … It is really the first important step for students to learn in medicine, they must study carefully and make familiar. Some later doctors do not understand the 12 jing luo, they made mistakes when they said something or did something, they were so ignorant, it is a pity.") This indicates further that the jing luo theory is directly applicable clinically. The early Qing dynasty Dr Yu yia yan also said, "fan zhi bing bu ming zang fu jing luo, kai kou dong shou cou." ("When treating disease if you don't understand zang fu and jing luo, you will make mistakes when you talk and do something"). In addition there are such as, "Bu qiong jing luo yin yang, duo feng ci jin, ji lun zang fu xu shi, xu xing jing xun ("*Biao you fu*) ("if you don't completely understand the jing luo and yin and yang, you will meet some problems you shouldn't, even if you are talking about zang fu and deficiency and excess, you should look for them from the point of view of the jing luo.")

"Bu zhi shi er jing luo, bu bian xu shi biao li han re wen liang cha zhi hao li, miu zhi qian li, ju shou bian cuo" (*Yi xu zhi gui*) " ("if you don't understand the 12 jing luo you cannot tell deficiency and excess, exterior and interior, coldness and heat, warm and cool, a slight difference can result in a significant mistake and you will make mistakes whenever you want to do something.") These kinds of statements and warnings can be found anywhere in Chinese medicine documents.

The Chinese medicine School of Jiang su province once wrote a book titled *Zhen jiu xue*. In the introduction they wrote "jing luo theory is the main basis for the construction of Chinese medicine as one of the superior theories. It and yin yang, wu xing, zang fu, ying wei qi xue, etc. make up the whole system of Chinese medicine, spreading to all aspects of anatomy, nutrition, pathology, diagnosis, and treatment etc. It holds supreme position, from theory to practice;" this opinion is quite appropriate.

Section 3
The generation and development of jing luo theory

The source and the generation process of jing luo theory

Jing luo theory was generated by the common people during the long period of struggle for the production and the practice of medicine. It is from the observation of anatomy and physiology and the theory of disease, as well as acupuncture's observation of certain principles that after a long time, hypotheses and conclusions were formulated in order to generate concepts, and summarisations upon which these kinds of academic theories were developed. It is the result of the earliest books of medicine in China like the *Nei Jing*, that jing luo theories have become a very complete natural theory. If the Nei Jing was written in the Chun (Spring) Chiu (Autumn) zan guo (period), so then the jing luo theories may well have been generated earlier in the Spring and Autumn times of perhaps even earlier. From the material now available regarding the generation of the jing luo theories, we now know that there were three methods responsible for the generation these are the source of the jing luo theories.

(1) The first one is from gui na (experimental results) i.e. from the surface of the body's reaction points and from the paths of sensation after needling, the discovery

and development of acupuncture treatment generated the basis of jing luo theory. In other words, the basis of acupuncture is there xue wei (acupuncture points), and it is the surface reaction points which are the important criteria upon which to select these acupuncture points, (the surface reaction points of course including the pain incurred by the patient him or herself, (pressing pain (ya tong), sensitivity (guo min), things felt under the skin, or even skin colour changes). Just like in the *Ling shu bei shu* which said, "yu de er yan zhi, an qi chu, ying zai zhang er tong jie." ("if the internal organs have some sicknesses you can press the reaction points, at some place on the body so the pain will be decreased.") Also in the Ling shu Jiu zhen shi er yuan, it is said "wu zang you liu fu, liu fu you shi er yuan, shi er yuan chu yu si guang wu zang you ji ye, ying chu shi er yuan. … ming zhi qi yuan, du qi ying, er zhi wu zang zhi hai yi" ("you can find the reaction points in the four limbs for the sicknesses in the internal organs, the relationship between the reaction points in the body and the internal organs is the source of the theories regarding the jing luo's internal and external connections").

As a result of a long time of medical practice, people know that this doctrine is not only concerned with the relationships of the internal organs but also has some regulatory considerations. The medium of this connection is the mai qi of course, the key of acupuncture is to get the qi. The book the *Ling Shu jiu zhen shi er yuan* said, "ci zhi er qi bu zhi, wu wen qi shu, ci zhi er qi zhi nai qu zhi, wu fu zhen" ("If you needle and the qi doesn't come, you cannot count it. If you needle and the qi comes then you can take the needle out and you don't need to do it again"). "Wei ci zhi yao, qi zhi er you xiao, xiao zhi xin, ruo feng zhi chui yun, ming hu ruo jian cang tian, ci zhi dao bi yi ("or needling, the important thing, if the qi comes, is to have some effect, if like the wind on the clouds you can see in the sky, you can finish the needling"). "Qi zhi" means de qi when you needle, this is the feeling of the patient of suan (soreness/ sourness), ma (numbness), zhang (fullness), and zhong (heaviness). These feelings are around certain paths of the mai qi, and these transportation paths are the basis for the conception of jing luo. From the observation of de qi ancient doctors made a summarisation of these paths and the regulatory effects of needling them. Hence they were then able to make conclusions regarding the 12 meridians of the hands and feet and the circulation and distribution of the eight extraordinary meridians, the relationship between the internal organs and the 12 meridians, and the eight channels and their symptoms originally eminating from the organs jing luo, ultimately further aiding jing luo theories.

In recent years, experiments confirm that in the pathways of people's bodies, when needling according to this doctrine patients have needle feelings along the same areas as shown in ancient jing luo distribution. This then makes for a number of conclusions regarding needling transportation regulation. This is also the basis for the celebration of jing luo theories in ancient times.

(2) With regards to summarising the main properties of the xue wei (acupuncture points), ancient people knew these step-by-step over a long period of time. The procedure for this, from the not certain reaction points to the certain xue wei, from the treatment points in the body to the lines, and from the classification by the main properties of the xue wei to systems, was the generation of the jing luo theories. At first, people didn't know the xue wei in the body, only when at some time a person was especially touched or hit by something or burned by something and then as a result, the sickness was removed or decreased, did people come to know the special effect of some special positions. Hence the way for obtaining the xue (xue wei) generally was "yi tong, wei shu" ("depending on the pain depending on the shu to catch it"). The pain in these cases includes "zhi fa tong" (self pain) and "ya tong" ("press pain") so they hadn't any specific or definite positions, also there were no names for the xue wei so the affected position could only be called "bian jiu chu" ("stone needle moxa area").

After people had accumulated more experience they knew that some special positions were good for some special sicknesses so they gave them names which in fact referred to their positions, their special properties and their correct placings. For example "ying xiang" (LI20) for the treatment of sicknesses of the nose, "and he gu" (LI4) between the bones of the hand.

Over the years and with the further observation of the needling conduction function of the xue wei, people got to know that the connection of the xue wei and the paths and the distribution of the connection paths, were like lines. In these lines there is "mai qi" running, so in the book the *Su wen* they called the "xue wei" the "mai qi suo fa" ("the source of the mai qi") and the "qi xue" ("the qi points"). Later they called the xue wei "shu xue". This refers to the transportation position of the qi and blood and the hole xue (Kong xue). Because the xue wei in the same limbs have the same functions so people used the limbs as a basis to classify the xue wei. This helped people to make progress in their understanding and knowledge of the xue wei. Therefore even though people now have still not seen the xue wei as individual real points we think of the relationship between different xue wei and their many functions. Hence the jing luo theories include the relationship between the xue wei and the whole system.

For example, the xue wei in the hand tai yin lung meridian. Generally it can have the main functions of treating the sicknesses of the lungs, the bronchials, throat and surface of the body (ti biao). On the other hand, as the indications of the hand tai yin lung meridian, out of the 12 meridians, reflect the same treatment uses as the xue wei on this jing mai line, there is clearly a relationship between the jing mai and the xue wei.

(3) With regards to summarising anatomy and physiology: the theory of jing luo and the generation of the source of jing luo theory, all came from the anatomy of the body and the observation of human physiology by ancient people.

In China the sciences of anatomy and physiology go back quite a long way e.g. from the Jia gu wen (i.e. a very old language in ancient times) we can see even prior to 1400 years BC, there were words for ear (er), eye (mu), mouth (kou), nose (bi), head (shou), and also names for people's organs. The descriptions also show that at that time people used special words for the different parts of organs and their functions. In the *Shi ji* it describes "Yi fu" (a person's name) cutting the abdomen to treat sickness. In this particular book Bian que cang gong i.e. in Bian que's biographical records it said, "chen wen shang gu zhi shi, yi you shu fu, zhi bing bu yi tang ye, li sa, chan shi, jiao yin, an wu, du yu; yi ba jian bing zhi ying, yin wu zang zhi shu, nai ge pi, jie ji, jue mai, jie jin, niao sui nao, she huang, zhua (zhao) mu, jian huan chang wei, shu di wu zang, lian jing yi xing" ("in very, very old times there was a doctor called Yi fu, he didn't use medicine soups for sicknesses, he used to cut the skin, or puncture superficially with a stone needle, or massage and encourage physical breathing exercises, or massage and exercise the limbs, or specifically to find the cause of the disease, he would check the 5 zang's shu points, cut the skin, separate the muscles, part the tendons, hold the marrow and the brain, and where the disease had attacked the vitals, he would wash the stomach and intestines, rinse and wash the five viscera or change the patient's outlook.") This paragraph described how this ancient doctor did anatomy at that time. The *Nei jing* describes the observation of people's organs when doing anatomy. Some of them are nearly to the level of the modern anatomy results. The *Ling shu jing shui* said, "ruo fu ba chi zhi shi, pi rou zai ci, wai ke du (or duo); liang qie xuan er de zhi, qi si ke jie pao er shi zhi, qi zang zhi jian cui, zang zhi da xiao; gu zhi duo shao, mai zhi chang duan, xue zhi qing zhuo, qi zhi duo shao … jie you da shu" ("a person is here, you can see his skin and muscles outside, if he dies you can do an anatomy and see his organs, what condition his organs are in and how large or small his organs are and whether his vessels are long or short, clear or turbid blood, how much qi, you can see approximately all this."). So this is saying that anatomy is a procedure following certain requirements and needs a certain approach. The *Ling shu chang wei* gave an example of anatomy: Yan men "zhi wei chang yi chi liu cun, wei yu qu qu, shen zh, chang er chi liu cun,. ... chang wei suo ru zhi suo chu, chang liu zhang si cun si fen" ("from the throat to the stomach is 1 chi and 6 cun long, if the stomach were straight it would be 2 chi 6 cun long, from the input to the output of the stomach and intestines it is in total 6 zhang 4 cun 4 fen long"). This says the ratio of the oesophagus and the large and small intestines will be equal to 1/35, this is just like the modern anatomy results. The *Su wen ci jin lun* also said, "zang you yao hai bu ke bu cha,.. ... ci zhong xin yi ri si, ci tou zhong nao hu, ru nao li si. ... ci ji jian zhong sui wei yu,. ... ci yin gu zhong da mai, xue chu bu zhi,. ... ci ying zhong xian zhong fei, wei chuan ni yang xi" ("you must know the importance of the organs,. ... if you pierce the heart it will die within one day, ... if you pierce the head, and inside the brain it will die immediately,. ... if you pierce the spine you won't be able to walk, ... if you hurt the da mai (the major blood vessels) of the inside of the thigh, the bleeding won't be able to stop, ... if you pierce the chest, you could break through the lung, and there will be panting adversely and longing to breathe.") This shows that the ancient people had knowledge of the blood vessels (xue mai) and the muscles and bones, and the organs from direct observation. This is to say, anatomy is a source of the generation of jing luo theories. The jing luo theories were generated by thousands of times of practice by the people of our country in their struggle with sickness and disease. They also came from experiments with body reaction points and needle feeling transfer, and from the main indications of the xue wei with regards to the observation of anatomy and physiology. From the combination of these three areas, people were able to summarise the principles and come to the conclusions of jing luo theories. Up to and including now, it has given direction to the practice of Chinese medicine. The generation of these theories over two thousand years ago is a great achievement in Chinese medicine.

2. The development of the jing luo theories

The first description of jing luo theory can be seen in the *Nei Jing*. The *Nei Jing* includes the *Su Wen* and the *Ling Shu*. The main contents of jing luo theories according to these two works include the following:

A description of the paths of the twelve jing mai, including their internal parts and external parts, and which organs they belong to;

A description of when the functions of the organs and the twelve jing mai are abnormal and their symptoms, and a description of the sicknesses each jing mai controls and their respective points;

A description separately listing the twelve jing bie the fifteen luo mai, and the twelve jing jin etc, their distribution and their functions;

A description of the qi jing ba mai distribution and functions;

A description of the relationships from top to bottom, internal and external, and between the twelve jing biao ben and the gen jie (roots/ foundations);

A description of whole bodies xue wei, their "numbers" and their names, and which part of them determines the length between a person's bones. It is the standard for the xue wei;

A description of the distribution of the ying, wei, qi, and xue of a body, whether they are running inside or outside the jing luo, and the protection of them and by them, affecting all the organs and organisational systems.

The above seven makes for the basis of jing luo theories.

The medicine book the *Nan Jing* also produced some developments re jing luo theory. For example, "shen jian dong qi" ("the qi runs between kidneys") is the source of the jing luo mai qi. This describes how the "ming men" can play a main part in jing luo physiology. At the same time, the twelve jing mai are running through the body, the luo mai are permeating through the whole body. The qi jing ba mai has the function of controlling qi and blood, which is given to the zang, fu, qi and blood, jin, mai, gu, sui, and ba hui points. The above have very important reference value when it comes to needling. They are the developments from the concepts of jing luo found in the *Nei Jing*. Besides these, the *Nei Jing* also developed the wei qu shang jiao ying qu zhong jiao theories Saying, "xin zhe xue, fei zhe qi, xue wei ying, qi wei wei" ("The heart controls the blood, the lungs control the qi, blood is from the transformation of nutrition for the organs, qi the guard/protector"). This gives credence to the warm sickness (wen bing) theories of the Qing dynasty using wei qi ying xue methods. They are also examples of the development of jing luo theories in application. In the *Nan Jing* it also describes, "shi er jing jie you dong mai" ("the 12 jing all have moving mai") "du qu cun kou" ("press here for feeling the mai"). This makes the basis for the later mai theories.

In the latter period of the Han dynasty, there were some new developments in jing luo theories. In the Eastern Han, Zhang Zhong jing's *Shang Han Lun* combined the same name jing in the hands and feet and called them the "liu jing" ("6 jing"). The summarising creation identification, and treatment of the "liu jing" in turn made for the conclusions of the rules regarding the ba gang including yin yang, biao li, xu shi and han re. They are not only the diagnostic basis for the treatment of external affects heat diseases but they also made a very big development contribution to internal medicine.

Huang Fu mi of the Jin dynasty wrote a book called the *Zhen jiu Jia yi jing*, in it he described the development of the jin luo jing xue. This book summarised the achievements of acupuncture jing luo (understanding) of the Jin dynasty. It is very important for the development of acupuncture medicine theories. (In addition, there was a very big development in channel (mai) theories in the Jin dynasty. In ancient medicine books, the jing luo theories almost all use the mai as their basis. Hence Jing luo is equal to jing mai plus luo mai. The ancient people noticed that whether a pulse was fast or slow or in some other abnormal state, was due to sicknesses of the jing luo and their organs. Wang Shu he in his book the *Mai jing* summarised and developed the applications of diagnosis using jing luo theories. In his book it described how different kinds of sickness will have different kinds of pulse. It summarised all the experiments in taking the pulse (qie mai) prior to the Jin dynasty. This is the basis of qie zhen (pulse taking diagnosis) in Chinese medicine. It is said that in Chinese medicine there are four diagnostic methods, qie zhen is one of them.

The original draft for the charts showing the jing luo xue wei, from our history, is recorded as beginning in Jin and Sui dynasties, at which time they were known as the "Ming tang jing". In the Tang, the charts of the jing luo xue wei were described by use of five colours. It was more detailed than before, this shows the transformation of zhen jiu xue wei, it made organisation out of the xue wei of the whole body based on the distribution position of the jing mai. From modern document research, it has been found that charts also began turning up in the Sui period. The book the *Huang Di Nei Jing Ming Tang* is an early book that made the whole body's xue wei belong to jing luo lines.

In the Tang dynasty, jing luo theory also had some new things to say, along with further developments of old ideas. For example, in the *Qian Jin Fang* it mentioned the selection of "a shi" points and their application, and expanded the range of acupuncture points, showing the detailed application of luo-mai, jing-jin, and skin parts etc. from jing luo theory. It gave inspiration and meaning to the later continuous discovery of strange new acupuncture points outside the channels.

Based on the summarisation of the acupuncture jing-luo points of people who come before him, Wang Wei yi of the Tang dynasty wrote the book *Tong Ren Shu Xue Zhen Jiu Tu Jing (Copper Man Acupuncture Points Acupuncture Charts)* and also made two human acupuncture models made of copper. This book and the copper men not only have important positions in our country's acupuncture development history, the acupuncture copper men also had significant influence in politics and international affairs.

Hua Bo ren of the Yuan dynasty summarised previous doctors' experiences, and wrote a book called the *Shi Si Jing Fa Hui (The Application of the 14 Jing)* in which it was mentioned again that the twelve jing mai and ren mai and du mai of the 8 extraordinary meridians should together be called the 14 meridians ("shi si jing"). He furthermore made some new developments in the circulation principle of qi and blood in the jing-luo and also made a quite detailed discussion about the shi si jing mai and the circulation, distribution and disease symptoms of the qi jing as well as the acupuncture points of the shi si jing. Zhang Yuan su of the Yuan dynasty also developed the yao wu gui jing theory and started the theory of combining herb applications with jing luo theory which in turn became the theoretical guide for making prescriptions by some medical doctors.

Li Shi zhen of the Ming dynasty wrote the *Qi Jing Ba Mai Kao* in which he made a study of the circulation position and the related acupuncture points of the qi jing. He additionally claimed the paths connecting the qi jing and the shi er jing mai's mai qi have the function to control the main disease symptoms of the qi jing. Zhang Jie bin wrote the *Lei Jing* and *Lei Jing Tu Yi* and also made some more developments regarding the jing luo. Loua ying on the other hand wrote the *Yi Xue Gang Mu* further promoted many opinions about the theory of jing qi circulation. Finally, Yang Ji zhou wrote the *Zhen Jiu Da Cheng* and made some contributions to the development of acupuncture. He held a number of views such as" shou wei zhu yang zhi hui, bai mai zhi zong" ("the head is a place where every yang goes it is the origin master of the 100 vessels") and ning shi qi xue, wu shi qi jing; ning shi qi shi, wu shi qi qi ("it would be better to lose a point, than to lose the jing; it would be better to lose the right time than to lose the qi"), all have constructive meanings.

The statements about the jing - luo in the Qing dynasty generally lacked new content. Only the *Jing Mai Tu Kao* discussed the acupuncture point positions with reference to the whole body bone structure and discussed the method of selecting points by touching the bone which made a more specific reference for acupuncture point determination. In addition, the *Tu Shu Ji Chang Yi Bu Quan Lu* also recorded the statements about the jing luo given by medical doctors of various generations which serves as the reference for study and research re jing luo theory.

From the Qing dynasty and until the Liberation, because of the reactionary control of the controlling class and imperialist invasion, Chinese medicine received a lot of damage to its reputation and the application and development of jing luo theory was greatly limited.

With regards to other countries, as early as the 6th century, jing luo theory and acupuncture treatment had spread to many oriental countries such as Korea and Japan, etc. Later, in about the 17th century, it spread to Europe and received attention from many countries throughout the world.

When new China was founded, the Party and the government paid attention to medical work, and the exploration and improvement of the Chinese medicine "treasure-trove" entered a new stage. The medical workers and scientific researchers used modern scientific knowledge and methods such as anatomy, histology, neurophysiology, electrophysiology, molecular biochemistry, histochemistry and biochemistry etc., and conducted a wide, deep research into jing luo theory and acupuncture principles, including a survey of jing luo sensitivity phenomena, the observation and determination of points (anatomical skin electro-potential, electro-resistance etc.), and the effects of acupuncturing jing points on the internal organ activities as well as its transmission paths, and research into acupuncture anaesthesia, such that ultimately there was a significant increase in the knowledge about the quality of jing luo and its importance in clinical practise.

CHAPTER 2
On each of the jing luo systems

Section 1
The twelve jing mai

The twelve jing mai is an important part of the jing mai system. It is the main body of the jing bie, qi jing and luo mal of the jing luo system. The effect produced is one of mutual cooperation. The main characteristics of the jing mai are:

the distribution position of each jing mai has certain rules;

each jing luo has internally related zang fu and is externally connected to the limbs and joints;

each jing luo belongs to an internal organ with a relationship of biao (fu), li (zang), mutually belonging to each other and connected;

when the jing qi has pathological changes, each jing luo has its own specific system group indications;

each jing luo has its distribution of shu points on the exterior. The twelve jing mai have extremely important regarding on the maintenance of human life activities, i.e. the treatment of various kinds of disease, the regulation of deficiency and excess in the body etc. The systematic observation opinion and dialectic treatment method of chinese medicine is formed by combining jing luo theory, in which the twelve jing mai is the main body, and zang fu theory.

The circulation lines and characteristics analysis of the twelve jing mai

The circulation lines of the twelve jing mai

(1)   The Lung Channel
Course

The Lung Channel of Hand-Taiyin originates in the middle warmer, the portion between the diaphragm and the umbilicus of the body cavity, running downwards to communicate with the large intestine. Turning back, it goes along the orifices of the stomach (the pylorus and the cardia), then upwards through the diaphragm into the pertaining organ, the lung.

From the pulmonary series (including the trachea, throat,) it comes transversely to the armpits (out of point Zhongfu, L1). It then descends along the medial aspect of the upper arm, and passes in front of the Heart Channel of Hand-Shaoyin and the Pericardium Channel of Hand-Jueyin, down to the middle portion of the elbow. From there it runs along the anterior border of the radius on the medial aspect of the forearm and goes into Cunkou, the place on the wrist over the radial artery where a pulse is felt. Then it arrives and then it runs along its border and emerges from the medial side of the tip of the thumb (point Shaoshang, Lu11).

The branch of the channel runs directly from the proximal aspect of the wrist (point Lieque, Lu7) into the radial side of the tip of the index (point Shangyang L11), in which it with the Large Intestine Channel of Hand-Yangming connections with zang fu containing channel points.

Connections with zang fu:

belongs to the lungs, luo communicates with the large intestines, and connects with the stomach and kidneys etc. systems.

Pertaining Channel points:

zhong fu (Lu 1), yun men (Lu 2), tian fu (Lu 3), xia bai (Lu 4), chi ze (Lu 5), kong zui (Lu 6), lie que (Lu 7), jing qu (Lu 8), tai yuan (Lu 9), yu ji (Lu 10), shao shang (Lu 11), altogether 11 points

(2)   The Large Intestine Channel of Hand-Yangming
Course

Lists channel starts from the tip of the radial side of the index (point Shangyang, LI1). It runs upward along the radial side of the index and passes between the ossa metacarpalia I and II, goes into the depression between the tendons of m. extensor pollicus longus and brevis, then along the anterolateral aspect of the forearm to the lateral side of the elbow (point Quichi, LI11) along the anterior border of the lateral side of the upper arm, it seems to the highest point of the shoulder (point Jianyu,

LI 15) and then goes along the anterior border of the acromion up to the seventh cervical vertebrae (point Dazhui, Du 14), from where it comes downwards into the supraclavicular fossa and communicates with the lung. Descending into the diaphragm, it enters its pertaining organ, the large intestine. The branch channel from the supraclavicular fossa runs upward to the neck, passes through the cheek, and enters into the lower teeth and gum. Then it curves around the lips and meets at point Renzhong (Du 26), or philtrum, the vertical groove on the middle line of the upper lip. From there the channel of the left side turns right, while the right side channel turns left. They go upwards to both side of the wings of the nose (point Yingxiang LI20) and connect with the Stomach Channel of Foot-Yangming.

Connections with zang fu:

Belongs To the large intestines, luo communicates with the lungs, connects with the stomach system.

Pertaining channel points:

shang yang (LI 1), er jian (LI 2), san jian (LI 3), he gu (LI 4), yang xi (LI 5), pian li (LI 6), wen liu (LI 7), xia lian (LI 8), shang lian (LI 9), shou san li (LI 10), qu chi (LI 11), zhou liao (LI 12), shou wu li (LI 13), bi nao (LI 14), jian yu (LI 15), ju gu (LI 16), tian ding (LI 17), fu tu (LI 18), he liao (LI 19), ying xiang (LI 20)

Meeting Points

Bing feng (Hand-taiyang), da zhui (du)

(3)   The Stomach Channel of Foot-Yangming
Course

This channel starts from the side of the nose (point Yingxiang L120), and descends to the root of the nose, meeting the Urinary Bladder Channel (at point Jingming, UB 1). Then it descends along the lateral side of the nose and enters into the upper gum. Emerging and curving round the lips, it passes downwards and connects with the symmetrical channel at Point Chengjiang (Ren 24) in the sulcus mentolabialis. And it runs along the posterior - inferior side of the parotid gland, through point Daying (St5), and point Jiache in (St6) succession, and then descends in front of the ear, through point Kezhuren, i.e. Shangguan (GB 3), the point of the gallbladder channel of Foot-Shaoyang. And finally, it runs along the hairline and reaches the forehead (point Touwei, ST 8).

One of its branches sprouts in front of Daying (ST 5), descends to Renying (ST 9), and goes along with throat into the supraclavicular fossa. From there it descends through the diaphragm, enters into its pertaining organ, the stomach, and communicates with the spleen.

A straight branch from the supraclavicular fossa descends into the medial border of the papilla mammae. Then it makes its descent along the side of the umbilicus and enters into point Qijie i.e., Qichong (ST 30).

One of the branches starting from the pylorus descends through the abdominal cavity, and joins the straight branch at Point Qijie (ST 30). From there it descends through Point Biguan (ST 31), Futu (ST 35), to the knee. Along the anteriolateral aspect of the tibia, it goes towards the dorsum of the foot, and then to the lateral side of the tip of the second toe (point Lidui ST 45).

Another branch sprouting from the region 3 individual *cun* below the genu (point Zusanli, ST 36), descends to the lateral side of the middle toe.

The branch sprouting from the dorsum of the foot (point Chongyang, ST 42) descends into the medial margin of the hallux and through its tip (point Yinbai, SP one), connects with the Spleen Channel of Foot Taiyin.

Connections with zang fu:

belongs to the stomach, luo connects with spleen, helps the heart, large intestines, and small intestines systems.

Pertaining channel points:

cheng qi (ST1), si bai (ST2), ju liao (ST3), di cang (ST4), da ying (ST5), jia che (ST6), xia guan (ST7), tou wei (ST8) ren ying (ST9), shui tu (ST10), qi she (ST11), que pen (ST12), qi hu (ST13), ku fang (ST14), wu yi (ST15) ying chuang (ST16), ru zhong (ST17), ru gen (ST18), bu rong (ST19), cheng man (ST20), liang men (ST21), guan men (ST22), tai yi (ST23), hua rou men (ST24), tian shu (ST25), wai ling (ST26), da ju (ST27), shui dao (ST28), gui lai (ST29), qi chong (ST30), bi quan (ST31), fu tu (ST32), yin shi (ST33), liang qiu (ST34), du pi (ST35), zu san li (ST36), shang ju xu (ST37), tiao kou (ST38), xia ji xa (ST39), feng long (ST40), jie xi (ST41), chong yang (ST42), xian gu (ST43), nei ting (ST44), li dui (ST45), totalling 45 points.

Meeting points:

ying xiang (Hand-yangming), jing ming (Foot-taiyang), shang guan, xuan li, han yan (Foot-shaoyang), ren zhong, shen ting, da zhui (du), cheng jiang, shang wan, zhong wan (ren).

(4) The Spleen Channel of Foot-Taiyin
Course

The channel starts from the tip of the medial side of the great toe (Yinbai, SP one). From there it runs along the junction of the red and white skin of the medial aspect of the great toe, passes the posterior surface of "Hegu", the nodular process on the medial aspect of the first metatarsophalangeal joint and descends in front of the medial malleolus to the medial aspect of the calf. It makes its way along the posterior border of the tibia, descends in front of the Liver Channel of Foot Jueyin, goes through the anterior medial aspect of the knee and thigh, and into the abdominal cavity, then enters its pertaining organ, the spleen, and communicates with the stomach. From there it goes through the diaphragm, and upwards along the two sides of the throat, reaches the root of the tongue and spreads over its lower surface.
The branch of the channel sprouts from the stomach, goes upwards through the diaphragm, disperses into the heart and with the Heart Channel of Hand-Shaoyin.

Connections with the zang fu:

belongs to spleen, luo communicates with stomach, connects with heart, lungs and large and small intestines systems.

Pertaining channel points:

yin bai (SP1), da du (SP2), tai bai (SP3), gong sun (SP4), shang qiu (SP5), san yin jiao (SP6), lou gu (SP7), di ji (SP8), yin ling quan (SP9), xue hai (SP10), ji men (SP11), chong men (SP12), fu shi (SP13), fu jie (SP14), da hong (SP15), fu ai (SP16), shi dou (SP17), tian xi (SP18), xiong xiang (SP19), zhou rong (SP20), da bao (SP21), altogether 21 points.

Meeting Points:

zhong ji, guan yuan, xia wan (ren), ri yue (Foot-shaoyang) qi men (Foot-jueyin), zhong fu (Hand-taiyin).

(5)   The Heart Channel of Hand-Shaoyin
Course

This channel starts from the heart, comes out of the cardiac system (the large vessels connecting with the other viscera) and descends through the diaphragm to connect with the small intestine.

The branch of the channel sprouts from a cardiac system, runs upwards along the side of the throat, and joins the ocular connectors (the structures connecting the eyeball with the brain), including blood vessels and optic nerves.

The original channel ascends from a cardiac system to the lungs descends to the axilla. And then it travels along the posterior border of the medial aspect of the upper arm, passes behind the Lung Channel of Hand -Taiyin and the pericardium Channel of Hand -Jueyin, goes downwards and reaches the cubicle fossa.

It continues to run along the posterior border of the medial aspect of the forearm, and arrives at the capitate bone proximal to the palm. It travels via the posterior border of the medial aspect of the palm, and then along the medial side of the little finger, reaches the tip (point Shaochong H9) and finally connects with the Small Intestine Channel of Hand-Taiyang.

Connections with zang fu:

Belongs to heart, luo communicates with small intestines, connects with lungs and kidneys systems.

Pertaining channel points:

ju quan (H1), qing ling (H2), shao hai (H3), ling dao (H4), tong li (H5), yin xi (H6), shen men (H7), shao fu (H8), shao chong (H9), altogether 9 points.

(6)   The Small Intestine Channel of Hand - Taiyang
Course

This Channel starts from the tip of the ulna side, of the little finger (point Shaoze, ST 1), and follows the ulna border of the dorsum of the hand, ascends to the wrist, and then through the styloid process of the ulna and posterior border of the forearm, finally passing between the olecranon of the ulna and the epicondyle of the humerus. It continues to travel along the posterior border of the lateral aspect of the upper arm, and out of the shoulder joint. Then circling around the shoulder blade, it meets the Du Channel at point Dazhui (Du 14).

From there it goes forward into the supraclavicular fossa and then connects with the heart.

Ascending along the oesophagus, it passes the diaphragm, reaches the stomach, and enters its pertaining organ, the small intestine.

One of the branches of this channel emerges from the supraclavicular fossa, and ascends along the neck to the cheek. From there it reaches the outer canthus of the eye, and then goes into the ear (at Point Tinggong, SI 19).

The other branch of the channel, which is separated from the cheek, ascends into the infraorbital region (point Quanliao, SI 18), reaches the lateral side of the nose and terminates at the Inner canthus. Then it is distributed obliquely over the zygoma and connects with the Urinary Bladder Channel of Foot-Taiyang.

Connections with zang fu:

Belongs small intestine, luo communicates with heart, connects with stomach system.

Pertaining channel points:

shao ze (SI1), qian gu (SI2), hou xi (SI3), wan gu (SI4), yang gu (SI5), yang lao (SI6), zhi zheng (SI7), xiao hai (SI8), jian yu (SI9), nao shu (SI10), tian zong (SI11), bing feng (SI12), qu yuan (SI13), jian wai shu (SI14), jian zhong shu (SI15), tian chuang (SI16), tian rong (SI17), quan liao (SI18), ting gong (SI19), totalling 19 points.

Meeting points:

da zhui (du), shang wan, zhong wan (ren), jing ming, da zhu, fu feng (Foot-tai yang), he liao (Hand-shaoyang), tong zi liao (Foot-shaoyang).

(7)   The Urinary Bladder Channel of Foot-Taiyang
Course

This channel commences from the inner canthus, ascends to the forehead and joins its symmetrical channel at the vertex (point Baihui, Du 20).

One of its branches splits off the vertex and goes into the upper aspect of the auricle. The original channel leaves the vertex for the brain where it re-emerges and runs downward to the back of the neck. Continuing along the medial side of the scapula, it travels parallel to the vertebral column and reaches the lumbar region;

passing the paravertebral muscles, it communicates with the kidney and enters into its pertaining organ, the urinary bladder.

The branch from the lumbar region runs downwards parallel to the vertebral column (1.5 individual cun lateral to the back midline), through the gluteal region and into the popliteal fossa.

Another branch emerges from the original channel at the back of the neck, from the medial side of the scapula passes through the scapula, and runs downward parallel to the vertebral column (3 individual cun lateral to the back midline). Then it runs through the trocanter major of the femur, downwards along the posterior border of the lateral side of the thigh where it meets the branch descending from the lumbar region in the popliteal fossa. From there it makes its way down through the musculus gastrocnemius, emerges from the posterior aspect of the external malleolus, runs along point jinggu (UB 64) to the lateral side of the tip of the small toe (point zhiyin, UB 67), where it connects with the Kidney Channel of Foot-Shaoyin.

Connections with zang fu:

Belongs to urinary bladder, luo communicates with kidneys, connects with the brain and heart systems.

Pertaining channel points:

jing ming (UB1), can zhu (UB2), mei chong (UB3), qu cha (UB4), wu chu (UB5), cheng guang (UB6), tong tian (UB7), luo que (UB8), yu zhen (UB9), tian zhu (UB10), da zhu (UB11), feng men (UB12), fei shu (UB13), jue yin shu (UB14), xin shu (UB15), du shu (UB16), ge shu (UB17), gan shu (UB18), dan shu (UB19), pi shu (UB20), wei shu (UB21), san jiao shu (UB22), shen shu (UB23), qi hai shu (US24), da chang shu (UB25), guan yuan shu (UB26), xiao chang shu (UB27), pang guang shu (UB28), zhong gu shu (UB29), bai huan shu (UB30), shang liao (UB31), ci liao (UB32), zhong liao (UB33), xia liao (UB34), hui yang (UB35), (UB36), yin men (UB37), fu xi (UB38), wei yang (UB39), wei zhong (UB40), fu feng (UB 41), po hu (UB42), gao huang shu (UB43), shen tang (UB44), yi xi (UB45), ge guan (UB46), hun men (UB47), yang gang (UB48), yi she (UB49), wei cang (UB50), huang men (UB51), zhi shi (UB52), bao huang (UB53), zhi bian (UB54), he yang (UB55), chong jin (UB56), cheng shan (UB57), fei yang (UB58), fu yang (UB59), kun lun (UB60), pu shen (UB61), shen mai (UB62), jin men (UB63), jing gu (UB64), shu gu (UB65), tong gu (UB66), zhi yin (UB67), totalling 67 points.

Meeting points:

qu bin, shuai gu, fu bai, tou qiao yin, wan gu, tou lin qi, huan tiao (Foot-shaoyang), shen ting, bai hui, nao hu, da zhui, tao dao (du).

(8) The Kidney Channel of Foot-Shaoyin

The Kidney Channel of Foot-Shoyin starts from the plantar surface of the little toe, and runs obliquely towards the centre of the sole of the foot (point Yongquan, K 1). Emerging from point Rangu (K 2) (at the interior aspect of the tuberosity navicular bone) it runs behind the medial malleolus, and reaches the heel. Then it ascends along the medial side of the Musculus Gastrocnemius and emerges from the medial side of the popliteal fossa. Ascending continuously along the medio-posterior aspect of the thigh, it runs through the vertebral column. From there it enters its pertaining organ, the kidney, and communicates with the urinary bladder.

Its direct branch re-emerges from the kidney, runs straight up through the liver and diaphragm, into the lung, from which it travels along the throat and terminates at the root of the tongue. Another branch of it exits from the lung, with the heart, and is distributed over the thoracic cavity is to meet with the Pericardium Channel of Hand-Jueyin.

Connections with the zang fu:

Belongs to the kidneys, luo communicates with urinary bladder. Connects with liver, lungs and heart, etc., systems.

Pertaining points:

yong quan (K1), ran gu (K2), tai xi (K3), da chong (K4), shui quan (K5), zhao hai (K6), fu liu (K7), jiao xin (K8), zhu bin (K9), yin gu (K10), heng gu (K11), da he (K12), qi xue (K13), si man (K14), zhong zhu (K15), huang shu (K16), shang qu (K17), shi guan (K18), yin du (K19), tong gu (K20), you men (K21), bu lang (K22), shen feng (K23), ling xu (K24), shen cang (K25), yu zhong (K26), shu fu (K27), totalling 27 points.

Meeting Points:

san yin jiao (Foot-tai yin), chang qiang (du), guan yuan, zhong ji (ren).

(9)   The Pericardium Channel
Course

This channel commences from the chest where it exits from its pertaining organ, the pericardium. Then it descends through the diaphragm and links up with the triple warmers in the upper, the middle and the lower portions of the body cavity. One of its branches runs along the chest, through the costal region at a point 3 individual cun below the armpit, and ascends to the axilla. From the medial aspect of the upper arm, it makes its way downwards between the Lung channel and the Heart channel, and reaches the cubital fossa. From there it runs still further downwards to the forearm between the tendons of m. Palmaris longus and m. flexocarpi, and enters the palm. It runs along the middle finger to its tip (Point Zhongchong, P 9).

Connections with zang fu:

Belongs to pericardium luo, luo communicates with triple heater (san jiao).

Pertaining points:

tian chi (P1), tian quan (P2), qu ze (P3), xi men (P4), jian shi (P5), nei guan (P6), da ling (P7), lao gong (P8), zhong chong (P9), totalling 9 points.

(10) The Triple Heater Sanjiao Channel of Hand-Shaoyang
Course

The Triple Heater Channel of Hand-Shaoyang starts from the ulna side of the tip of the ring finger (point Guanchong, TH1.), and runs upward between the two fingers i.e., the fourth and fifth metacarpal bones. Along the dorsum of the wrist, it travels to the dorsal side of the forearm between the two bones or the radius and ulna. It goes upwards through the olecranon, along the lateral aspect of the upper arm, to the shoulder region, where it meets the Gall Bladder Channel of Foot-Shaoyang, and afterwards leaves its posterior aspect for the supraclavicular fossa. From the fossa it descends further, is distributed to point Shanzhong (Ren 17) and ascends to the supraclavicular fossa, from where it goes upwards to the nape of the neck. From the posterior border of the ear, it makes direct descent through superior aspect of the auricula, curves down to the cheek, and then reaches the infraorbital region.
Another branch originates in the retro-auricular region and passes into the ear. Emerging in front of the ear, it runs in front of Kezhuren or Shangguan point

Shangguan (GB 3), crosses the above-mentioned branch at the cheek and reaches the outer canthus where it connects with the Gall Bladder Channel of Foot-Shaoyang.

Connections with zang fu:

Belongs to the triple heater, luo communicates with the pericardium.

Pertaining points:

guan chong (TH1), ya men (TH2), zhong zhu (TH3), yang chi (TH4), wai guan (TH5), zhi gou (TH6), hui zong (TH7), san yang luo (TH8), si du (TH9), tian jing (TH10), qing leng yuan (TH11), xiao luo (TH12), nao hui (TH13), jian liao (TH14), tian liao (TH15), tian you (TH16), yi feng (TH17), qi mai (TH18), lu xi (TH19), jiao sun (TH20), er men (TH21), er he liao (TH22), si zhu kong (TH23). Totalling 23 points.

Meeting points:

bing feng, quan liao, ting gong (Hand-taiyang), tong zi liao, shang guan, han yan, xuan li, jian jing, (Foot-shaoyang), da zhui (du).

(11) The Gall Bladder Channel of Foot-Shaoyang
Course

This Channel starts from the outer canthus of the eye, runs upwards to the corner of the forehead, and curves downward to the retro-auricular region. Then it runs along the side of the neck in front of the Triple Warmer Channel to the shoulder. Turning backwards it goes behind the Triple Warmer Channel of Hand-Shaoyang, and enters the supraclavicular fossa.

One of its branches originates in the retro-auricular region, passes through the ear, re-emerges in front of the ear and then reaches the posterior aspect of the outer canthus of the eye.

Another branch leaves the outer canthus for point Daying (ST 5), and meets the Triple Warmer Channel of Hand-Shaoyang again. From there it reaches the infra orbital region, then descends through point Jiache (ST 6) to the neck, from where it passes into the supraclavicular fossa and meets the original channel. Then it continues to travel through the chest, the diaphragm, the liver, and then to the gallbladder. It then travels though the inside of the hypochondrium, through point Qijie or Qichong (ST 30), around the margin of the public region, transversely into point Huantiao (GB 30).

A third straight branch descends from the supraclavicular fossa to the axilla, where it continues its descent along the lateral aspect of the chest, through the hypochondrium, to Huantiao (GB 30), it goes down along the lateral aspect of the thigh, emerges from the lateral side of the knee, and continues its downward travel along the anterior aspect of the fibula, and straight to Juegu, i.e., a hollow in the low part of the fibula and 3 individual cun above the external malleolus. Along the dorsum of the foot, it finds its terminus at the lateral side of the tip of the 4th toe.

A fourth branch leaves the dorsum of the foot, makes its way first between the first and second metatarsal bones, then through the distal portion of the big toe, back into its nail and finally out of the hair portion proximal to it, and communicates with the Liver Channel of Foot-Jueyin.

Connections with zang fu:

Belongs to gall bladder, luo communicates with liver, connects with heart system.

Pertaining points:

tong zi liao (GB1), ting hui (GB2), shang guang (GB3), han yan (GB4), xuan lu (GB5), xuan li (GB6), qu bin (GB7), shuai gu (GB8), tian chong (GB9), fu bai (GB10), qiao yin (GB11), wan gu (GB12), ben shen (GB13), yang bai (GB14), tou lin qi (GB15), mu quang (GB16), zheng ying (GB17), cheng ling (GB19), feng chi (GB20), jian jing (GB21), yuan ye (GB22), zhe jin (GB23), ri yue (GB24), jing men (GB25), dai mai (GB26), wu shu (GB27), wei dao (GB28), ju liao (GB29), huan tiao (GB30), feng shi (GB31), zhong du (GB32), yang guang (GB33), yang ling quan (GB34), yang jiao (GB35), wai qiu (GB36), guang ming (GB37), yang fu (GB38), xuan zhong (GB39), qiu xu (GB40), zu lin qi (GB41), di wu hui (GB42), xia xi (GB43), zu qiao yin (GB44). Totalling 44 points.

Meeting points:

tou wei, xia guan (Foot-yangming), yi feng, jiao sun, he liao (Hand-shaoyang), ting gong, bing feng, (Hand-taiyang), da zhui (du), zhong men (Foot-jueyin), shang liao, xia liao (Foot-taiyang), tian chi (Hand-jueyin), tian rong (Hand-taiyang).

(12) The Liver Channel of Foot-Jueyin
Course

The Liver Channel of the Foot-Jueyin starts from the border of the hair behind the great toe, passes the dorsum of the foot and reaches region one individual cun in front of the medial malleolus. From there, it ascends 8 individual cun above the medial malleolus where it crosses the Spleen Channel of Foot-Taiyin, then runs behind the channel up to the medial border of the popliteal fossa. It continues its descent along the medial side of the thigh, to the pubic region where it curves around the external genitalia and enters the lower abdomen. From there, it runs upward via the stomach into its pertaining organ, the liver, and communicates with the gall bladder. Further upward, it passes through the diaphragm, is distributed to the hypochondrium, and ascends along the posterior aspect of the larynx to the nasopharynx, where it connects with the surrounding tissues of the eye, then emerges from the forehead, and finally meets the Du Channel at the vertex.

One of the branches originates in the tissues connecting the eyeball with the brain, goes downwards into the cheek and curves around the inner surface of the lips. Another branch originates in the liver, passes through the diaphragm and penetrates to the lung, where it connects to the Lung Channel of Hand-Taiyin.

Connections with zang fu:

Belongs to the liver, luo communicates with gall bladder, connects with lungs, stomach, kidneys, and brain systems.

Pertaining points:

da dun (LIV1), xing jian (LIV2), tai chong (LIV3), zhong feng (LIV4), li gou (LIV5), zhong du (LIV6), xi guan (LIV7), qu quan (LIV8), yin bao (LIV9), wu li (LIV10), yin lian (LIV11), ji mai (LIV12), zhang men (LIV13), qi men (LIV14).

Meeting points:

san yin jiao, chong men, fu she (Foot-taiyin), qu gu, zhong ji, guan yuan (ren).

(2) The analysis of the correct circling paths of the twelve jing mai

1. The relationship between the directions and the sequences and the connections of the 12 jing mai and the organs.
    (1) The regulation of the twelve jing mai is hand three yin jing (including the Hand-taiyin lung channel, Hand-jueyin pericardium channel, and the Hand-shaoyin heart channel), from the zang organs, chest through to the hand. The hand three yang jing (including the Hand-yangming large intestine channel, the Hand-shaoyang triple heater

channel, and the hand tai yang small intestine channel) from the hand up to the head. The three yin jing (including the foot tai yin spleen channel, the foot jue yin liver channel, and the foot shao yin kidney channel) from the feet through the abdomen (chest). The foot three yang jing (including the foot yang ming stomach channel, the foot shao yang gall bladder channel, and the foot tai yang urinary bladder channel) from the head goes through to the feet.

(2) The flow injection order and the connection of the 12 zheng jing. The twelve jing mai are the main channels for qi and blood circulation and the qi and blood are transported by the jing mai. It's transformed from the qi of water and grain in the middle heater so jing mai accept the essence of the grain qi at the zhong jiao (middle heater) and transport to the lungs and from the lungs its starts to transfer to the foot jue yin liver and back to the lungs again forming the cycle of the 12 jing. The flow injection order of the 12 jing is hand tai yin lung channel, hand yang ming large intestine channel, foot yang ming stomach channel, hand tai yang small intestine channel, foot tai yang urinary bladder channel, foot shao yin kidney channel, hand jue yin pericardium channel, hand shao yang triple heater channel, foot shao yang gall bladder channel, foot jue yin liver channel back to the lungs.

Qi and bood according to the flow injection order of the 12 jing mai, cycles and transfers like a sealed ring continuously flowing. During the process of the flow injection of the 12 jing mai, the transfer of the mai qi is mainly in two forms:

(1) Inside the body there is a relationship of shu belonging or pertaining luo, networking or communicating of the organs. Mai qi is connected with this.

(2) Outside the body it is connected by zhi mai or luo mai to the next channel along. For example the hand tai yin lung channel internally pertains to the lungs and communicates with the large intestine outside the body "ji zhi zhe cong wan zhi chu ci zhi nei lian chu qi duan" (it's branch comes out from the wrist straight out to the second finger inner side to the tip).

(3) The relationship between the 12 jing and zang fu: each jing mai out of the 12 jing mai, inside the body is connected to zang fu forming a relationship of shu luo. Each yin channel belongs to organs, each yang channel belongs to bowels. Between yin

jing and yang jing, zang (organs) and fu (bowels), an exterior and interior relationship is formed. Such as the hand tai yin lung channel, a yin channel belongs to the lung organ and communicates with or is connected to the large intestine bowel. The Hand-yangming large intestine channel, a yang channel, belongs to the large intestine bowel and communicates with or is connected to the lungs. The zang and fu, ie. the lung and large intestine form a relationship of exterior and interior. In terms of distribution position outside the body, the exterior and interior jing also form a pair or relationship with each other's luo mai and are thereby able to connect with one another. The exterior and interior relationship of the 12 jing are as follows:

Exterior: LI ⇨ ST   SI ⇨ UB   TH ⇨ GB
            ⇧   ⇩   ⇧   ⇩   ⇧   ⇩
Interior: LU   SP ⇨ H   K ⇨ P   LIV

Explanation: The flow direction of the flow injection order of the jing mai is an agreed upon law or rule according to the principle of "yin shang yang jiang" (yin goes upwards, yang sinks), it doesn't mean it is the only form of circulation of qi and blood. Here, the purpose is to explain the close relationship of the jing mai in the upper and lower, left and right positions on the body exterior, and to show how the limbs and body and the internal zang and fu have a relationship of internal and external body and the internal zang and fu have a relationship of internal and external connections. In the past, the circulation of jing and wei and qi and blood in the jing luo was believed to circulate according to the above order and direction of the jing mai distribution lines, one channel after another channel circulating endlessly throughout the body. In fact, this is only one kind of statement about the theory of jing mai circulation made by ancient medical doctors.

Jing qi circulates in the body by many paths and many forms of circulation. Ying and qi circulates in the mai (vessels) according to the direction of the 12 jing mai and travels along the channels themselves. Wei qi travels outside the mai, travels in the yang in the day, travels in the yin at night, and travels in a circle. The jing bie gives emphasis to this internal circulation of external and internal channels. The luo mai give emphasis to the random distribution on the body exterior and at the same time the jing jin (tendon and muscular channels) etc. have a function of helping the jing qi circulation to collect at the centre or heart; also the qi jing extra ordinary channels help to control the circulation of jing qi by a form of overflow storage and regulation. They all have both systematic differences and a close connection. They all make for a whole jing qi circulation system with the 12 jing mai as the main body of that system.

2. The local anatomy of the circulation lines of the 12 jing mai: any of the natural sciences receive certain philosophical directions during their development processes. Formation of jing luo theory into a really quite complete theoretical system is itself not independent of basic ancient dialectics (e.g. yin yang wu xing theory). The *Su wen-jin gui zhen yan luo* said: "Yan ren zhi yin yang, ze wai wei yang, nei wei yin: yan ren shen zhi yin yang, ze bei wei yang fu wei yin" ("when we are talking about yin and yang, then the exterior is yang, and the interior is yin. When referring to the yin and yang of the human body, the back is yang, the abdomen is yin. About the yin yang of the human body's zang fu, the zang … are yin, the fu bowels are yang"). The circulation distribution and its belonging to or pertaining to relationship with the zang fu of the 12 jing mai are obeying yin yang theory and show the above principle of how yin yang characterisation can be seen.

    (1) The upper limbs explanation: according to the characterisation principle yin yang i.e. nei wei yin, wai wei yang (the inner side is yin, the outer is yang) the boundary is the line between red and white flesh. The three yin channels of the hand travel on the inner side, the three yang channels of the hand on the outer side. On the yin side (inner side), the hand tai yin lung channel travels in the front (radial bone side), the hand jue yin pericardium luo channel circulates in the centre between the two tendons (radius bone side between the flexi carpi radialis and the palmaris longus), the hand shao yin heart channel travels in the rear to this on the side, and the yang side surface, i.e., the external side, the shou san yang jing (the hand three yang channels), according to the relationship of external and internal channels, circulate and distribute at corresponding positions. So the hand yang ming large intestine channel travels on the outer side of the arm upwards, the radial side along the musculus brachioradialis

(upper boundary), the hand san jiao triple heater channel travels along the arm outer side centre line between the radius and the ulna. The hand tai yang small intestine channel travels on the outside of the arm ulna side, goes upwards along the humerus bone inner side between upper end process of the ulna's olecranon.

(2) The lower limbs: for convenience the description of the lower limbs has been separated into anterior, posterior, medial and lateral four sections. The foot three yin channels will be described in the following under the medial section and the foot yang ming stomach channel will be described in the following under the interior section. The foot shao yang gall bladder channel, will be described in the following under the lateral section. The foot tai yang urinary bladder channel will be described in the following under the posterior section. The foot three yin channels in the medial section can furthermore be separated into two sections from the medial ankle bone 8 cun and below the foot shao yin travels in front, the foot tai yin travels in the middle, and the foot shao yin travels behind, 8 cun above the medial ankle bone. The foot tai yang meets the jue yin and crosses in front from this place 8 cun above the medial ankle bone, the foot spleen channel travels in front, the foot jue yin liver channel goes in the middle and the foot shao yin kidney channel goes behind. These circulatory distribution positions correspond with the upper limbs and also they have a relationship with the organs' and the limbs' positions, and so have the same named channels in the hand and the feet. They have a relationship called tong qi xiang tong (same qi they are able to connect), this is the main background for the generation of luo jing bian zheng 6 channel differentiation and diagnosis. The 12 jing mai travelling and following along the four limbs can be shown in the following table: Table 5.

Table 5: The 12 Channels 4 Limbs Circling Parts External

		Yin	(Internal)	(External)	Yang		
Upper limbs (arms internal side)	Front	Hand tai yin	Lungs	Large intestines	Hand yang ming	Front	Upper limbs (arms external side)
	Middle	Hand jue yin	Pericardium	Triple heater	Hand shao yang	Middle	
	Behind	Hand shao yin	Heart	Small intestines	Hand tai yang	Behind	

Lower limbs (internal side surface)	Front	Foot jue yin	- foot tai yin governs spleen	Stomach	Foot yang ming	Front	Lower limbs (front external back surface)
	Middle	Foot tai yin	- foot jue yin governs liver	Gall bladder	Foot shao yang	Middle	
	Behind	Foot shao yin	Kidney	Urinary bladder	Foot tai yang	Behind	

(3) The head surfaces and neck: the 12 jing mai external circulating lines on the head surfaces can be summarised as the front or anterior surface is governed by the yang ming channel; the lateral surfaces are governed by the shao yang channel, the posterior surface is governed by the tai yang channel; the head crown position is governed by the foot tai yang channel; and the foot jue yin's mai qi goes up through to the crown. This can be seen in table 6.

Table 6: The 14 Channels External Travelling Head Parts Route Phase

Head Face Parts	Governs Cycling Parts Channels
Front Face	Foot yang ming stomach channel, hand yang ming large intestines channel; ren, du channels
Side Head	Foot shao yang gallbladder channel, hand shao yang triple heater channel, hand tai yang small intestines channel
Head Top	Foot tai yang urinary bladder channel; du channel, foot jue yin channel (channel qi through to the crown)
Head Back	Foot tai yang bladder channel; du channel

If we only view the distribution channels from the perspective of the head and face jing mai external parts, then the channels in the head and face position mainly yang Channels. Yin channels generally don't go up to the head, only the foot jue yin liver channel goes up to the crown top, and the hand shao yin heart channel goes up and connects with the eye system. However, from the whole Chinese medicine theory system viewpoint and jing luo theories, the head and face play a very important part. This is because except for the 14 jing mai external distribution parts, the head and face also have other types of channel cycling paths. Not only do the yang channels go through to the head, the foot three yin channels after connecting with the yang channels, also reach the face. Furthermore, the hand three yin channels go from the armpit (ye wo) and into the internal organs, afterwards going through the throat, to connect with the head and face. Finally, the extra-ordinary channels and the jing jin etc. related systems have many kinds of connections too. Altogether this enables the jing qi of the body to pass through the channel qi circulation and accumulate in the head, brain, face, and the five sense organs (wu guan) positions. So, in the qi pathway theories they place the concept that the head qi belongs to the pathway, in a very important position. The book *Ling Shu-xie qi zang fu bing zang* points out that the "shi er jing mai, san bai liu shi wu luo, qi xue qi jie shang yu mian er zou kong qiao. Qi jing yang qi shang zou yu mu er wei jing. Qi bie qi zou yu er wei ting. Qi zong qi shang chie bui er wei xiu. Qi shuo qi chu yu wei, zou chun she er wei wei. Qi qi zhi jin ye, jie sheng xun yu mian". ("The 12 jing mai, the three hundred and sixty-five luo and all the blood and qi go up to the face and through the empty openings (orifices). The jing yang qi, the human essence of yang qi, goes up through to the eyes for seeing. The bie qi goes through to the ears for hearing. The zong qi (pectoral qi) goes up to the nose for smelling, the zhuo qi (turbid qi) goes from the stomach, through to the tongue for tasting, and the qi ye (fluids) all go up to the face.") This describes the reason why the head, face and empty openings are important locations for the accumulation of jing qi. The later doctors paid great attention to developing these theories and came up with the conclusion that "shou wei zhu yang shi hui bai mai zhi zong" ("the head is the meeting place for all the yang and is the source of or the master of the one hundred mai or vessels").

The distribution of external paths in the neck and throat and nape of neck positions mainly includes the yang channels. The hands and feet three yang channels mai qi, all connect at the back of the nape of the neck at da zhui point (GV 14) and then go up through to the head.

The distribution of the paths of the 12 jing mai in the neck, throat and nape of neck positions can be described as below:

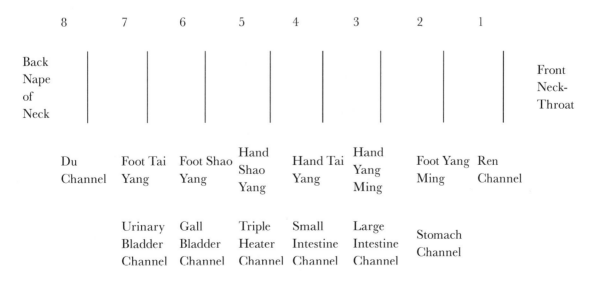

	8	7	6	5	4	3	2	1	
Back Nape of Neck									Front Neck-Throat
	Du Channel	Foot Tai Yang	Foot Shao Yang	Hand Shao Yang	Hand Tai Yang	Hand Yang Ming	Foot Yang Ming	Ren Channel	
		Urinary Bladder Channel	Gall Bladder Channel	Triple Heater Channel	Small Intestine Channel	Large Intestine Channel	Stomach Channel		

(4) The body positions: the paths of the twelve jing mai in the body
basically follow bei wei yang (back is for the yang), fu wei yin (the
abdomen is for the yin), yin and yang distribution principle. Only
one channel is exempt from this distribution principle. It is the foot
tai yang ming stomach channel. It belongs to the yang channels, but
it passes through the abdomen on either side of the abdomen centre
line (zhong xian) the foot yang urinary bladder channel goes through
the sides of the back while the foot shao yang gall bladder channel
goes through both sides of the rib positions. The foot three yin
channels travel through the abdomen position using the central line
of the abdomen or ren mai, as a standard, 0.5 cun beside of which is
the foot shao yin kidney channel, and 4 cun beside which is the foot
tai yin spleen channel; the foot jue yin liver channel also can be found
going from the pubic bone joint connecting the last 2.5 cun below at
ji mai (Liv 12) point and then going up to the seventh floating rib, i.e.
to zhang men point (Liv 13) and ending between the two ribs under
the breast at qi men point (Liv 14). The 12 jing mai distribution in
the abdomen position can be seen in the following figure 1:

Figure 1

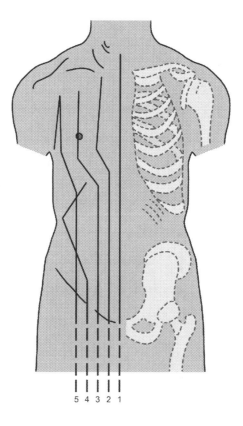

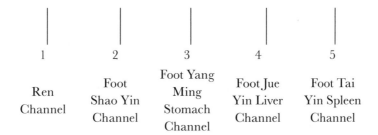

1	2	3	4	5
Ren Channel	Foot Shao Yin Channel	Foot Yang Ming Stomach Channel	Foot Jue Yin Liver Channel	Foot Tai Yin Spleen Channel

Section 1

With regards to the analysis of sickness, from the book the *Ling Shu-Jing Mai* it is said, each jing mai bing hou of the twelve jing can be separated into "shi dong" "suo shen bing" two parts. For the meaning of "shi dong" and "suo shen bing" this will be the special topic of discussion in another time in this book. This section is really based on the *Ling Shu-Jing Mai* from its original writings for the purpose of analysis. Some of the jing mai bing hou has reference from *Nei Jing*. The twelve jing bing hou have an idea of "qi sheng you yu: ("too much qi") "qi xu" ("qi deficiency") - this is the same as "shi zheng" ("excess condition") and "xu zheng" ("deficiency condition"). Although there are deficiency and excess conditions listed for all the organs, only the first three sections are given i.e. the kidney jing has the most commonly quoted proof of the kidney deficiency solely existing. To analyse the meanings from the original documents, each jing's bing hou are listed by way of separation into external jing bing hou and internal organ's bing hou two parts.

(1)   12 channels bing hou (problems emitted by the channel) theory separated

1.   Hand tai yin lung channel: *Ling Shu-Jing Mai* said shi dong then illness lungs distended stuffy, ha ha sound, and panting and coughing, supraclavicular fossa pain, extreme then meets both hands and du, all becomes bi jue. Governs lung suo sheng bing, cough, raising of qi, panting and thirst, upset, chest stuffy, pain adverse down inside front shoulder and upper arm, hands inside hot …

    (1)   The external jing bing hou: doesn't like cold, fever, no sweating or sweating, nose is blocked, headache, clavicle bone (i.e. supraclavicular fossa) pain, chest painful, or shoulder and back painful, hand and arm cold and painful.

    (2)   Internal organ bing hou: cough, asthma (xiao chuan), qi urgent or panting (qi ji), chest parts feeling full and stuffy, vomiting phlegm, throat feeling dry, colour of urine changes, upset, (xin fan), or maybe

43

saliva has blood, centres of the hands are hot. Sometimes can also be seen the abdomen feels distended and stuffy and the stools loose.

(3) Too much qi - excess condition: shoulder and back pain, if damage by the wind and cold, there will be some sickness with self-sweating etc., attacked by wind symptoms, or maybe the urine will be frequent but the quantity will be little.

(4) Not enough qi - deficiency condition: shoulder and back painful and doesn't like cold, breathing short and hurried, the urine colour will have abnormal change.

2. Hand yang ming large intestine channel: *Ling Shu-Jing Mai* said, "Shi dong ze bing chi tong, jing zhong. Shi zhu jing ye suo sheng bing zhi, mu huang, kou gan, bi (zhi bi sai duo ti) nü, hou bi, jian qian, ru tong, da zhi ci zhi bu yong. Qi you yu ze dang mai suo guo zhi re zhong; xu ze han li bu fu. ("shi dong sickness then tooth pain, the neck swelling, if the problem comes mainly from the fluids suo sheng bing the eyes will be yellow, the mouth dry and the nose (will be blocked and much mucous and bleeding), the throat feeling sore and blocked, the front shoulder and upper arm painful, the big finger and second finger cannot be used. If too much qi, where the channel passes through, it will hot and swollen [causing swelling] if deficient, there will be cold and feeling chilly.

Analysis of bing hou:

(1) External jing bing hou: fever, mouth feels dry and thirsty, throat is painful and the nose is bleeding, tooth pain, eyes red and painful, neck swollen, shoulder and scapular and upper arm painful, or red swelling and feeling hot, or have cold feeling, the second finger cannot move easily.

(2) Internal organs bing hou: Umbilicus and abdomen (qi fu) pain or the abdomen painful is not in a fixed place, intestinal sounds, the stools are loose (diarrhoea) or maybe have yellow sticky stools. Some patients may also have qi ji (i.e. panting) and chuan ni (dyspnea).

(3) Too much qi and excess condition: the place the jing mai goes through will have fever and swelling.

(4) Not enough jing qi, deficient condition: feeling cold, chilly, not easy to return to warmth.

3. The foot yang ming stomach jing: The book *Ling Shu Jing Mai* said, "shi dong ze bing sa sa zhen han, shan yin, su qian, yan hei, bing zhi ze ren yu huo, wan mu sheng ze ti ran er jing, xin yu dong, du bi hu sai you er chu, shen ze yu shang gao er ge, qi yi er zou, pen xing fu zhang, shi wei gan jue. Shi zhu xue suo sheng bing zhe, kuang, nue, wen yin, han chu bi nü, kou wo chun zhen, jing zhong, hou bi, da fu shui zhong, xi bin zhong tong, xun ying ru, qi jie, gu, fu tu, gan wai lian, zu fu shang jie tong, zhong zhi bu yong. Qi sheng ze shen yi qian jie re, qi you yu yu wei, ze xiao gu shan ji, niao se huang; qi bu zu ze shen yi qian jie han li, wei zhong han ze zhang men". "When shi dong the sickness will show as feeling cold as if lying in water on body, likes to groan, frequently yawns, the face (frontal skin) colour is black, the patient doesn't like to see people and fire, upon hearing wood sounds the patient will feel nervous, the heart likes to move, likes to live by himself and close the door, in serious cases will like to go up and sing songs or abandon clothing and walk about, borborygmus, the abdomen feels distended, this is all called gan jue. If the patient has suo sheng bing from the main blood: madness, malaria, febrile diseases, sweating out, nose bleeding, mouth deviation, lips have papules, neck swelling, throat pain, big abdomen edema, knee cap swelling and pain circling in the pectoral muscle and breast, the groin qi above the patella, sides of the tibia, the thigh (femur), the feet back upper surface feeling painful, involves the sides of the groin, the middle toe cannot use. For too much qi, the front of the body feels hot and for others, the qi is in the middle of the abdomen, so good digestion and feeling hungry, and has a yellow colour to urine; for the one who doesn't have enough qi, the front of the body feels cold and chilly, inside the stomach is cold and feeling full.

The analysis of bing hou:

(1) External jing bing hou: seriously high fever, or malaria, red face, sweating out, coma, delirium, crazy and impatient, some of them have a feeling of not liking cold; or the eyes painful, the nose dry and bleeding, the lips have ulcers (papules), the throat painful, the neck (throat) swollen, or the mouth and lips are deviated and the chest feels painful, the leg and feet red and swollen and painful, or the leg and feet feeling cold.

(2) Internal organs bing hou: abdomen expanded big and feeling full and stuffy, edema, and feeling not good when lying down, or depressed and crazy. It can be seen as good dysentery and easily hungry. The colour of the urine is yellow.

(3) Too much qi – excess condition: front of the chest abdomen position fever, the stomach has too much heat so has good strong digestion, easily hungry, the colour of the urine is yellow.

(4) Not enough jing – deficient condition: the chest and the abdomen position at the front of the body feels cold and chilly. If the stomach's central yang becomes deficient and has cold, the water and grains will stop and stagnate in the middle heater and create a feeling of fullness and stuffiness.

4. The foot tai yin spleen jing: In the book *Ling Shu-Jing Mai* it says, "shi dong ze bing shi ben qiang, shi ze ou, wei wan tong, fu zhang, shan yi, de hou yu qi, ze kuai, ran ru shuai, shen ti jie zhong. Shi zhu pi suo sheng bing zhi, shi ben tong, ben bu neng dong yao, shi bu xia, fan xin, xin xia ji tong, tang jia xie, shui bi, huang dan, bu neng wo, qiang li, gu xi nei zhong, jue, zu da zhi bu yong." ("If shi dong then the sickness will show tongue stiff, when eats gets vomiting, the gastric cavity is painful, abdominal distention, flatulence and frequent eructation which may be alleviated after moving the bowels and breaking wind, the body feeling heavy. If the patient's suo sheng bing caused by the spleen, the tongue root will feel painful, the body cannot move, cannot eat, upset (irritable), below the heart there is tense pain, stools loose, difficulty in passing urine, jaundice, cannot lie down, standing inflexible (or difficult), internal thigh and knee internal side swelling, jue condition, big toe cannot be used.

Analysis of the bing hou:

(1) External jing bing hou: head heavy, body heavy, body feeling hot, limbs feeling tired and no power, or painful in cheeks and forehead, tongue stiff and is not easily moved out, or four limbs muscles become atrophied and smaller (thinner), feeling internal side of the knee is cold feeling, or the leg and the feet have edema (dropsy).

(2) Internal organ bing hou: gastric cavity painful, stools loose, or not complete digestion of grains, intestines sounds (borborygmus), vomiting, hard lumps (masses) in the abdomen, and eating decreases,

46

or jaundice, or the abdomen stuffy, swollen and distended, urination doesn't flow.

5. Hand shao yin heart meridian
    In the *Ling Shou-Jing Mai* chapter it says "shi dong ze bing yi gan, xin tong, ke er yü yin, shi wei bi jue. Shi zhu xin suo sheng bing zhi, mu huang, xie tong, nao bi nei hou lian tong, jue, zhang zhong re tong." ("shi dong then there are sicknesses such as dry throat, heart pain, thirsty and likes to drink, all these things are bi jue. If a suo sheng bing associated with the heart, there will be yellow eyes, pain in the sides of the ribs, and the upper arm and forearm internal side are painful, and hot and painful in the centre of hands").

    Bing hou analysis:

    (1) External jing bing hou: body feels hot, headache, eye pain, chest and back are painful, dry throat, thirsty, likes to drink, hot and painful in the middle of hands, or feels adverse cold in the hands and feet, or shoulder blade (scapular) and inside of forearm painful.

    (2) Internal organs bing hou: heart pain, chest and sides of ribs stuffy and painful, under the ribs painful, upset (irritable), and breathing quickly (qi ji), not calm when lies (cannot sleep well), or dizziness and stupor, or nerves not well (i.e. nerves not normal).

6. Hand tai yang small intestine meridian
    In the *Ling shu-jing mai* chapter it says "shi dong ze bing yi tong, han zhong, bu keyi gu, jian shi ba, nao shin zhe. Shi zhu ye suo sheng bing zhe, er long mu huang, jia zhong, jing, han, jian, nao, zhou, bi wai hou lian tong." ("shi dong then there will be a feeling of throat pain, chin (jaws) swelling, you can't turn neck, shoulder feels as if being pulled, upper arm feels as if broken, if suo sheng bing from liquids (fluids) then deafness, yellow eyes, cheeks (jaw) swelling, neck, chin (jaws), shoulder, upper arm, elbow, external side of forearm have pain.

    Bing hou analysis:

    (1) External jing bing hou: mouth and tongue sodden (erosion, festering), pain in chin (jaws) and cheeks, throat pain, a lot of tears, neck (throat)

and the nape of the neck inflexible and straight, the shoulder and the external side of the forearm painful.

(2) Internal organ bing hou: the lesser abdomen feels distended and painful, and this pain connects (or extends) to the waist, lesser abdomen pain which connects with testes, stools very loose (diarrhoea), or with dry stools, constipation and stools won't pass.

7. Foot tai yang urinary bladder meridian:
In the *Ling shu-Jing mai* chapter it says "shi dong ze bing chong tou tong, mu shi tuo, xiang ru ba, ji tong, yao shi she, bi bu ke yi, guo ru jie, chuai ru lie, shi wei huai jue. Shi zhu jin suo sheng bing zhe, zhi, nüe, kuang, dian ji, tou bu xiang tong, mu huang, lei chu, bi nü, xiang, bei, yao, kao, guo, chuai, jiao jie tong, xiao zhi bu yong." "If shi dong then chong channel headache, feels pain in the eyes as if going out, pain in nape of the neck as if pulled up, backbone pain, waist feels broken, thigh cannot bend, spasm of popliteal fossa tendons, all this is huai jue. If suo sheng bing and is connected to the tendons, then there will be haemorrhoids, malaria, madness, depression, fontanel area headache and nape of neck painful, yellow eyes, eyes watering, nose bleeding, nape of neck, back, waist, buttocks, back of knees, fibula, calf, and feet all painful, small toe cannot use.

Bing hou analysis:

(1) External bing hou: feels cold and hot, headache, nape of neck inflexible, waist and spine painful, blocked nose, eyes painful and a lot of tears from eyes, or thighs, knees and back of knees, shanks (gastrocnemius muscle) and foot all painful.

(2) Internal organ bing hou: lesser abdomen feels distended and painful, urine doesn't flow, dysuria (long bi), or bedwetting (yi niao), or lose control of one's mind, or can be seen as opisthotonos.

8. Foot shao yin kidney meridian
In the *Ling shu-jing mai* chapter it says, "shi dong ze bing ji bu yu shi, mian ru qi cai, ke tuo ze you xue, he he er chuang, zuo er yu qi, mu huang huang ru wu suo jian, xin ru xuan ruo ji zhuang. Qi bu zu ze shan kong, xin ti ti ru ren jiang bu zhi, shi wei gu jue. Shi zhu shen suo shen bing zhe, kou re, she gan, yan zhong, shang qi, yi gan ji tong, fan xin, xin tong, huang dan, chang pi, ji gu nei hou lian tong, wei, jue, shi wo, zu xia re er tong". ("If shi

dong then hungry but doesn't like to eat, face looks like lacquer, coughing with blood, bronchial wheezing, when sits wants to stand up, when look at something cannot see it (i.e. blind and can't see), heart feels suspended (i.e. as if hanging) and not comfortable. If qi is not enough then will have palpitations with fearfulness, (susceptibility to fear) feels as if somebody will arrest one, all this is gu jue. If illness comes mainly from the kidney and suo sheng bing, then mouth hot, dry tongue, throat swollen, qi goes up, throat dry and painful, upset (annoyed), heart pain, jaundice, bloody stools, intestinal pi (dysentery or bloody stools) spine feels painful, limb atrophy, likes to lie, soles of feet feel hot and painful.")

Bing hou analysis:

(1) External bing hou: back and spine painful, waist painful, both feet feel adversely cold, feet atrophy and no power, or mouth dry, throat painful, or thighs (or hips) and legs back painful, and can be seen that the soles of feet are painful.

(2) Internal organ bing hou: dizziness, face part swelling, face looks dark grey (ie ashen), can't see things clearly, shortness of breath, urgent or rapid breathing, likes sleeping, or upset (i.e. irritable), loose stools, or long time diarrhoea, or stools difficult and not smoothly passing, also it can be seen that there is abdominal distention, vomiting badly or impotency.

(3) Qi deficient and not enough – deficient condition: usually feels frightened and heart palpitation like someone will arrest one.

Explanation: from this jing bing hou, only say qi is not strong but don't say too much qi, however regarding the foot shao yin kidney jing it can also be confirmed that there is an excess condition explained in the Mai Jing's *Ling Shu-ben shen* chapter where it is said: "shen qi xu ze jue shi? zang" ("kidney qi weak will have jue, and kidney qi if too strong will feel distended"). And the *Ling shu-jing mai* chapter said: "zu shao yin zhi bie … qi bing qi ni mi ze fan men, shi ze bi long, xu ze yao tong" etc. ("If the foot shao yin is deficient … its illness will cause qi adverse upset, too strong will have dysuria, deficiency then will have waist pain etc). We also meet some examples in kidney illness of edema (shui zhong) and can confirm these things in addition to kidney hot condition of xiang huo pian kang (mutual fire too strong) but in order to cure these things always attack the evils by treating the evils of other zang fu. So you can obtain the clearing of the kidney analysis, the majority of the conditions belong to weakness. Most of doctors treat foot shao yin jing illness as deficiency (conditions), like for example *Shang han lun's* shao yin illness's <u>si ni tang</u>, <u>zhen wu tang</u> etc. all belong to transform the cold conditions, all this comes from yang deficiency. <u>Huang lian e jiao tang</u>, <u>zhu ling tang</u> these are for transforming hot conditions and belong to yin deficiency; warm illness (wen bing) later stage, when the heat stays a long time, true yin has been stolen. Mainly these are caused by liver and kidney yin deficiency. In internal medicine, with the exception of xu lao (consumption), they specifically show self-sweating and night sweating (dao han), dizziness, tinnitus, and palpitations, can't sleep, dry throat, breathing with panting, (chuan xi), waist painful, seminal emission, impotency etc., conditions. Most of them are caused by kidney deficiency, others like diarrhoea, edema, high blood pressure and other illnesses they use up a lot of jing qi, to a degree they all affect the kidney especially some illnesses which are chronic illnesses, after a long time they always involve kidney deficiency. Kidney yin deficiency always presents itself like a hot condition. Kidney yang deficiency always presents itself like a cold condition. Just like Zhang jin you explained, "shui kuai qi yuan, ze yin xu zhi bing die chu; huo shuai qi ben, ze yang xu zhi zheng die sheng"("water hasn't got the source then yin deficiency illness, yin will go out and fire will lose its basis then yang deficiency will go out") *Lei ying fu yi.* These are the different illness weaknesses of foot shao yang kidney jing and other any zang-fu; all doctors are always concerned with kidney channel characteristics in illness mechanisms. As Li Dong yuan said, "shen ben wu shi, bu ke xie" ("kidney origin is not strong, you cannot sedate (or reduce)") *Li gao shi shu.* Also like Li Ying said, "shen wu shi, bu ke xie, gu wu xie shen zhi yao …" ("kidney is not too strong, it cannot release so there is no meridian for the release of kidney") *Shen jing tong kao.* From all this we know, the differentiation curve of foot shao yin kidney jing illness is from the inner mechanism of kidney illness, which could be deficient or excess but mainly is deficient. Therefore from this curve we should mainly tonify (i.e. strengthen or reinforce). Of the twelve meridian illnesses, only the foot shao yin kidney jing emphases deficiency and not excess. And this indicates kidney illnesses are more of a deficient nature, this is an important illness mechanism for consideration, and can give direction when it comes to treatment application.

9. Hand jue yin pericardium luo meridian:

In the *Ling Shu-jing mai* chapter it says, "shi dong ze bing shou xin re, bi zhou wan ji, ye zhong, shen ze xiong xie zhi man, xin zhong zhan zhan da dong, mian chi, mu huang, xi xiao bu xiu. Shi zhu mai suo shang bing zhe, fan xin, xin tong, zhang zhong re" ("If shi dong then illness will present hot in centre of the hands, arms and elbows spasmed, swelling under the armpits, fullness in the chest and hypocardium regions, heart palpitations, red face, yellow eyes, laughs without stopping. If illness comes from the vessels suo sheng bing, upset (irritable), heart pain, hot in the middle of the hands.")

Analysis of bing hou

(1) External jing bing hou: head and nape of neck inflexible and straight, hands and feet convulsions, red face or eyes painful, swelling under the armpits, arms and elbows are restricted, spasmed and can't bend flexibly, or hot in middle of the hands.

(2) Internal organs bing hou: incoherent talk (i.e. delirium), fainting (or falling into a coma), upset (irritable), chest and hypocondrium full and stuffy, tongue cannot speak or palpitations which won't calm down, or heart pain, also can be seen as laughing continuously without stopping, i.e. spirit abnormal symptoms (jing shen yi chang).

10. Hand shao yang triple heater meridian:

"shi dong ze bing, er long hun hun tun tun, yan zhong, hou bi. Shi zhu qi suo sheng bing zhe, han chu, mu rui zi tong, jia tong, er hou, jian, nao, zhou, bi wai jie tong, xiao zhi ci zhi bu yong" ("If shi dong then illness will show as deafness, can't hear clearly (ie auditus depression, hypoacusis), throat swollen, sore throat. If the illness comes mainly from qi suo sheng bing, sweating out, eye corners painful, jaw (cheek) pain, back of ear, shoulder, upper arm, elbow, and external side of arm all feel painful, small finger and ring finger cannot use.")

Analysis of bing hou:

(1) External jing ing hou: swelling and pain in throat, cheek position painful and eyes red and painful, or deafness, or can be seen as painful at the back of ear and external side of shoulder and arm.

(2) Internal organ bing hou: abdominal parts feel distended and full, lower abdomen hard and full, urine will not pass, urinates a lot and urgent urination, skin deficiency swelling (xu fou), edema or bed wetting.

11. Foot shao yang gall bladder channel:

In the *Ling shu-jing mai* chapter it says, "shi dong ze bing kou ku, shan tai xi, xin xie tong, bu neng zhuan ce, shen ze mian wei you jian, ti wu gao ze, zu wai fan re, shi wei yang jue. Shi zhu gu suo sheng bing zhe, tou tong, han tong, mu rui zi tong que pen zhong zhong tong, ye xia zhong, ma dao xia ying, han chu zhen han, nue, xiong, lie, bi, xi, wai zhi jing, jue gu, wai huai qian ji zhu jie jie tong, xiao zhi ci zhi bu yong." ("If shi dong then there will be illnesses such as mouth bitter, frequently deep sighing, heart and hypocondrium region painful, cannot turn the body, and in extreme cases the face is slightly painted and the face dusty and body is not oily and bright (i.e. is grey), feet external side feel hot, all them belongs yang jue, illness comes mainly from the bones suo sheng bing, there will be headache, chin (or jaw) pain, corner of the eye pain, supraclavicular fossa swollen and painful, swelling under the armpit, ma tuberculosis (i.e. a series of scrofula) of lymph nodes (in supraclavicular fossa or upper shoulder to hypochondrial regions), goitre, sweating out and shivers with cold, malaria, chest and hypocondrium and ribs, thighs (or buttocks, hipbone) and external side of the knee to fibula, GB39 area, in front of the external ankle and all (i.e. numerous, various) the joints feel painful, small toe and fourth toe cannot use.")

Bing hou analysis

(1) External bing hou: hot and cold comes and goes, headache, malaria, face is ashen grey (dark), eyes painful, chin (or jaw) painful, swelling under armpit, scrofula, deafness, thigh parts or leg, knee and fibula parts feel painful.

(2) Internal organ bing hou: hypocondrium region and ribs painful, vomiting, mouth bitter, and chest painful.

12. Foot jue yin liver channel:

In the *Ling shu-jing mai* chapter it says, "shi dong ze bing yao tong bu ke yi fu yang, zhang fu kui shan, fu ren shao fu zhong shen ze yi gan, mian chen, tuo se. Shi zhu gan suo sheng bing zhe xiong man, ou ni, sun xie, hu shan, yi niao, bi long" ("If shi dong then illness will show waist pain so that you can't bend facing downwards or upwards, kui hernia, less abdomen swelling in women, in serious cases dry throat, face painted and the face looks dirty and has lost its colour, if suo sheng bing with illness coming mainly from the liver, there will be chest fullness, vomiting, diarrhoea with undigested food, inguinal hernia (hu hernia), bed wetting, dysuria")

Bing hou analysis

(1) External bing hou: headache, dizziness, can't see things clearly, tinnitus, or fever, feet and hands shaking (spasms, convulsions), waist painful to the testes.

(2) Internal organ bing hou: ribs and hypocondrium region feel distended, full and painful, has pi kuai (i.e. abdominal masses), feels full and stuffy in chest and gastric cavity areas, abdominal pain, vomiting, or jaundice, or can be seen as mei he qi (globus hystericus), diarrhoea with undigested food, smaller abdomen pain, hernia, bed wetting, dysuria, yellow urine.

The above is the 12 jing and each jing bing hou is explained.

Apart from special bing hou for each jing, some illness can be presented in a variety of different jing mai illness. Now, I will provide a summary below:

1. Huang dan (jaundice): in the 12 channel bing hou, jaundice if presented in the body, this means it involves the foot tai yin spleen channel and the foot shao yin kidney channel. If mu huang (yellow eyes) are presented, this means hand yang ming large intestine channel, hand shao yin heart channel, hand tai yang small intestine channel, hand jue yin pericardium channel and foot tai yang urinary bladder channel, all together 7 channels.

2. Nüe (malaria): if malaria is present this means the involvement of the foot tai yang urinary bladder channel, foot yang ming stomach channel, foot shao yang gall baldder channel, 3 channels.

3. Kuang (madness): it shows involvement of the foot yang ming stomach channel, foot tai yang urinary bladder channel, hand jue yin pericardium channel; they (i.e. these patients) are always laughing without stop, all this belongs to the craziness area.

4. Chuan (panting): it shows up in the hand tai yin lung channel and foot shao yin kidney channel, 2 channels.

5. Xie (watery discharge, diarrhoea): it shows up in the foot tai yin channel, foot shao yin kidney channel and foot jue yin liver channel, three channels.

6. Nu (nose bleeding): it shows involvement of the hand yang ming large intestine channel, foot yang ming stomach channel, foot tai yang urinary bladder channel, three channels.

7. Ou (vomiting): it shows involvement of the foot tai yin spleen channel, and foot jue yin liver channel.

8. Hou bi (inflammation of the throat): it shows involvement of the hand yang ming large intestine channel, foot yang ming stomach channel, hand shao yang triple heater channel, foot shao yin kidney channel; other channels like the hand shao yin heart channel and foot jue yin liver channel also have symptoms like yi gan (condition of dry throat). (Hou bi – inflammation of the throat - includes can't swallow things smoothly, dry, and swollen, painful, etc.

9. Han tong jia zhong (Chin or jaw painful and cheeks or jaw swollen): it shows involvement of the foot shao yang gall bladder channel, hand tai yang small intestine channel, and hand shao yang triple heater channel. The foot yang ming stomach channel shows swelling of the neck illnesses (chin or jaw painful and cheeks swollen), it normally shows as surgical diseases such as pyogenic infections and ulcers (chuang yong), mumps, and fa yi (a tuberculosis-like swelling on one side of the cheek) etc., illnesses.

10. Jue: "jue normally means fingers, toes, hands and feet feel cold and not warm, this type of illness, but in the 12 channel bing hou bi jue (cold arms) (hand tai yin channel, hand shao yin channel), gan jue (due to perverted qi of the Yang channel) (foot yang ming channel), huai jue (cold sensation in the ankle) (foot tai yin channel), gu jue (syncope of bone), (foot shao yin channel), yang jue (yang type syncope) (foot shao yang channel), 5 different jue concepts (including 6 channels). Their meaning still needs research.

With regards to others in the 12 bing hou, each channel described shows presentation of symptoms according to the main channels' circulation and distribution. From here we can then also make the rule "sheng ze xie zhi xu ze bu zhi, re ze yi zhi, han ze liu zhi, xian xia ze jiu zhi, bu sheng bu xu, yi jing qu zhi" ("excess should be reduced, deficiency should be tonified, hot should be cured with cold, and cold should be hot. If there is concave down, then moxa it, not excess, i.e.

deficient, not all get from the channels"), all this is the rule of cure and treatment. This has an important meaning in the treatment process with the differentiation curve, and acupuncture cure.

(2) The twelve jing bing hou as the basis of Chinese medicine theory and the foundation of the differentiation curve

Chinese medicine characteristics can be seen as a differential curve. In differentiation practice, there are yin yang, biao li (external, internal), han re (cold, hot), xu shi (deficiency, excess) ba gang differentiations and there are also 6 jing differentiations of the *Shang han lun* and the wei qi ying xue and the san jiao (triple heater) of the wen bing school etc. differential methods. The doctors using these schools have agreeance in the treatment of illness and they summarise their experiences and carry out developments on these original bases. Although these differential methods have different conformations, they have common characteristics, their analysis of illness mechanisms from what illness symptoms are told and examinations by doctors give a lot of insights into present illnesses. In other words, to explain further, the differential curve mainly relies on the total characteristics of the illness. The 12 jing bing hou explains the symptoms of illnesses perfectly and in a detailed systematic fashion. These illnesses and their symptoms are zang fu jing luo effect with regards to illness change (bing bian), etc., [i.e. the zang fu jing luo change caused by illness]. This is based on practical experience obtained by the People in the treatment process of a lot of illnesses over time, then confirmed by a lot of examples and finally by the records. It is not only a systematic summary of complex symptoms but also reveals a very important thing – that there are external connections when an illness is in different stages and all of the illnesses are presented at the same time, which leads to a connection with illness mechanism and treatment process. This is very important. Even if people only know the symptoms and connections of each symptom they can start from that point, i.e. according to the external presentations of symptoms to reach an understanding of the internal illness mechanism so that one can treat and research the illness from a holistic perspective. In this way, the differential curve has some basic principles, otherwise there would be no connections and would be regarded as single symptoms and occasionally would be presented as such and therefore it will not be a differential curve and therefore just a guide to show people that: headache, treat the head; foot pain, treat the foot; cure the outside not the inside. From the above we can understand the "ba gang" ("eight conditions"), "liu jing" ("six channels"), "wei qi ying xue" (protective qi, qi level, nutritive level, blood level), "san jiao" (triple heater), etc., important differentiation methods which is very important, i.e., treatment process in the Chinese medicine. These are fundamental mechanisms and the 12 jing bing hou has connections which cannot be separated.

From the above, the major points of 12 jing bing hou external jing bing hou and internal organs bing hou are classified as xu-shi concepts, they are different and require different treatment process routes, etc. They are the basis of Chinese medicine, they are also very useful in the development of the Chinese medicine differentiation curve theory system.

The 6 jing differentiation is a development from the 12 jing symptoms

The method of 6 jing differentiation can be seen as important proof of Chinese medicine's ability to treat illness from the external pathogens, and it is also suitable for many internal medicine diseases. Six is the whole of six types of illness. The differentiation methods of the six jing were developed on the basis of 12 jing bing hou founded by the doctor Zhang Zhong jing. Now we will list the major symptoms of six jing then analyse their connections with and transformations from the process of the twelve jing symptoms:

1. Tai yang illness:
    (1) Jing symptoms: e han (afraid of the cold), fever, headache, tongue coating is thin white, pulse floating. This kind of symptom normally presents as the first stage of external illness. For example, it shows sweating (han chu) and afraid of wind, pulse floating moderate (huan), these people belong to more of attack by wind evil (feng xie). If someone has no sweating but joints painful, cough and panting, pulse floating tense symptoms this shows attack by cold evil is more prevalent (han xie).
    (2) Bowel illness (fu bing) symptoms: afraid of cold, fever, head and neck rigid and painful, etc. external conditions. If very thirsty, when drink gets vomiting, urine is not very good, upset and impatient (fan zao) etc. symptoms, this is called "qi sui zheng" ("qu sui condition") ["water inside condition"]. If smaller abdomen ji jie (tense and hard) and impatient and mad (zao kuang), urination is good, this is called "yu re zheng" (stagnant heat condition).

2. Yang ming illness:
    (1) Jing illness symptoms: high temperature, a lot of sweating, thirsty, likes cold drinks, red face, and impatient and upset, yellow tongue coating and pulse surging big (hong da). These symptoms are mainly presented in a hot illness stage, when evil heat goes awry.
    (2) Bowel illness symptoms: hot and never cold, impatient and upset, and constipation with blockage or stools like water (diarrhoea) and abdomen distended and painful and don't like to be touched and sometimes is unclear and dizzy (shen hun), delirium (with incoherent talk) (zhan yu) yellow tongue coating which is dry and sticky, pulse sunken, excess and forceful (chen shi you li).

3. Shao yang illness:
    (1) Jing illness symptoms: cold and hot comes and goes, chest and sides of trunk (from armpits to ribs) distended full or painful, doesn't like to eat and drink, e xin (nausea), vomiting, or mouth bitter, dry throat, blurred vision, yellow tongue coating, pulse xuan (bowstring).
    (2) Bowel illness symptoms: fever or cold and hot comes and goes, chest full, stuffy and sides of trunk full and painful or pi ying (distention and fullness or mass in abdomen or hypochondrium with hardness), vomiting, constipation with blockage, or diarrhoea and not well, yellow sticky tongue coating, pulse xuan shi you li (bowstring, excess and forceful).

4. Tai yin illness:
    Main symptoms: abdomen distended and full feeling, doesn't like to eat or drink, stools thin and watery, always feel abdomen painful, white slippery and sticky tongue coating, pulse ru ruo wu li (soft, weak, and without force) or chi huan (slow and moderate).

5. Shao yin illness:
    (1) Xu han (deficiency cold) type symptoms: afraid of cold, likes to sleep huddled up or curled up, or four limbs adversely cold, very tired, likes to sleep, tongue bland, pulse wei xi (indistinct and thin), or vomiting, diarrhoea (or dysentery) grains can't transform, urine clear and long, sometimes sweating and the yang dies (wang yang).

(2) Xu re (deficiency heat) type symptoms: irritable or upset (xin fan), insomnia, mouth and tongue dry, throat painful, tongue crimson red, pulse thin rapid (xi shu).

6. Jue yin illness:
   (1) Cold and hot come together symptoms: thirsty, feels like the qi is coughing up into the chest, stomach and gastric cavity painful and burning hot, very hungry but doesn't like to eat, when eats food then vomiting out, or vomiting out roundworms, and when he feels painful, feet and hands also feel adverse cold. Patients sometimes quiet (an jing), sometimes upset, hot or sometimes vomiting, sometimes diarrhea, when eats food, vomiting immediately, etc., conditions.
   (2) Jue hot triumphing in return (sheng fu) symptoms: feet and hands adverse cold but has a fever, jue more and hot less means have a heavy sickness, jue less but hot more means light illness, blood deficiency cold jue it shows externally as hands and feet jue (adverse) cold, pulse xi (thin) and almost stops or dies (yu jue).

The six jing have the same names as the channels of the 12 jing (shou zu tai yang, shou zu yang ming, shou zu tai yin, shou zu shao yin, shou zu jue yin). According to the mechanism relating to the same name jing and "tong qi xiang tong" ("same qi will go together"), these jing are combined into the six jing so they give the 6 jing described symptoms. Normally use shou or zu and then use the same name jing along with the symptoms of the 12 jing but here they are simply added together. Because the twelve jing symptoms include the jing luo's internal organ illnesses and the external illnesses (wai gan bing), many illnesses, as the six jing differentiation explains, treat external illness instead of simplifying the 12 jing symptoms to include internal illness. For example, in the 12 jing symptoms, normally there are feet and hand jing luo symptoms listed, but here the external illnesses emphasise whole body symptoms so with the jing luo symptoms there are shoulder, arm, waist, leg, knee, feet, fingers and toes, etc., painful and swelling symptoms as well as mouth and lips distorted (i.e. slanted), deafness, cheek (or jaw) painful, edema (shui zhong), depression and craziness (dian kuang), thirstiness, scrofula (luo li), hernia (shan qi), bedwetting, etc., internal sicknesses; in other words, many external illnesses reflect the whole body's condition. On this basis, the 6 jing classification has added some symptoms which come from external illness. If we try to analyse the 6 jing symptoms three yang (tai yang, yang ming, shao yang), we see that tai yang illness means headache and inflexible neck, waist painful, from which we can add symptoms of fever, afraid of wind-cold, pulse floating, etc., all these make up tai yang illness jing illness whole symptoms. We also can add symptoms of bowel (fu) illness. Shao yang, on the other hand, has sweating, shaking with cold, malaria or nüe (cold and hot come and go), mouth bitter, chest and side of trunk (i.e. armpits to the ribs) stuffy, to which we can add dry throat, blurred vision, irritable or upset, likes to vomit, pulse bowstring, etc., conditions. Yang ming illness, also in the original book had very high temperature (gao re), sweating, crazy (and delirium, incoherent talk), thirsty and attracted to drinks, abdomen distended, etc., symptoms, to which we can add constipation, abdomen pain which refuses touch, and pulse surging big (hong da) or sunken excess (chen shi you li) symptoms. This shows the continuation of symptoms of yang ming jing illness and bowel illness. Re the three yin (tai yin, shao yin, jue yin) symptoms, their basis is also the same as that of the three yang. Therefore, here we don't need to discuss further. From all this we know that symptoms classified according to the six jing are not separate from the symptoms of 12 jing, and that jing differentiation used in the treatment indicates the importance of jing luo bing hou. So, 6 jing differentiation is also a development of the 12 jing bing hou in the treatment of illness.

Wei qi ying xue differentiation is the development of jing qi theories

The wei qi ying xue differentiation is the method of differentiation in external warm hot sicknesses. It is the main concern of Qing dynasty's doctors. It was developed from the wen bing xue and based on jing-luo study and jing-luo theories. It has some differences from the six jing differentiation in the classics method. This is more complex. It believes the important basis of chinese medicine treatment is in hot diseases. Now, firstly is the classification of the zheng-hou group and the description of the relationship between this and the jing-qi theories:

1. Conducting symptoms of the zheng-hou of the wei fen (level): fever, a little afraid of the cold, headache, cough, thirstiness, painful throat, no sweating, or have some sweating but not fully, or vomiting. The coating on the tongue and the colour is white and a little yellow. The pulse is floating countable (mai fou shu).

2. Zheng-hou group of the qi fen:
    (1) Too much heat and the fluids are injured: high fever hates heat but doesn't hate cold, more sweating, easily angered, mouth thirsty and likes to drink, strong qi, the urine colour is yellow and red.

The coating of the tongue is yellow and dry. The pulse is hong da (surging big).

(2) Accumulation of dampness-heat: the body temperature is sometimes high, sometimes low, the four limbs are tired, the chest is heavy' a little vomiting, thirsty but doesn't like to drink, or likes to drink hot drinks, stools loose or incomplete defecation, urine short and small. The coating of the tongue is white and sticky or yellow. The pulse is ru shu (soft and rapid) or hua shu (slippery rapid).

(3) Accumulation of heat in the intestinal path: high fever, constipation, the abdomen feels full and painful. If serous, the spirit shows dizziness, and talking nonsense, the coating of the tongue is yellow and sticky and thick or burnt black (jiao hei). The pulse is sinking but has power (chen shi you li).

3. Zheng-hou group of the ying fen: the body is hot and at night time will become more serious, cannot be quiet, the spirit is not very clever, sometimes talks nonsense, the mouth is dry but not drinking a lot and maybe appears some spot papules (ban zhen), the tongue is atrophied, the limbs jue. The tongue is crimson red, the pulse is thin rapid (xi shu)

4. The zheng-hou of the xue (blood) fen
   (1) Excess heat of the blood level: high temperature in the evening (wan shang), spot papules the colour of purple and black, the spirit is easily angered, and maybe vomiting blood and the nose bleeding or the root of the teeth also bleeding, stools bleeding, urine with blood, for women will have too much period, if serious the spirit will show dizziness and talking nonsense, and jing jue (convulsions or spasms), and dong feng (moving wind). The tongue is crimson red, and the pulse is sunken rapid (chen shu).

   (2) Deficiency heat at the blood level: the body is hot continuously, the spirit is dry (ie. not good) withered, the mouth is dry and the throat dry, the lips broken, the teeth are coated, deafness, the centres of the hands and feet are hot, for serious cases the tongue will be stiff and talk will be abnormal (atrophied), the fingers shaking, following the clothes and touch the bed (?). The tongue has a crimson colour and is dry or the quality of the tongue is dim (zhi) and a little purple black, the pulse is thin and indistinct (xi wei) or deficient big rapid (xu da er shu).

According to the above, there is a close relationship between the wei qi ying xue and the jing luo theories. Because the distribution of the wei qi ying xue in the human body is through the jing luo and distributed to the whole body, so it has a close relationship with the jing luo. Based on the description of the wen bing theories, "fei zhu qi wei wei, xin zhu xue wei ying" ("the lungs control the qi and belong to the wei, the heart controls the blood and belongs to the ying") (this is from the book *Wai gan wen re pian*. The warm evil attacks, generally the wei will have a sickness first, "wei zhi hou fang yan qi, ying zhi hou fang yan xue" ("after the wei you can say qi, and after the ying you can say blood"). This basic principle of the wen bing is based on the jing luo theories, the cycling of ying wei qi and xue in the jing luo; they have the difference of deep and shallow, internal and external and they have their own special connection to the internal organs. In the jing luo theories, they said wei qi "xian xing pi mao" ("circling the skin and hair"), the skin and hair are the combination of the lung, also said the "wei qu shang jiao" ("the wei is out of the upper heater'), this is the basis of the lungs controlling the qi and belonging to the wei. And also said "rong jue ying qi, shi wu suo bi, shi wei mai" ("rong keeps the ying qi, and doesn't allow it to escape or as much as can be avoided, and is the so-called vessels"), the pericardium can become sick from the main "vessels", the heart controls the blood the blood has a close relationship with the pulse so the sickness at the ying level, generally has evil surrounding the pericardium. This is the source of the theory that the heart controls the blood and belongs to the ying.

In the wen bing theories, generally they use the differential zheng-hou group of wei qi ying xue to analyse the sickness evil, and how deep the evil is injuring the body. This is also the process of the jing qi theory in the jing luo theories. In jing qi theory, it is said, "wei qi zhi, suo yi wen fen rou, chong pi fu, fei chou li, shi kai he zhi ye" ("the wei qi, so the warmth separates in the muscles, feeling in the skin, affects the chou li, the? openings and combines?") (from the *Ling shu-ben zang*). And ying qi is mainly for "he tiao you wu zang, sa chen you liu fu" ('makes balance in the five viscera, feeds the six bowels" (the *Su wen-bi lun*). This describes the differences in the qi of their ying wei, circulating and distributing in their bodies. This is the theory basis for the warm evil first the wei, then the ying. From the reasons of the sicknesses of the wei qi or ying xue and their different theories, so "wei zhi hou fang yan qi, ying zhi hou fang yan xue" ("after wei you can say qi, after ying you can say blood"). Therefore, they have the separated 4 zheng- hou groups of wei qi ying xue. In fact, the classics of zheng-hou have clearly described the ying wei theories in terms of the jing luo, for example they said the wei qi has the functions of warming and feeding the skin and separating the muscle (fen rou) and cou li. We can also say if the wei qi is surrounded by evil then there will be abnormal changes in the skin, fen rou, and cou li. This summarizes the zheng-hou groups of the wei level and the qi level. If the skin is in combination with wei and also belongs to the range of the tai yang jing, the fen rou is in the range of the yang ming jing, and cou li belongs to the range of the shao yang jing, so the zheng-hou group at present for the wei are nearly the same as the tai yang. The symptoms of the qi level and too much heat and heat accumulation in the intestines zheng-hou group are nearly the same as the jing bowel fu zheng in the yang ming sickness, the symptoms of the qi level zheng-hou group are exactly the symptoms of the shao yang sickness. In the wen bing theories, they have many clear descriptions, for example, in the book *Wai gan wen re pian* it said, "qi bing you bu chuan xue fen, er xie liu san jiao, yi ru shang han zhong shao yang bing ye" ("the qi sickness if not transferred to the blood level, and if the evil stays in the triple heater, it is like the *Shang han's* shao yang sickness"). The zheng-hou group of damp-heat staying in the triple heater is called the evil in the qi level. It is based on "san jiao chu qi" ("the san jiao generates qi") in the jing luo theories and "zhu qi so sheng bing" ("the control qi sickness of the triple heater theory"). So from the above, we can see there are many symptoms the same from the six jing differentiation and the wei qi ying xue differentiation in many zheng-hou groups desciptions of the zheng-hou group of the ying xue. It was more complicated and completed the 6 jing differentiation. This is the development of the jing luo theories in the differentiation treatment area.

Summarizing the above, the wei qi ying xue differentiation and the 6 jing differentiation all belong to the classification of zheng-hou in chinese medicine, and the differentiation of wei qi ying xue are mainly used for the differentiation of warm heat sicknesses. It is based on the development proceedure of the wai gan warm and hot sicknesses. The dfferent appearences of the wei qi ying xue damage by the warm heat evil and the theories of sickness, and the depth of sickness positions from external to internal, summarizing the four kinds of zheng hou, these are the four steps to the development of warm hot sickness as their differential basis. The basis of the generation of these theories is mainly from the jing qi theories in the jing luo theories, so wei qi ying xue differentiation is the development of jing luo theories in the classical use.

The twelve jing bing hou improving the generation and the development of zang fu differentiation and ba gang differentiation.

The internal organs bing hou in the twelve jing bing hou is the basis of organ differentiation and in later development it continuously contributed to the contents of the jing luo bing hou and the classics system. The characteristics and the system of evil and good, from the up and down of that evil and good, and the deficiency and excess of cold and heat according to the classics and the systems of characteristics are the generation of the methods of organ differentiation. The following has differentiation methods of one internal zang (viscera) as an example describing the relationship between it and the twelve jing bing hou. For example, the spleen organ deficiency generally can be separated into several main sections:

1. Spleen qi deficiency and weak (xu ruo): when it appears the appetite decreases and the digestion is weak, after eating the abdomen is full and heavy, the stools are not excess, the muscles are thin, the four limbs have no power, or there is prolapse of the anus and uterus prolapse (tuo sui), and the abdomen has a sinking and full feeling.

2. The spleen yang is not strong (bu zu): it is an injury (sun) and the wan abdomen is always feeling full and there is some unclear pain with a cold feeling, likes heat and likes pressure, the stools are loose and has some undigested food, the intestines have sounds, and the four limbs are not warm.

3. Water dampness accumulates in the spleen: it appears as abdominal fullness, vomiting, the face and feet are swelling with oedema (fou zhong), or maybe the whole body is fou zhong, the body is heavy and the food consumption decreases, the stools are loose, the urine is short and less, and the limbs feel tired and have no power.

4. The spleen cannot control the blood: when it appears the stools are bloody, too much periods, and continuously beng lou, and on the skin appears dark bruises, the face colour is not bright, the spirit is tired and there is dizziness, one eats less and has no power.

You can compare the above spleen organ differentiation to the spleen jing bing hou in the twelve jing: "shi ben zhuo, shi ze ou, wei wan tong, fu zhang, sai yi, de hou you qi, ze kuai ran ru shuai, shen ti jie zhong … shi ben tong, ti bu neng dong yao, shi bu xia, xin fan, xin xia ji tong, tang jia xie, shui bi, huang dan, bu neng wo, qiang li, gu xi nei zhong, jue, zu da zhi bu yong" etc. ("tongue root stiff, eats then vomits, gastric cavity painful, abdomen distended, likes to burp, after passing stools passes gas, then fast feeling like weak, the body heavy … .tongue painful, the body cannot sway, the body cannot eat because food sitting there, upset, under the centre acute pain, uterine masses causing the stools to be loose, water blockage, jaundice, can't lie down, stiff standing?, internal knee swelling, collapse (jue), feet big toe can't use etc."). The bing hou of the spleen jing closely includes the main contents of the spleen viscera differentiation, and the blood (xue) zheng-hou group due to the spleen cannot control the blood which is also based on "ying chu zhong jiao" ("ying comes from the central heater"), and "pi zang ying" ("the ying stores in the spleen") in the jing luo theories. The close relationship between ying and blood and the large luo of the spleen shows that the spleen can control the luo, ie. the "luo luo zhi xue" ("the blood belongs to the luo of the whole body"), and generates the concept from clinical experience. In addition, in the area of the spleen viscera such as spleen-lung sickness at the same time, spleen stomach not in harmony, liver spleen lose balance, the heart and spleen loses, and the spleen and kidney yang is deficient all have a close relationship re jing luo theories.

The ba gang differentiation is the most basic differentiation principle in chinese medicine diagnosis and treatment. Ba gang is yin, yang, biao, li, han, re, xu, shi (yin, yang, external, internal, cold, hot, deficiency, excess). It is the summarizing of the different kinds of differential methods. Ba gang is a concept formed by summarizing and analysing the contents of the jing luo theories such as Zhang Jing yue said, "yi shi er jing fen yin yang, ze liu yang si fu wei biao, liu yin si zang wei li, … er san yang zhi jing, ze you yi tai yang wei yang zhong zhi biao, yang ming wei yang zhong zhi li, shao yang wei ban biao ban li" ("separate yin and yang from the twelve jing and 6 yang will belong to the bowels as biao, 6 yin belong to the viscera as li, … .and the jing of the three yang and the tai yang is biao of the yang and the yang ming is the internal of the yang, and the shao yang is half external half internal." (*Jing yue quan shu*). This is the source of the yin yang biao li differentiation. In the twelve jing bing hou, there are descriptions of zheng-hou such as "qi sheng you you" ("qi is too strong and too much") and "qi bu zu" ("not enough qi"), and points out "sheng ze xie zhi, xu ze bu zhi, re ze yi zhi, han ze liu zhi" ("if too strong lose it, if deficiency tonify, if heat cure it, if cold keep the same") and this is the principle and method for the differentiation of treatment. Based on this, many doctors and their families completed the development of the zheng-hou of yin yang, biao li, han re, and xu shi and generated the treatment methods of ba gang differentiation.

Summarizing all the above, the ba gang differentiation and the viscera and bowels differentiation are like the 6 jing differentiation; they are all based on the close connection with the twelve jing bing hou. From this, we can see the jing luo theory is very important in the creation of all the treatment methods in Chinese medicine. Or, you can also say, the differentiation treatment principle and all the different treatment methods in Chinese medicine are all generated and based on the introduction of the jing luo theories, and are completed and developed from the jing luo bing hou combined with the viscera theory.

<u>The twelve jing bing hou is the summarizing of the main treatment areas of the jing and the xie (pts).</u>

All the treatment methods, whether taking herbal medicine or needles or tui na (massage) are all intended to create balance in the zang fu of the jing luo and to reach the target re treatment of illness. Needle points are called yu xue (injection and accumulation places of qi) in the jing luo theories, yu points lead to the human body's jing luo's viscera and bowels, so they are also called qi points (qi points).

Each point has certain special functions for many viscera positions. Re functions, they have special connections; for example, the organ sickness in the head and face you can take he gu (LI4), for the urine and genital system sickness you can use san yin jiao (SP6), for the stomach and intestinal system sickness you can use zu san li (St 36), and the connection between the points and the viscera and bowels is the jing luo. So, all the common relationships between reaction points and internal organs are all based on the distribution of the jing luo circulation. Distribution, because its jing mai belongs to the jing points and re main treatment of sickness they have a lot of consensus. In other words, "jing mai suo guo, zhu zhi suo ji" ("the paths of the jing mai have treatment for the organs they pass"). Summarizing the above, it can be shown below:

1. The hand three yin jing:
    (1) The main treatment range and the action positions of the hand tai yin jing points: chest position, throat, trachea, nose, and lung sicknesses
    (2) The main treatment range and the action positions of the hand jue yin jing points: chest position, stomach, heart, and spirit sicknesses.
    (3) The main treatment range and the action positions of the hand shao yin jing points: chest position, tongue, heart, and spirit sicknesses.

2. The hand three yang jing:
    (1) The main treatment range and the action positions of the hand yang ming jing points: head and face, eyes, ear, nose, mouth, and teeth, throat, intestines and hot sicknesses.
    (2) The main treatment range and the action positions of the hand shao yang jing points: head and tou nie (temple), eyes, ear positions, throat, chest, ribs, and hot sicknesses.

(3)   The main treatment range and the action positions of the hand tai yang jing points: head, top, eyes, ear positions, throat, hot sicknesses, and spirit sicknesses.

3.   The foot three yang jing:
   (1)   The main treatment range and the action positions of the foot yang ming jing points: head and face, nose positions, mouth and teeth, throat, stomach and intestines, heat sicknesses, and spirit sicknesses.
   (2)   The main treatment range and the action positions of the foot shao yang jing points: head and sides of head, nose, eye system, throat, chest, ribs, and hot sicknesses.
   (3)   The main treatment range and the action positions of the foot tai yang jing points: the head and top, nose, eye system, waist and back, hot sicknesses, spirit sicknesses.

4.   The foot three yin jing:
   (1)   The main treatment range and the action positions of the foot tai yin jing points: umbilicus and abdomen, stomach, intestines, urinary and generative systems sicknesses.
   (2)   The main treatment range and the action positions of the foot jue yin jing points: ribs, abdomen, lesser abdomen, generative and urinary systems, and head part position sicknesses.
   (3)   The main treatment range and the action positions of the foot shao yin jing points: waist, abdomen, generative, urinary systems, throat, and spirit sicknesses.

5.   Ren mai and the du mai:
   (1)   The two mai of the ren and du mai, their jing points have the same commonality in treatment functions: it is the jing points in the chest and back positions, generally they can treat all the sicknesses of the lungs, heart and pericardium, the jing points in the abdomen and back positions, generally they can treat the diseases of the liver and gall-bladder, spleen and stomach, the jing points in the lesser abdomen and waist vertebrae generally they can treat sicknesses of the kidneys, urinary bladder, large intestines, and small intestines.
   (2)   The different points and main treatment actions of the jing points of the ren and du mai: the reaction points of the du mai can mostly treat sicknesses in the head and brain, backbone, waist and legs and

hot sicknesses but the reaction points of the ren mai mostly can treat the sicknesses of the throat, chest, abdomen, umbilicus and generative and urinary systems. As well as the digestive tract and cold sicknesses.

From the analysis of the above main treatment actions of the fourteen jing and their points, the main treatment for sicknesses of the different jing mai, have a close connection with each jing mai's distribution positions and internal organs. At the same time, all the jing points will have treatment actions for all the sicknesses of their circling order positions of the jing mai. This is the theory basis for needling and the acupuncture clinical principle "yuan dao qu xue" ("far away from the disease is a reaction point") and "ji bu qu xue" ("only have the reaction point in one place is ok"). Summarizing all of this, is based on the "xun jing qu xue" ("along the jing to have the reaction points").

The twelve jing bing hou is the summarizing of the zheng-hou group for each jing mai distribution circulation and their positions and their connection with the viscera and bowels. So, the relationship between the jing luo bing hou and the main treatment of jing points can be seen as the summary of the twelve jing bing hou i.e. is the main treatment range of the jing points in the classics.

(3) The research for "shi dong" and "suo sheng bing".
     The book the *Ling shu-jing mai* chapter is a special chapter for discussing the twelve jing mai. The description of the bing hou for each jing mai is separated into "shi dong" and "suo sheng bing" two parts. But as to the meaning of "shi dong" and "suo sheng bing" different people have different descriptions. Up to now, there are still different descriptions for them. It is an unresolved problem in accordance in Chinese medicine.

For deep research into the jing luo theories, the analysis of "shi dong" and "suo sheng bing", not only helps us understand the twelve jing bing hou but also has an important meaning in the use of jing luo theories in the clinical use. So, from the references from the papers in medicine, we have the following analysis for "shi dong" and "suo sheng bing":

1. Different doctors at different times had different understandings of "shi dong" and "suo sheng bing". The first reference to "shi dong" and "suo sheng bing" can be seen in the *Nan jing*. Later, there were many different meanings for "shi dong" and "suo sheng bing". The chinese doctors in

Japan also have their own understanding. Now, we will choose the most important ones and give the examples as follows:

(1) Zan guo (Zan country), Chen Yue ren in the *Nan jing-er shi er nan* believed, "shi dong zhi, qi ye; suo sheng bing zhi, xue ye. Xie zai qi, qi wei shi dong; xie zai xue, xue wei suo sheng bing. Qi zai zhu ke zhi, xue zhu ru zhi. Qi liu er bu xing zhe, wei qi xian bing ye; xue rong er bu ru zhe, wei xue hou bing ye. Gu xian wei shi dong, hou suo sheng ye". ("the shi dong one is qi, those suo sheng bing blood. The evil at the qi, qi is shi dong; evil at the blood, blood is suo sheng bing. Qi controls those warm, blood controls those moist. The qi keeps and cannot go circling, is first the sickness of the qi. The blood cannot keep circling, the blood is the later sickness. So, the first is shi dong, the later is suo sheng bing.")

(2) In the Tang dynasty, Yang Xuan chao in the book *Nan jing ji zhu* said, "shi dong, xie zhong you yang, yang wei qi, gu qi xian bing, yang qi zai wai gu ye. Suo sheng bing, ruo zai yang bu zhi, ze ru yu yin zhong, yin wei xue, gu wei xue hou bing, xue zai nei gu ye." ("shi dong, the evil is in the yang, yang is for qi, so the sickness is first in the qi, yang qi is in the outside. Suo sheng bing if not treated in the yang, the evil will go into the yin, yin is for blood, so the blood is the later sickness, and the blood is inside (or internal)."

(3) In the Song dynasty, Yu duo in the book *Nan jing ji zhu* said, "shi dong, mai dong fan chang, xie zai qi ye. Suo sheng bing, qi shou xie, chuan zhi xie, gu xue wei suo sheng bing." ("shi dong, the vessels moving adversely, the evil is in the qi. Suo sheng bing, the evil damages the qi and transfers to the blood, the blood is suo sheng bing.")

(4) In the Song dynasty, Li guang wrote the *Nan jing zhu jie*, where he said, "shi dong, xie zhong yu yang, qi xian shou re, xing zhi yu mai. Suo sheng bing, qi bing chuan xue, xue rong bu run, bing suo you sheng. Qi shou re ze ye yi wang xing gu ye shi dong. Qi chuan zhi you xue, fu shou ze feng, gu xue rong bu ru er bing." ("shi dong, the evil is in the yang, qi is hot first and then can be seen in the vessels, the yang qi moves the vessels. Suo sheng bing, the sickness of the qi transfers to the blood and the blood is not so smooth and the sickness generates from this. The qi has been heated so is surrounded but not regularly so this is called shi dong, the qi transfers to the blood and then meets the wind so the blood is not smooth and sickness.")

(5) In the Yuan dynasty, Hua sou in the book the *Nan jing ben yi* said, "shi dong, qi zhu zhu zhi, wei qi xi xu ran lai, zun zang you pi fu fen rou ye. QI liu er bu xing, wei qi bing, suo sheng bing, xue zhu ru zhi, wei xue ru run jing gu, hua li guan jie, rong yang zang fu ye. Xue yong er bu ru, wei xue bing. Ran xie yi you zhi zai qi, yi you jing zai xue zhi, you bu ke yi xian hou zhu ye." ("shi dong, qi controls zhu zhi?, it is said the qi will steam the skin and fen rou. If the qi stays and doesn't surround it, is the sickness of the qi. Suo sheng bing, the blood controls the ru zhi?, it is said the blood will feed the bone and the jin gu (tendons and bones), smooth the joints (guan jie), and feeds the viscera and bowels. If the blood is not cycling, it is a sickness of the blood, if the evil not only is in the qi, but also in the blood, it can not be separated into the former or the latter.")

(6) In the Ming dynasty, Ma shi in the book *Ling shu zhu zheng fa wei* said, "suo sheng bing, shi jia x jing suo sheng zhi bing er. "("suo sheng bing, is some sickness from some jing."), he thinks "nan jing yi shi dong wei qi, suo sheng wei xue, zhi 'dong sheng' er zi, fen wei qi xue, ren 'Nan jing' zhi yi shuo er" ("the *Nan jing* thinks shi dong is qi, suo sheng bing is blood, these are two words 'dong sheng' separated into qi and blood, this is the meaning from the book the *Nan jing*".)

(7) Also, in the Ming dynasty, Zhang Jing yue in the *Lei jing:* "shi dong, dong yan bian ye, bian ze bian chang er wei bing ye. Ru yin yang yin xiang da lun ru, zai bian dong wei wo, wei sui zhi lei, ji ci zhi wei." ("shi dong, it means the change of dong, The change is usually as the sickness such as the yin yang shapes appear, it controls the changes and classically the sui, it says this.") He thinks "fan zai wu zang, ze ge yan zang suo sheng bing, fan zai liu fu, ze huo yan qi, huo yan xue, huo mai, huo jin, huo gu, huo jing ye. Qi suo sheng bing, ben ge you suo sheng, fei yi qi xue er zi, tong yan shi er jing zhi ye, *Nan jing* zhi yan, yi fei jing zi". ("if in the 5 viscera, the suo sheng bing can be said to be in each viscera, if it is in the 6 bowels maybe said to be in the qi or in the blood or in the pulse/vessels (mai) or in the tendons or in the bones or in the fluids (jing ye). The suo sheng bing maybe has different causes, cannot only use qi and blood two words to include the whole twelve jing, the results in the *Nan jing* is not so clear.")

(8) Once again in the Ming dynasty, Zhang Xie xian in the book *Tu zhu nan jing ba shi yi nan bian zhu* wrote, "shi dong, qi bai xie qin ze liu

zhi er bu xing, qi zhi bing suo yi xian jian yuan. Qi liu ze han. Suo sheng bing, xue xing jia fu qi ye, qi tuo bu xing, xue bu de yi zi xing, ze yong zhi er bu ru, yi chong er bing yan. Xue zhi ze re. Shi gu xian bing wei shi dong, hou bing wei suo sheng ye." ("shi dong, if the qi is hurt by evil and cannot srround, so the sickness of the qi can be seen first, the qi cannot surround so it will be cold. Suo sheng bing, because the surrounding of the blood cannot surround automatically (by itself) so the blood will stay and cannot surround so the blood will be sick, the blood cannot surround so it will be hot. So, the shi dong is the sickness first and suo sheng is the sickness later.")

(9) In the Qing dynasty, Zhang Zhi cong in the book the *Ling shu ji zhu*, shi dong, bing zai san yin san yang zhi qi, er dong jian you ren ying, qi kou, bing zai qi er bu zai jing. San yin san yang zhi qi xuan zhuan bu xi, gu ri shi dong. Bing yin yu wai. Suo sheng bing, wei shi er jing mai ren zang fu zhi suo sheng, zang fu zhi bing, wai jian yu jing zheng ye. Jing mai sheng yu zang fu, gu rou suo sheng. Bing yin yu nei. Fan bing you yin yu wai zhi, you yin yu nei zhi, you yin yu wai er ji yu nei zhi, you nei wai zhi jian zhe. Zhi bing zhe dang sui qi suo jian zhi zheng, yi bei nei wai zhi yin, you bu bi xian wei shi dong, hou ji suo sheng, er bing zheng zhi bi zhu ye." ("shi dong, the sickness in the qi of the triple yin and the triple yang, the dong can be seen in the ren ying, qi kou, the sickness is in the qi but not in the jing. The qi of the triple yin and the triple yang surround and cannot stop so it is called shi dong. The reason for the sickness is from the outside. The suo sheng bing, it is said the sickness of the viscera and bowels because the twelve jing mai are generated by them from outside it can be seen in jing zheng. The jing mai are generated from the viscera and bowels so it is called suo sheng. The reason for the sickness is from the inside. If the reason is from the outside, have reasons from the inside, the reason outside, inside and outside inside, inside outside, all are both inside and outside. So, the doctor must be following the zheng, he can see and sererate it whether it was caused by inside or outside, it is not necessary to separate it into shi dong first and later suo sheng, but the bing zheng is all."

(10) Qing dynasty, Xu Da chen in his book the *Nan jing jing shi*, it is recorded, "shi dong zhe bing, re ben jing zhi bing. Suo sheng zhi bing, ze yi lei tui, er pang ji ta jing zhe," ("It should be said all the

sickness of shi dong are the sickness of the jing itself, the sickness of suo sheng bing can be concluded from the classics, and connects with the other jing.") He thinks "jing wen bing wu qi xue fen xu zhi shuo." ("jing is not separated by qi and blood").

(11) Qing dynasty, Xue xue in the book the *Yi jing yuan yi* wrote, "shi dong, dong yan bian ye, bian chang er wei bing ye. Suo sheng bing, yin jing, ben zang shou sheng bing ye. Yang jing, jin ye qi xue ding suo sheng bing." ("shi dong, the chang of dong, the change from the normal is sickness. Suo sheng bing, yin jing, the sickness of th viscera and the pulse/vessels. Yang jing, the sickness of the fluids, qi and blood.")

(12) Qing dynasty, Ding jin in the *Gu ben nan jing can zhu* said, "shi dong, qi zhe xue zhi sui ye, mai zhe qi zhi cong ye, qi xian bing mai zi ying zhi, xie zai qi ji jian mai. Suo sheng bing, xue bing bi you yu qi bing, xue hou bing, bing hou yan zhi. Xie zai xue, you jian yu bing. Qi xian liu er bu xing, ran hou xue zhi er bu ru, gu qi xian wei shi dong yu mai, er xue hou suo sheng yu bing ye." ("shi dong, is in the lead re the blood, the mai is the qi's feeling, if the qi is sick the problem will respond, the evil if in the qi can be seen in the mai (pulse/vessels). Suo sheng bing, the blood sickness certainly must be caused by the sickness of the qi, the blood sickness later. The sickness can be seen coming from the blood. The evil in the blood can be seen coming from the sickness, the qi cannot surround first and the then the blood stays and cannot surround so the qi's shi dong first can be in the mai (pulse/vessels) and then the blood later suo sheng bing.")

(13) Qing dynasty, Ye lin in the book *Nan jing zheng yi* said, "shi dong, xie zai qi, qi wei shi er dong, mai zhi dong zhe, qi wei zhi. Suo sheng bing, xie zai xue, xue wei suo sheng bing, suo sheng bing zhe, xue wei zhi." ('shi dong, the evil in the qi, the qi is dong and the pulse/vessels is the moving one is caused by the qi. Suo sheng bing, evil is in the blood, the blood is the suo sheng bing, suo sheng bing one, is caused by the blood.") He also added, "qi bing chuan xue, gu yi mai bian wei er bing ye". ("the sickness of the qi transfers to the blood so one mai (pulse/vessel) becomes two sicknesses".)

(14) Japan, Gong ben yi bao, in his book the *Shi si jing fa hui he yi chao* claimed that "shi dong, qi jing luo bian dong suo sheng. Suo sheng bing, qi zang fu suo sheng bing." ("shi dong is generated from the

changes of the jing luo, suo sheng bing is the sickness of the viscera and bowels.")

2. The interpretation and analysis of the different academic groups, from the interpretation of the above it can be classified into three groups:

    (1) The *Nan jing group*: this group is based on the qi is first and the blood later. This group includes Yang Xian chao, Jin shi, Li guang, Zhang Xie xian, Ding jin, and Ye lin.

    (2) Disagree with the *Nan jing* group: this group disagrees with the basis of first qi and later blood. It includes Ma shi, Zhang Zhi cong, Xu Da chen, Xue xue, and Gong ben yi yao.

    (3) The group between the *Nan jing* group and the disagree-with-the-Nan *jing* group: they are based on the celebration of qi and blood and they disagree with the former and the latter of the *Nan jing* group such as Hua sou.

The evaluation of the *Nan jing* group:

    (1) Qin Yue ren wrote the book *Nan jing-er shi er nan* and said, "qi zhu zhu zhi, xue zhu ru zhi" ("the qi controls the zhu zhi, the blood controls the ru zhi"). The cause of the not circling of the blood and qi, and the reason there is evil in the qi and cannot circulate, the qi is sick first. There is evil in the blood, the blood cannot cycle, therefore there is blood sickness later. So, suo sheng bing is a development from shi bing. It must be shi dong first, and you can say suo sheng bing and shi dong belong to the sickness of the qi, while sheng bing belongs to the sickness of the blood. Based on this, compared with the original papers of the twelve jing bing hou in the book *Ling shu-jing mai*, it is not clear in many places. For example, the shi dong of th hand tai yin "fei zhang men, pang pang er chuan ke, que pen zhong tong", ("lung full and stuffy, hacking sounds and panting and coughing, painful in the clavicular fossa"). This can be seen as the sickness of the qi but the panting and the coughing in the suo sheng bing, it can also be seen as the sickness of the qi. Why would you need to interpret this as a blood sickness? Also, in the shi dong of the zu shao yin it says, "ke qiu ze you xue, he he er chuan" ("when coughing has blood, when drink? there is panting"), this is seen as the sickness of the qi but why is "shang qi" in suo sheng bing and is seen as a sickness of the blood.

The *Su wen-ni tiao lun* said, "yang qi xu ze bu ren, wei qi xu ze bu yong, yang wei ju xu, ze bu ren qie bu yong." ("The deficiency of the yang qi will bu ren?, and the wei qi cannot be used. If both the yang and the wei are deficient, they will be bu ren and cannot be used.") The wei is yang, belongs to the qi, so the sickness of bu rong must belong to the sickness of the qi. But, from the suo sheng bing of the twelve channels, the hand yang ming has "da zhi chi zhi bu yong" ("cannot use the first and second fingers"), the foot yang ming has "xing ying ru, qi jue, gu, fu tu, gan wai lian, fu tu shang jie tong, zhong zhi bu yong". ("along the chest breast the qi street, femur, shin, gu leading edge and the foot upper all painful, the central toe cannot be used.") In the foot tai yin, it has "zu da zhi bu yong". ("the foot big toe cannot be used"). The foot tai yang has "xiao zhi bu yong" ("the small toe can't be used".) The hand shao yang has " ... zhou, bi wai jie tong, xiao zhi chi zhi bu yong". (" ... the elbow, the outside edge of the forearm are all painful, the small finger and the 2nd last finger cannot be used".) And the foot shao yang has " ... wai huai qian ji zhu jie jie tong, xiao zhi, chi zhi bu yong". ("in the external ankle front all the joints are painful, the small toe and the 2nd last toe cannot be used".) These are not the sicknesses of the blood. How can you say the suo sheng bing is the sickness of the blood?

The *Su wen-ju tong lun* said, "han qi ru jing er xia chi, qi er bu xing, ke yu mai wai ze xue shao, ke yu mai zhong ze qi bu tong, gu zi ran er tong". ("The cold qi into the jing makes it delayed and cannot surround it, if it is the action in the outside of the mai, so the blood will decrease, if its action is inside the mai, the qi will not go through it so will be painful"). This makes the qi not circulate and it will be painful. In the book *Su wen-yin yang ying xiang da lun* it said, "qi shang tong." ("qi that has been hurt will cause pain"). So, the pain will belong to the sickness of the qi. In the book *Su wen-sheng qi tong tian lun* it also said, "ying qi bu cong, ni yu rou li, nai sheng yong zhong". This is to say, "ying qi ben lai shi liu xing yu jing mai zhi zhong de, ru guo han qi ru yu jing mai, ying qi bu neng shun cong ying zou de dao luo yun xing, er zuo ni yu ji rou zhi zhong, ri jiu bian cheng yong zhong". ("the ying qi surrounds around the jing mai, if the cold qi enters the jing mai, the ying qi cannot surround along this path, so it will accumulate in the muscles a long time and this will cause a yong zhong (boil or carbuncle swelling)". So, the yong zhong should belong to the sickness of the blood. If based on "qi shang ze tong, xue ni sheng zhong" ("if the qi has been hurt it will be painful, blood adverse creates swelling"). Analyse and compare the twelve jing bing hou, it will be found:

i   In shi dong, the hand yang ming "neck swelling". The hand tai yang has "han swelling". The hand jue yin has "armpit swelling". The hand shao yang has "yi swelling". The foot jue yin has "women's lesser abdomen swelling" etc. parts belong to blood fen illnesses, and aren't qi fen illnesses.

ii In "suo sheng bing", the hand tai yin has "ru bi nei qian lian tong". ("the internal side of the forearm has pain"). The hand yang ming has "jian qian ru tong". ("the front of the shoulder is painful"). The foot yang ming has "xi bin zhong tong … zu fu shang ju tong". ("the knee is swollen and the upper part of the foot is all painful"). The foot tai yin has "shi ben tong … xin xia ji tong". ("The tongue is painful … below the heart is acutely painful") The hand shao yin has "xie tong, ru bi nei hou lian tong". ("ribs painful, the arm internal side is painful".) The hand tai yang has "jing, han, jian, ru, zhou, bi wai hou lian tong". ("the neck, jaws, shoulder, arm, elbow, forearm external side are painful".) The foot tai yang has "xiang tong … jiao jie tong". ("the nape of the neck is painful … all of the feet are painful".) The foot shao yin has "yi gan ji tong, xin tong, ji gu nei hou lian tong, zu xia re er tong". ("the laryngopharynx dry and painful, the heart painful, the internal back side of the spine is painful, the feet under are hot and painful".) The hand jue yin has "xin tong". ("heart pain".) The hand shao yang has "mu rui ci tong, shuai tong … bi wai jie tong". ("the canthus of the eyes painful, the cheeks (xia) painful … the external side of the arm painful".) The foot shao yang has "tou tong, han tong, mu rui ci tong … .wai huai qian ji zhu jie jie tong". ("headache, jaw painful, the canthus of the eyes painful … external ankle front and various joints all painful".) All of these are the branch sicknesses of the qi, they are not the branch sicknesses of the blood. If one considers that "shi dong" is the branch sickness of the qi, "suo sheng bing" is the branch sickness of the blood. So

74

in the twelve jing mai will know that the bing hou of any jing mai should agree with this.

Also, we will therefore discuss "qi xian bing, xue hou bing" ("the qi sickness first, the blood later"). It is described here that the "shi dong" sickness comes first, and "suo sheng bing" later. This is the relationship between "shi dong" and "suo sheng bing" ie. one of transfer and change: first the cause is "shi dong" and the result is "suo sheng bing". This kind of understanding is not suitable in practice. For example, the shi dong of the hand tai yin: "fei zhang man, pang pang er chuan ke, que pen zhong tong" ("lungs are distended and stuffy, there are noises and panting and coughing, the centre of the clavicular fossa is painful"). In this section this is the serious step-up to dyspnoea, but in the "suo sheng bing" there is "ke shang qi chuan ge" ("coughing and the qi goes up, and panting and thirsty"). This is the light step in the case of dyspnoea. The first sickness is the heavy one, the later sickness is the light one; this kind of transfer is seldom seen in disease. So, qi is "shi dong", blood is the "suo sheng bing", and yet the first sickness of the qi is "shi dong", the later sickness of the blood is "suo sheng bing". Surely, we cannot get people to agree with this?

(2) The interpretation of Yang Xian chao's advantages and disadvantages: Mr, Yang first pointed out "shi dong, bing zai yu wai, suo sheng bing, bing zai nei". ("shi dong, the sickness is outside, suo sheng bing, the sickness is in the inside".) He used the inside and outside concept to separate "shi dong" and "suo sheng bing". It is quite reasonable and can give later generations some new ideas. This is his advantage. But, his theory includes the first and the later of the *Nan jing's* qi and blood theory and also uses the external is in the qi and is the first sickness, and internal is in the blood and later sickness relationship mixed together, without any analysis. This is his disadvantage.

(3) The interpretation of Yu duo (Jin shi): this can also be seen in terms of advantage and disadvantage. He says: "mai dong fan chang, xie zai qi" ("abnormal pulse/vessels, the evil is in the qi") is shi dong, and "qi shou xie, chuan zhi yu xue" ("the qi has been hurt by evil, transferred to the blood") is suo sheng bing. He has also borrowed the concept of the first and later of qi and blood of the *Nan jing*, but

the sentence "mai dong fan chang" ("abnormal pulse/vessels") can give a big new idea for future generations. This is his advantage.

(4) The interpretation of Li guang: he says "qi shou re ze zuo lan wang xing, gu rou shi dong. Qi chuan zhi yu xue, fu shou ze feng gu xue rong bu ru bing ke you sheng", ("the qi has been hurt and surrounding not regular, this is called shi dong. The qi transfers to the blood and is hurt by the wind and the blood cannot circulate and then there is sickness generation.") This also uses the concept of first qi, and later blood in the *Nan jing* but has the concept of "yang yin xie er dong" ("the yang qi is moved by the evil") is shi dong, and "xue rong bu run er bing" ("the blood cannot circulate and causes sickness") is suo sheng bing. This gives some ideas for later generations.

(5) The interpretation of Zhang Xie xian, who also got the ideas from Li guang. He used the relationship of qi and blood and how they cannot circulate as his basis and the first and later relationship of qi and blood to describe shi dong and suo sheng bing. The unreasonable places for unsatisfactory interpretations is the same as the *Nan jing*.

(6) The interpretation of Ding jin, he used the idea that "xie zai qi, yi jian mai" ("the evil in the qi, can be seen in the mai") is shi dong, and "xie zai xue, you jian yu bing" ("evil in the blood, can be seen in the sickness") is suo sheng bing. Also, he points out, "qi xian bing, mai zhi ying zhi, xue hou bing, bing ke yan zhi." ("the qi sickness first, the pulse/vessels respond, the blood sickness later, the sickness can be examined"). From this interpretation, not only has it got the concept from the *Nan jing*, it also discusses the changes of pathogens (bing ji) and the symptoms of the bing hou separately. This is his advantage, but he also said the evil is in the qi and is when it has the sickness in the jing mai, otherwise when there is evil in the blood it has the symptoms of the bing hou. This is not in agreement with the shi dong which is described in th twelve bing hou.

(7) The interpretation of Ye lin, it is a little more completed compared to the "mai dong fan fan chang" ("abnormal pulse/vessels") of Mr. Zhang bu does also follow the qi sickness transfer to the blood of the *Nan jing*. No new discussions, so is not enough to use.

The evaluation of the disagree with the *Nan jing* group:

(1) The interpretation of Ma shi: he points out that suo sheng bing is the sickness of some jing, and is critical saying, the "*Nan jing* yi shi dong wei qi, suo sheng wei xue, yi dong sheng er zi, fen wei qi xue, nai *Nan jing* zhi yi shou er", ("*Nan jing* used shi dong as qi, and suo sheng bing as blood. The two words of 'dong' and 'sheng' can be separated into 'qi' and 'blood'. This is my own personal idea regarding the *Nan jing*.") This is a good idea but unfortunately he didn't describe the meaning of shi dong. Therefore, this a non-completed point.

(2) The interpretation of Zhang Jie bin: he received the "mai dong fan chang" ("abnormal pulse/vessels") from Yu duo. He thinks shi dong is "mai qi bian chang er wei bing" ("the mai qi is abnormal in sickness") and criticized the *Nan jing* zhi yan, shi fei jing zhi" ("what is said in the *Nan jing* is not correct"). It only described the meaning of shi dong from words. This also gives us some understanding of shi dong, but it doesn't describe anything about suo sheng bing. Therefore, this is also not complete.

(3) The interpretation of Zhang Zhi cong: he was critical of "zang fu jing mai nei wai chuan bian shou", ("viscera and bowels and the jing mai can transform each other from internal to external"). This is not only limited in the classics to blood and qi and the first and latter transfer, but it is more clever than first and latter of blood and qi of the *Nan jing* group. On the one hand, he interprets shi dong as the "bing yan yu wai" ("the reason for the sickness is from outside") and suo sheng bing as "bing yan yu nei" ("the course of the sickness is from internal"). On the other hand, he explains "bing you yin yu wai er ji yu nei zhe, you yin yu nei er ji yu wai zhe". ("the sickness may be caused from external and reaches internal, and from internal and reaches to external, and also both of them internal and external"). This avoids any incomplete understanding. This interpretation not only agrees with the jing mai and the pathogenic transfer of the internal viscera but also agrees with the bing hou of the twelve jing mai.

(4) The interpretation of Xu Da chen: he thinks shi dong is of all the sicknesses is the sickness of the jing itself, suo sheng bing is the development of it and the extension of other jings. He also points

out they are not separated into qi and blood. This is his advantage, but his understanding of suo sheng bing and shi dong is limited to the sickness of the jing itself or other jing's and therefore not reasonable. For example, in the shi dong of the twelve jing mai, the foot yang ming has "san yin, su qian, yan hei" ("likes to groan, frequently yawns, black visage"), the symptoms of kidney sickness. The foot shao yin has "ke qiu ze you xue, ke ke er chuan" ("coughing with blood, and panting urgently") are the symptoms of lung sickness. In suo sheng bing, nearly each jing has its own bing hou and has no more description of the bing zheng than for the other jing, and no more description of the bing hou than the other jing. None. Such as, for example, the hand tai yin, hand yang ming, foot yang ming, hand tai yang, foot tai yang, shou jue yin, hand shao yang, foot shao yang as far as the suo sheng bing are concerned, they all have no bing hou of other jing's and other viscera and bowels. So, is not completely believable for this purpose.

(5) The interpretation of Xue xue: he got his ideas from Zhang Jie bin and Ma shi. He has the same description of shi dong as Zhang Jie bin, and has the same description of suo sheng bing as Ma shi ie. "yin jing de suo sheng bing shi ben zang de suo sheng zhi bing" ("the suo sheng bing of the yin jing's is the sickness of his belonging viscera.") But his "yang jing de suo sheng bing shi jin, ye, qi, xue, jing, gu deng suo sheng zhi bing" ("the suo sheng bing of the yang jing are the sicknesses of the jin ye (fluids), qi, blood, tendons, and bones is different from Ma shi. In Mr. Xue's understanding, the foot yang ming jing is controlled by blood, this includes "kuang, nue, wen yu, han chu, xiu qiu, kou wo, chuan zhen, jing zhong, hou bi, da fu shui zhong, xi bin zhong tong, xing ying ru, qi jie, gu, fu tu, gan wei lian, zu fu shang jie tong, zhong zhi bu yong "deng, ("crazy, malaria, epidemic pestilence, sweating out, nose bleeding, mouth deviated, lips have papules, neck/throat swollen, throat bi, big abdomen oedema, knees swollen painful, along the chest breast, qi jie, thigh, calf, femur outside edge, foot upper surface all have pain, middle toe can't use" etc.). This will all become the sickness of the blood. Also, in the hand shao yang jing if it is controlled by the qi, "han chu, mu rui ci tong, xia tong, er hou, jian, ru, zhou, bi wai jie tong, xiao zhi chi zhi bu yong" deng ("sweating out, canthus of the eye is painful, cheek painful, ear

behind, shoulder, upper arm, elbow, external part of the forearm all painful, small finger and 2nd last finger can't use" etc.) This is all the sickness of the qi. If, as described above, how can we have some separation of sickness of the blood and sickness of the qi? Maybe, Mr. Xue cannot answer this part. Also, in the foot shao yang, "shi zhu gu suo sheng bing zhi" ("controls the suo sheng bing of the bone") its "tou teng, han tong, mu rui ci tong, que pen zhong zhong tong, ye xia tong, ma dao xia ying, han chu zhen han, nue, xiong, xie, lei, bi, xi wai zhi jin, jue gu, wai huai qian ji zhu jie jie tong, xiao zhi chi zhi bu yong" deng, ("headache, jaw pain, canthus of the eyes pain, internal hollow of the clavicular fossa pain, underarm pain, ma dao xia ying (scrofula), sweating out shivering like cold, malaria, chest, ribs, hypochondriac region, hips, the external side of the knee to the shins, the point at jue gu, the external ankle bone front and all the various joints are painful, the small toe and the 2nd last toe can't use" etc. But, not all is the sickness of the bone. The hand yang ming controls the jin ye (body saliva and fluids), and the hand tai yang controls the ye (fluids), while foot tai yang controls the tendons. If using the interpretation of Mr. Xie, he not only cannot connect all the systems but also has many other problems. So, the interpretation from Mr. Xie is not complete. The judgement of the middle -of the- road group of the main group, the interpretation of Hua sou is to think the evil qi if hurt people, then this is only in the qi; some of them will be in the blood, they cannot be separated into first and later. This negates the viewpoint of the first and later of the *Nan jing*, this idea is quite suitable for practice in most clinics but it limited in the qi and blood of the *Nan jing* ie. this is not correct enough. This is his disadvantage.

The judgement of the viewpoint of the Japanese Han doctor is:

(1)   The interpretation of Gong ben yi yao: he thinks that shi dong is from the generation of changes of the jing luo, suo sheng bing is the sickness which is generated by the viscera and the bowels. If follow the description of the sickness of shi dong, there should not be sickness of the viscera and bowels. In the sickness of the suo sheng bing, there should not be the sickness of the jing mai. But in the comparison of the twelve jing mai bing hou, you can see:

i In the original writing of shi dong, the hand tai yin has "fei zhang men, pang pang er chuan ke" ("the lungs are distended and stuffy, make noises and panting and coughing"). In the hand tai yin, this is the sickness of the viscera and bowels. In the foot tai yin, it has "wei wan tong san yi" ("gastric cavity painful, flatulence"), the sickness of the spleen viscera and the stomach bowel. The hand shao yin has "xin tong" ("heart pain"), the sickness of the heart viscera. The shou jue yin has "xin zhong zang zang da dong" ("the heart always feels like it is moving") and "xi xiao bu xiu" ("smiling/laughing can't stop"), as the symptoms of pericardium luo sickness. While, the foot shao yin has "xi kong" ("always afraid/fearful"), as a kidney viscera sickness.

ii In the original writings of the suo sheng bing, the hand tai yin has "nao bi nei qian lian tong jue" ("internal front side of the shoulder and arm edge painful adverse"). the sickness of the jing mai. The hand yang ming has "jian qian ru tong, da zhi chi zhi bu yong" ("the shoulder front and arm painful, the big digit and 2nd finger can't be used"), the sickness of the jing mai. In the foot yang ming, it has "xun ying ru, qi jie, gu, fu tu, gan wai lian, zu fu shang jie tong, zhong zhi bu yong" ("along the chest breast, qi jie, femur, tibia, external edge of the fibula, foot surface all painful, the middle toe can't use"), the sickness of the jing mai. The foot tai yin has "gu xi nie zhong jue, zu da zhi bu yong" ("internal thigh and knee swollen adverse, the big toe cannot use"), the sickness of the jing mai. The hand shao yin has "ru bi nei hou lian tong, jue" ("the internal back edge of the shoulder and arm painful, syncope"), the sickness of the jig mai. The hand tai yang has "jing, han, jian, ru, zhou, bi wai hou lian tong" ("neck/throat, cheeks, shoulder, arm, elbow, forearm external back edge pain"), the sickness of the jing mai. The hand shao yang channel has "er hou, jian, ru, zhou bi wai jie tong, xiao zhi chi zhi bu yong" ("the back of the ear, the shoulder, arm, elbow forearm external all painful, the little finger and 2nd last finger can't use"), the sickness of the jing mai. And, the foot shao yang has "xiong, xie, lie, bi, xi wai zhi jin, je gu, wai huai qian ji zhu jie jie tong, xiao zhi chi zhi

80

bu yong" ("chest, ribs, the hypochondriac region, hip, external side of the knee to the shins, jue gu point, external front of the ankle and all the joints painful, the small toe and the 2nd last toe can't use"), are also sicknesses of the jing mai. From all the descriptions above, Gong ben yi yao only understood shi dong and suo sheng bing from the viewpoint of changes of the jing mai and suo sheng bing from the viscera and bowels. It is not reasonable, but the transfer series of the jing mai viscera and bowels may give some ideas to future generations.

(2) Other Han doctors in Japan, and those who haven't come up with new discoveries and creations: in the book the *Ling shu shi* written by Dan bo yuan jian, in his description, "shi dong and suo sheng bing only falls under the ideas formulated by Zhang Jie bin, Ma shi, and Zhang Zhi cong etc. He hasn't described, "Gai shi dong suo sheng, qi yi bu ming si, yi wei zhi shou shi". ("Gai is generated by shi dong, this meaning is not clear and not natural".) In the book the *Nan jing shu zheng* by Dan Bo yan, later writers feel he only makes a reference to Yu duo, Ding jin, Hua sou, and Xu Da chen. He hasn't added any other interpretations. The book the *Jing luo zhi liao jing huo* by Ben jian xiang bai says, "shi dong suo sheng bing, nai shi ge jing mai qi xue xun huan bian dong zhi bing zhuang, bing bu shi ge jing bing zheng zhi qian bu" ("the shi dong and the suo sheng bing are all the symptoms of the changes of the jing mai qi and blood circulation, not the total bing zhen of each jing".) It also uses the *Nan jing's* "shi dong nai qi bian dong zhi bing, suo sheng bing nai xue bian dong zhi bing" ("shi dong is the sickness of the qi changes, suo sheng bing is the sickness of the blood chang".) His interpretation belongs to the *Nan jing* group, so has no new good ideas which can be seen.

3. The viewpoint of shi dong and suo sheng bing in present times:
   (1) Abstracts from recent people's interpretations:
   Li Ji ying said, "in the tweve jing bing hou shi dong and suo sheng bing, they are connected. After describing each jing mai travelling paths, from the *Ling shu jing mai pian*, Li Ji ying makes the conclusion that 'shi dong' and 'shi zhu suo sheng bing' describe each jing mai changes and their symptoms and treatment process. In the twelve

jing mai, 'shi dong' and 'shi zhu suo sheng bing' two groups, there is no contradictory meaning. So, it can be concluded 'shi dong' and 'shi zhu suo sheng bing' are the same system, they are two groups of symptoms which have a connection to each other." (from *Shang hai zhong yi yao za zhi* 1962 vol. 6 p. 20).

Lu Shou yan said, "'shi zhu x' and 'suo shen bing' are two sentenses, that must be read separately and cannot be mixed together. Otherwise, it will result in complications when read in the old books. Nobody explained this and read it together so it has resulted in a misunderstanding. Xue xue talked about the meaning of the sickness, he thought the yang jing (yang channels) are the jin ye (saliva and body fluids) and qi and blood together etc. They cause the sickness, this is the fault right here." (*Ha bin zhong yi* vol. 75th edition 1962 p. 11).

Wang You quan said, "Lin qu originally said: shi dong then illness: yi gan (larynx pharanyx dry) ... becomes bi jue. Shi zhu: illness from the heart. Yellow eyes ... hot and painful in the hands. Explanation: the blood changes (unusual, not normal) will result in these symptoms; dry parched throat ... (etc. symptoms), this is called bi jue. This channel in charge: illness of the heart viscera. Yellow eyes ..., pain and hot in the hands. 'Shi dong' and 'suo sheng bing' they are not nouns in the *Jing mai pian*, they are also not illnesses associated with special nouns. The *Nan jing* treated 'shi dong' and 'suo sheng bing' as two independent special nouns and discussed this mechanism of illness. This is not only not suitable itself, but also it gives a very big false impression to later doctors. It leads doctors following him down the wrong path to study the mechanism of illness! 'Shi dong, then illness' and 'shi zhu' they are connected, you can only say one or two or two or one. They combine with each other. Like everybody knows 'shi dong then illness' etc. symptoms, is a series of symptoms which results from some illness and abnormal changes in each of the twelve channels jing mai. 'Shi zhu' etc. symptoms, its series of symptoms of each of the jing mai, can controll the illness. First, it includes serious symptoms of each channel jing mai abnormal changes and each channel 'shu' and 'luo' zang qi and each channel passes organs which result in some illness. Meanwhile, it also includes some illnesses which have connections with the ben (original) jing original organ and with other jing with other organs. Each channel 'shi dong, then illness' etc. symptoms and 'shi zhu' etc. symptoms, although they are two different parts, they have major parts to play based on the same symptoms of the jing mai themselves. In the two big groups of symptoms, they are internally connectected with each other. So, we say that they are two and one. But analysed correctly they still have differences. Each symptom includes parts, which still have wide and narrow differences so they are also one and two". (*Ha bin zhong yi* 1963 vol. 6 p. 55.)

(2) Typical opinions:

In the important works of modern society: *Zhen jiu xue jian pian*: "its called 'shi dong' illness because it is caused by the external factors invading the ben (original) channel. Its called 'suo sheng bing' when the illness is caused by the internal and the jing luo." (*China research institute* edited Beijing August 1976 2nd edition p. 10).

Zhen jiu xue, "'shi dong' mainly explains the illness that is caused by jing mai when it has unusual changes. 'Suo sheng bing" is explained when the illness that was caused by the original channel jing qi abnormality can be treated by the channel channel point. So, the symptoms of shi dong and suo sheng bing are almost the same. The original book describes the symptoms of jing luo from the phenomena of the illness mechanism of the jing mai and jing points treatment, two parts. These two parts are the same. (*Shang hai chinese medicine college*, Shang hai July 1974 1st edition p.38).

Zhen jiu xue jiang yi, "shi dong, is the illness caused by abnormal changes of the original channel's jing mai. Shi zhu suo sheng bing is the illness controlled by the original channel and the ben zang. Both of them explain the symptoms of each channel and the zang fu. They affect each other and change each other although they have differences in the jing mai and the zang fu, and the qi and blood. Because the jing mai, zang fu, qi and blood, and jing ye etc. they react with each other. (*Nan Jing Chinese medicine college acupuncture research and teaching group* Beijing 1961 1st edition p.8, this book republished in August 1964, it explained shi dong and suo sheng bing, simply called *zang fu jing mai symptoms (bing hou)*).

(3) Personal study opinion: shi dong explained to be the 'mai qi abnormal change' is quite suitable according to the olden doctors' explanation. Example: Li ji, Zhang Jie bin, Zhang Zhi cong, Xue xue, Ye lin etc.

all have this opinion. The meaning of shi dong can be explained as "mai dong abnormal", this is also explained in the original jing mai chapter example, "mai zhi zu ran dong zhe, jie xie qi she zhi" ('people, their channels if abnormal, they all belong to evil qi gets control"). The *Su wen - ci jin lun* chapter indicates that, "ci zhong xin ... qi dong wei yi, ci zhong gan ... qi dong wei yan, ci zhong shen ... qi don wei ti, ci zhong fei ... qi dong ke, ci zhong pi ... qi dong wei wei tun, ci zhong dan ... qi dong wei ou" etc. ("put acupuncture in/pierce the heart ... makes change for yi?, put it in/pierce the liver ... is for language, put it in the kidney ... is for sneezing, put it in the lung ... is for coughing, put it in the spleen ... is for eating (swallowing), put it in the gall bladder ... is for vomiting"). In here, the "dong" character is also to mean the change of zang fu qi. This is almost the same as the modern explanation that "shi dong" is the abnormal change of channel qi.

Re the explanation of suo sheng bing, Ma shi's explanation (is all x channels illness), is more reasonable. The *Ling shu-zhong shi* chapter said, "bi xian tong shi er jing mai zhi suo sheng bing, er hou ke de chuan yu zhong shi yi" ("if you want to know how to treat the patient, you will first of all need to know the illness that is caused by the twelve jing mai"). The "shi dong" and the "suo sheng bing" of the Jing mai chapter is the detailed part of the "shi er jing mai zhi suo sheng bing" in the Zhong ci chapter. It is not all cohesive. The *Ling shu-bai bing shi sheng* chapter, when it discussed the change of mechanism of illness, in the upper, middle, and lower three parts, it also indicates, "ci nei wai san bu zhi suo sheng bing zhe ye" ("this illness is caused by the internal and external three parts"). So, a person who gets an illness, they not only have an illness mechanism change in the organs (qi guan) and the twelve jing mai, but also have an illness in the organs. Therefore, according to the explanations given in the modernday and by Ma shi, "suo sheng bing is a description of the ben (original) channel and original zang etc. illness", is the same. When they explain the suo sheng bing, their opinions also have the same meaning: "suo sheng bing is an illness that is caused by the original jing jing qi abnormal change, which can be treated by this channel's channel points.

Zhang Zhi cong developed the theories of the internal and external transfer change of the zang fu jing mai. He discussed the "shi dong" and the "suo sheng bing" not only from the meaning of the characters, he explained them to be the "bing yin yu wai" ("the illness comes from the external") and "bing yin yu nei" ('the illness comes from the internal"). Then, he explained the connection of them and gave a differential opinion which is suitable for the practical phenomenon of the change in internal viscera (zang) mechasism of illness. Compared to the explanation of the difficult channel system, it seems better. The explanation from modernday and by Zhang shi that "shi dong shi you wai yin xun fan ben jing zhi jing qi er fa sheng de bing bian. Suo sheng bing shi you nei yin fa sheng de bing bian sha ji zhi jing luo er chu xian de bing zheng" ("shi dong is the illness that is caused by the external invaded original channel. Suo sheng bing is the illness that is caused by the internal factors and has a relationship with the jing luo".) Their opinions are almost the same.

In summary of the above, "shi dong" and "suo sheng bing", they are described as the jing mai illness change of the twelve jing zang fu jing mai. Both of them help each other. They describe the illness which is in change in the jing mai and with the zang fu jing luo together. They also explain the connection of the jing luo and the zang fu..

Section 2
Eight extraordinary channels

Introduction

The eight extraordinary channels are an important part of the jing luo system. The qi jing ba mai is the du mai, ren mai, chong mai, dai mai, yin qiao mai, yang qiao mai, yin wei mai, and yang wei mai, eight channels. The major characteristics of the qi jing ba mai is: it is not limited by the channels, and does not belong to its luo the zang fu. Its major action is adjusting qi and blood and allowing for the storage of zhen jing mai qi. So, the *Nan jing-er shi qi, er shi ba nan* described the zhen jing as channels, the qi jing as lakes (hu) and if the qi of the zhen jing is strong then they flow into the qi jing, In the 8 mai, except for the ren, du 2 mai, the points belong to the shu points of the ben (original) jing. In other words, the 6 mai all belong to the zhen jing. The qi jing ba mai connects with the zang fu by way of the twelve jing mai, but they have a circular road and special actions and, control illness themselves.

"Qi", has the meaning of "storage", "odd", "other", and "adjusting". Because, their actions and characteristics have differences from the twelve jing mai, they are called storage channels.

"Du" has the meaning of "leader and supervisor", "superintendent", "orderer", "together", and "all". It can also be explained as "central". The du mai controls the yang qi of the body, it is the key of the yang mai. The hand and foot 3 yang jing jing qi all meet at the du mai, ie. is the sea of the yang jing jing qi. Its major action are:

1. control the yang qi of the whole body,
2. maintains the yuan yang (source qi) of the whole body.

"Ren" has the meaning of "doing something", "pregnant", "look after the child", and "put up with/don't get angry with channel". It can also be explained as "hold". It controls the yin jing of the whole body ie. it's the sea of the yin mai. It has a pregnancy action, ie. it is also the basis of pregnancy. Its major actions are:

1. adjust the yin qi of the body,
2. gives some nutrition to the women when they have the baby (pregnant and after pregnant).

"Chong" has the meaning of "key road", "key road", "channel"; it can also be explained as "through". The chong mai flows from up to the head and down to the foot and the qi and blood of the twelve jing pass it, i.e. is the key road of control, controlling every channel's qi and blood, it is the sea of the twelve jing mai. Its major actions are:

1. connects the qi of the pre-natal and the post-natal, stores the zhen qiof the whole body,
2. is the sea of blood, in charge of blood illnesses.

"Dai" has the meaning of "limitation", or "wrap/band". The dai mai is around the waist like a band, limit's the yin yang each mai. Its major actions are:

1. limits and raises every mai, doesn't allow them to go down and lose their ways,
2. adjusts the mai qi, makes things clear.

"Yin qiao", "yang qiao": "qiao" and "stilts" have the same use and can also be explained as "shou that are made from straw" and also can be explained as "strong". Their major actions are:

1. the yin qiao controls the yin of the body, the yang qiao controls the yang of the body, they adjust the yin jing and the yang jing,
2. they control the switch of go and stop in the body

"Yin wei", "yang wei": "wei" has the meaning of "net" and "dimension". It is also explained by someone as "suburb" The "yin wei" controls the three yin jing travels the yin fen, it controls the internal part of the body. The "yang wei" controls the three yang jing and goes to the wei fen, it controls the external (surface) of the body. Their major actions are:

1. they control the surface and internal parts of the body together,
2. makes the yin yang jing qi change each other. They control and connect the twelve jing.

In simple words, if speak like west and east, the du controls the yang of the back of the body, and the ren controls the yin of front of the body. If speak like south and north, the dai mai limits every mai of the body. The chong mai, stores the qi and blood of the body. The yang wei goes to the wei fen, and it controls the surface of the body. The yin wei goes to the yin fen, and it controls the internal part of the body. Yin yang qiao controls the yin yang of the body together

Distribution road of the Eight extraordinary channels.

About the circle distribution road of the qi jing ba mai, the records in the olden days have different explanations and do not have system theories. According to the *Su wen*, the *Ling shu*, and the *Nan jing*, and other doctors' descriptions, one can make a summary below:

(i) Du mai
    1. Distribution road: there are four lines of the du mai:
        (1) From the private parts of the lower abdomen along the backbone, goes up distributed to the back of the neck feng fu point (GV16), into the brain, goes on top of the head along the forehead, and goes down to the nose.

(2)   From the middle abdomen bao, goes down to the private parts, from the wai lu bone, and out and around the bone, and meets the jing mai of the foot tai yang and meets the channel of the gu nui hou edge of the foot shao yin, then returns and goes through the backbone into the body to the kidney viscera.

(3)   From the inner corner of the eyes, with the foot tai yang mai goes to the forehead and meets at the top of the head and then goes down along the neck and the backbone to the waist and connects with the kidney viscera.

(4)   From the lesser abdomen, goes up past the umbilicus and connects with the heart, goes into the throat, out to the face, comes around the lips to the lower part of the eyes.

2.   About the shu points:
chang qiang, yao shu, yang guang, ming men, xuan qu, ji zhong, zhong qu, jin suo, zhi yang, ling tai, shen dao, shen zhu, tao dao, da zhui, ya men, feng fu, nao hu, qiang jian, hou ding, bai hui, qian ding, lu hui, shang xing, shen ting, su miu, shui gou, dui duan, yin jiao. Together 28 points.

Meeting points: feng men (foot tai yang), hui yin (ren mai) etc. points.

(ii). Ren mai

1.   Distribution road: there are two distribution roads of the ren mai:
(1)   From the lower part of the ji point in the lesser abdomen, goes down to the private parts, along the abdomen and the chest, goes up to the throat, then goes up to the cheek and then goes to part of the face and into the eyes.

(2)   From inside the bao and the organs and spine, goes up to the back.

2.   About the shu points:
hui yin, qu gu, zhong ji, guan yuan, si man, qi hai, yin jiao, shen jue, shui fen, xia wan, jian li, zhong wan, shang wan, ju jue, jiu wei, zhong ting, tan zhong, you tan, zi gong, hua gai, xuan ji, tian tu, lian qian, cheng jiang. Together 24 points.

Meeting points: cheng qi (foot yang ming), yin jiao (du mai) etc. points.

(iii) Chong mai

1. Distribution road: there are five distribution roads for the chong mai:
    (1) From inside of the abdomen part, goes out to the qi jie part, and goes parallel with the foot shao yin kidney channel passed the umbilicus to the centre of the chest and then spreads around.
    (2) After the chong mai spreads from the chest, it goes up and distributes to the mai, "kong sang" part (nei bone san qiao).
    (3) The mai qi transfers to the kidney from the lesser abdomen, goes out to the qi jie, along the inside of the yin gu into femur bone (guo wo) and passes along the inside of the shin bone, goes to the back of the internal ankle, to the bottom of the foot.
    (4) From along the inside of the shin bone, goes up the outside, then into the ankle, to the surface of the foot and distributes on the big toe.
    (5) Goes out from the bao of the lesser abdomen, goes up along the backbone, circles around the back.

    The below six mai all do not have ben jing shu points. "About (belong) shu points", means it depends on the zhen jing, the ben jing mai and the fourteen jing mai meeting points.

2. About shu points: hui yin (ren mai), qi chong (foot yang ming), heng gu, da he, qi xue, si man, zhong zhu, huang shu, shang qu, shi guan, yin du, tong gu, you men, (all of the above belong to the foot shao yin), yin jiao (ren mai).

(iv). Dai mai

1. Distribution road: the dai mai goes from the 14th vertebrae, from the 14th vertebrae to the hypochondriac ribs region, around the body goes along the waist and abdomen.
2. About the shu points: dai mai, wu qu, wei dao (the above are all foot shao yang), zhang men (foot jue yin).

(v). Yang qiao mai

1. Distribution road: yang qiao starts from the shen mai point (UB62) of the foot tai yang of the external ankle, along the external side goes up and extends passed the outside gu (thigh), distributes at the ribs, goes around outside of the shoulders, along the neck, to the mouth, and then

goes to the eyes, and then goes parallel with the tai yang-yin qiao mai, goes into the hair ji (the hairline), goes around the back of the ear to feng chi point (GB20), from the back of the neck, feng fu point (GV16) goes into the brain

2. About the shu points: shen mai, pu shen, fu yang (above points are all the foot tai yang), zhu miu (foot shao yang), ru shu (hand tai yang), ju gu, jian you (the hand yang ming), di cang, ju miu, cheng qi (above points are all the foot yang ming), jing ming (foot tai yang), feng chi (foot shao yang), feng fu (du mai).

(vi). Yin qiao mai

1. Distribution road: the yin qiao mai starts from the foot shao yin kidney jing along the zhao hai point (K6) under the ankle and then goes forewards to the internal leg and then extends past the private parts. It goes to the chest, goes up to the clavicle, along the throat to the front of the ren ying, from the internal cheek to the canthii of the eyes, and meets the tai yang-yang qiao mai, then goes up parrallel to the brain.

2. About the shu points: zhao hai, jiao xin (the above points are the foot shao yin), jing ming (the foot tai yang).

(vii). Yang wei mai

1. Distribution road: the yang wei mai starts from the meeting points of each and every jing. And its mai qi source is from jin men point (UB63) of the foot tai yang jing, goes up along the external side of the leg and hip parts, to the bi part, and then to the external of the lesser abdomen part, along the ribs goes up, goes up to the shoulder and then passes from the shoulder to the back of the shoulder. Then goes to the back of the ear, after reaching the forehead, then goes back to the top of the ear level bone position, directly to the feng fu point (GV16), which is at the back of the neck.

2. About the shu points: jin men (foot tai yang), yang jiao (foot shao yang), tian miu (hand shao yang), ru shu (hand tai yang), jian jing (foot shao yang), feng chi (foot shao yang), ya men, feng fu (these are all du mai), nao kong, chen ling, zheng ying, mu chuang, tou lin qi, yang bei, ben shen (all foot shao yang), tou wei (foot yang ming).

(viii). Yin wei mai

1. Distribution road: the yin wei mai starts from the meeting point of each and every yin jing. Its mai qi starts from zhu bin point (K8) of the foot shao yin jing, goes along the internal leg into the lesser abdomen parts, then from the ribs goes up connects with the chest and the two sides of the throat, and meets with the ren mai.

2. About the shu points: zhu bin (foot shao yin), chong men (foot tai yin), fu she, da heng, fu ai (all foot tai yin), qi men (foot jue yin), tian tu, lian qian (all ren mai).

The qi jing ba mai mainly adjusts and stores qi, blood. This type of adjustage is presented as a dynamic balance for the twelve jing qi and blood, but the qi jing also has its circle road and has its circling and transforming of jing qi. And the qi jing jing qi goes up and down, which exchanges or mixes together and makes for a strong connection for th twelve jing mai and the organs of the body.

Symptoms of the qi jing ba mai

(i) Symptoms of the du mai

backbone hard and cannot bend, jiao gong fu zhang (opisthotonos), pain because the lesser abdomen qi goes up, people can't pass excretion from the front and the back, "chong shan" ("chong hernia"), long, haemorrhoids, enuresis, yi gan (larynx and pharynx problems), women's infertility, hands and feet convulsions, shaking, spasms, stroke and can't speak, epilepsy, depressive state, madness (kuang), head part pain, eyes red swollen painful, a lot of tears, pain in the leg, knees, waist, back, the throat neck stiff and straight, shang han (typhoid or attack by cold), throat and teeth swollen and painful, hands and feet numb, night sweating, nerves abnormal, infantile convulsions etc.

(ii) Symptoms of the ren mai

men have qi shan (the seven hernias), women have red and white leucorrhoea, various blockages in the abdomen (jia ji), irregular menstruation, miscarriage, infertility, lesser abdomen tense and spasmed. Haemorrhoids, diarrhoea, dysentery, malaria, cough, vomiting blood, blood in the urine, teeth painful, throat swelling, urine influent, chest and abdominal cavity parts pain, hiccoughing, after give birth to a child have a stroke, waist pain, baby die in the body can't go out, umbilicus and abdomen have a cold chilly sensation, vomiting, nausea, breasts painful, uterine bleeding and dripping etc. symptoms.

explanation: there are different explanations for the "seven hernias":

1. The *Su wen* considered the seven hernias to be: chong hernia, hu (wolf) hernia, tui hernia, jue hernia, hernia jia, ji hernia, and long hernia.
2. Xiu Zhen fang considered the seven hernias as: jue hernia, zheng hernia, han hernia, qi hernia, pan hernia, fu hernia, and lang hernia.
3. Zhu Dan xi, Zhang Zi he thought the seven hernias are han hernia, shui hernia, jin hernia, xue hernia, qi hernia, hu hernia, and kui hernia.
4. Ma shi thinks the seven hernias are xin (heart) hernia, gan (liver) hernia, pi (spleen) hernia, fei (lung) hernia, shen (kidney) hernia, hu hernia, and tui hernia.

At present, chinese medicine judges hernias based on the seven hernias developed by Zhu Dan xi, Zhang Zi he. So, it has described their characteristics as below:

(1) Han hernia: the scrotum feels cold and hard, the testes feel painful, the waist is painful, the pulse is sunken and chi (slow).
(2) Sui hernia: the scrotum is painful, swollen and itchy, or yellow water comes out.
(3) Jing hernia: the penis is swollen and always feels something is pulling down, painful and itchy, or has something like semen flow out.
(4) Qi hernia: after angry and crying, then the scrotum swells, if stop getting angry and crying then the scrotum becomes smaller again.
(5) Xue hernia: injury flows down, testes injury, blood stops inside, swelling painful.
(6) Hu hernia: hernia can go out and come in, and when lay down the hernia comes in and the scrotum becomes smaller, and if stand up and go the hernia will reduce and the scrotum will become bigger.
(7) Tui hernia: men will find the scrotum swollen, not very painful, not itchy, and in women their private parts go out.

(iii) Symptoms of the chong mai

because "chong-ren-du three mai go up together but different ways, one source but three directions, all connect to dai mai" (*Ru men si qin-zheng fu ren dai xia chi bai chao fen han re zhang).* So, if there is some illness, need to be concerned with the ren-du together. This mai, major symptoms are: irregular menstruation, absence of periods, beng lou (too much period), little breast milk. It also has qi going up to the throat from the lesser abdomen and attacking the throat, panting and can't lie down comfortably, dong qi (active qi) in the abdomen, abdomen has a feeling of distension and acute pain, dead baby inside, lou tai (miscarriage), centre abdominal cavity painful, chest and abdominal cavity stuffy and full, jie xiong, adverse stomach, alcohol and food accumulation and lumps, intestinal noises, stools like slurry, yan ge (illness of the diaphragm and the oesophagus), ribs distended, umbilicus and abdomen pain, intestinal wind and bloody stools, malaria, retained lochia, after have a baby gets syncope etc.

(iv) Symptoms of the dai mai

   abdomen inside is stuffy and full, waist feels cold and not strong, sometimes feel like sitting in water. Leucorrhoea, uterus collapses, hands and feet stroke paralysis, hands and feet painful, numb and shaking, fever, head-wind headache, jaw swelling, eyes red and painful, teeth painful, throat swelling, light-headedness (tou xuan), deafness, skin rubella (feng zhen) and itchy, feels like someone is pulling at one's tendons and vessels uncomfortable, leg painful, feet atrophied can't use, ribs and hypochondriac region painful etc.

(v) Symptoms of the yin qiao mai

   epilepsy, spasms, paralysis, feet turned outwards, likes to sleep, inner corner of the eyes red and painful, men have yin hernia, women have lou xia. Throat painful, urine lin li (dripping), urinary bladder qi painful, intestinal sounds, intestinal wind and bleeding, vomiting and diarrhoea, adverse stomach (eructation), stools difficult, difficult to pass a baby, stupor (hun mi), intestines have lumps (ji kuai), chest and diaphragm burping, mei he qi (globus hystericus), jaundice etc.

(vi) Symptoms of the yang qiao mai

   depression, epilepsy, and madness (dian xian kuang), spasms, paralysis, feet turned inward, cannot sleep, waist and back stiff and straight, legs swollen, afraid of wind, spontaneous sweating, headache, sudden head-wind, head sweating, eyes red and painful, corner of eyebrow bone painful, hands and feet palsy and painful, shaking and convulsions, jue ni (syncope), blue milk (qui you), deafness, nose bleeding, swelling of the whole body etc.

(vii) Symptoms of the yin wei mai

if the yin wei mai cannot contain each yin jing, it will result in loss of concentration, or the nerves are not settled, when serious, will feel heart pain. Yin qi stops inside, it will result in chest pain, under the ribs feel stuffy, waist pain and inside the sexual organs pain etc. It also results in: intestinal noises, diarrhoea, prolapse of the rectum, eructation and problems with the diaphragm and oesophagus, blockages in the abdomen and horizontal stick-like objects, typhoid or attack by cold, malaria etc.

(viii) Symptoms of the yang wei mai

If the yang wei mai cannot control each yang jing, it will result in no force in the hands and feet, doesn't like activity (movement), when serious, will result in coldness and have fever. Yang too strong, it will show head and eyes dizziness, qi quan (out of breath panting), the shoulder raised up, skin painful and not sensitive. It also shows typhoid fever and spontaneous sweating, hands and feet (limbs) joints swelling painful, head and neck painful, the bone near the corner of the eye painful. Hands and feet hot, can't control, the back is twisted and the tendons and bones are painful, the four limbs paralysed, night sweating (dao han), tetanus (lockjaw), kness feel cold and have a chilly feeling, lower legs and heels swollen, eyes red and painful etc.

The actions of the qi jing ba mai

The qi jing ba mai is not only different from the twelve zheng jing, but is also different from the fifteen luo mai. They show characteristics of both jing mai and mai luo. They also have a special action in the human body jing luo system. I will describe this in 4 ways:

(i) Connecting action

The qi jing ba mai have a connecting action with the twelve jing mai, they make each jing mai connect with each other.

Example: The du mai connects the hand 3 yang channels and the foot 3 yang channels, ie. all the body's yang jing qi, all meet at da zhui point (GV14) of the du mai. The ren mai also includes the 3 yin jing mai qi, ie. The foot 3 yin channels all meet at zhong ji (CV3), and guan yuan (CV4) points of the ren mai. Another example, the chong mai connects the 5 zang and the 6 fu, ie. it's the sea of the twelve jing mai. Furthermore, the dai mai connects every jing mai which distributes throughout the body in an up and down direction. The yang wei and the yin wei have the actions of connecting the net like yin jing and the yang jing. The yin qiao and the yang qiao have the actions of connecting every jing mai. All these confirm that the qi jing ba mai have different connection characteristics with the twelve jing mai and re the zang fu.

(ii) Adjusting action

The qi jing ba mai is distributed and goes around between the twelve jing mai, when the twelve jing mai and the zang fu have strong qi and blood, ie. the qi jing can store them. And when the human body needs them, the qi jing can give them again. So, olden day's doctors said the twelve jing mai are like rivers, and the qi jing is like a lake. This shows the adjusting action of the qi jing ba mai re the twelve mai qi.

(iii) Combining action

Although, the twelve jing mai have different characteristics and relativity, they have some characteristics the same with the jing mai. The qi jing classifies the approximate-same actions of the jing mai, ie. it shows that the twelve jing mai have an organizing action which keep the same characteristics.

Example: the yin jing and the yang jing of the twelve jing combine together by way of the yang wei and the yin wei, the yin qiao and the yang qiao mai which makes the different and combined yin and yang of the left side and right side of the body, and the dai mai combine and limits every jing mai in the body and makes each jing mai in the lower part of the body have a strong connection. So, the qi jing has a classifying action on the different jing mai in the twelve jing mai, and have a combining action re the jing mai which have the same characteristics.

(iv) Major actions

The qi jing ba mai have actions not only in the connection and the adjusting and the combination of all the body's jing luo, but also have important actions which have a control action after it classifies the twelve jing mai. Example, the du mai is the summary of each yang jing mai in the human body, it also has a connection with the kidney and the brain in particular. It also has some effect on the foot jue yin liver jing. Likewise, it has an action on, and leads and controls the yang qi and is in charge of the zhong yuan. The ren mai has an action of adjusting and supporting the yin jing mai qi. In the human body, qi is yang and blood is yin. Pregnancy, having a baby, women's periods, and leucorrhoea etc. women's illnesses have an important relationship with the yin blood. Chen Zi ning called "ren zhu bao tai" ("the ren controls the uterus and babies") (*Fu ren liang fang*), it explains the major leading and controlling actions of the ren mai along with every other yin jing. The chong mai starts from inside the bao, so it is called the "xue hai" ("the sea of blood") (*Fu ren liang fang*) because it has an important effect on the twelve jing mai and the wu zang liu fu. In addition, it is also called the "shi er jing mai zi hai" ("the sea of the twelve jing mai"), the "wu zang liu fu hai" ("the sea of the 5 zang 6 fu") (*Fu ren liang fang*). The dai mai is in charge of every jing qi and blood, adjusts and makes the jing qi clear. The qiao mai and wei mai control the yang jing and the yin jing, in the left and the right, in the internal and the external of the body. All this indicates that the qi jing have a major leading action on the twelve jing mai. From the major roads in which the qi and blood are distributed and go around, the twelve jing mai are the major part of all the jing luo. If there is any concern re jing mai characterisation and actions, the qi jing ba mai is the leader and controller of the twelve jing mai so the twelve jing mai and the qi jing ba mai have the same importance in the jing luo theory.

Practical use meaning of qi jing theories

The qi jing ba mai combines and organizes several of the same characteristics of the jing mai, as mentioned above. Its major actions are connecting, adjusting, combining, and controlling this jing luo combination system. So, the symptoms of the qi jing mainly describes some together illness of the jing mai controlled illnesses which are controlled by each of the qi jing. In other words, the symptoms of the qi jing are classified as the symptoms of the twelve jing mai

The qi jing bing hou indicates importance - in the twelve jing mai, some jing mai have the above characteristics and have both internal and strong connections in the mechanism of illness. It tells the chinese medicine doctors: when treating an illness, should not only be concerned with the symptoms of the zang fu and jing luo, but also be concerned with the connections of the mechanisms of illness which have the same characteristics in the zang fu and jing luo. The more important is that it indicates people treat illnesses by analysis perfectly from all directions, it makes chinese medicine differential treatment on a higher level. Unfortunately, some doctors in the olden days, were not very concerned with qi jing theories. So, in this area, there is not a lot of experience and not a lot of system theories. It needs further study. Now, we will just describe the practical use meaning from the illness diagnosis, medicine treatment, and acupuncture three parts.

(i) The qi jing theories and the direct meaning of the illness diagnosis

The qi jing symptoms, in effect, are the together illnesses which come from jing mai which are controlled by every qi jing. So, in the practical sense, when several jing mai have illness changes at the same time, they present many symptoms. The qi jing bing hou can classify and combine these symptoms and analyse the mechanisms of illness in order to diagnose - indicating which major jing mai have an illness change.

This is suitable for normal illness. For some complex and difficult illnesses, it gives a very good diagnosis method in order to summarize the illness. In other words, some illnesses of the qi jing perhaps haven't complex symptoms, but this indicates that when concerned with the mechanisms of illness and analysis, it is necessary to be concerned with the jing mai and internal organs which have related characteristics, and avoid incorrect diagnoses. This has a very important direct meaning in the illness diagnosis.

In the women's disease area, from the physiology and mechanisms of illness, they all have a good connection with the chong, ren, and dai of the qi jing. Like the *Su wen - shang gu tian zheng lun* said, "e qi e tian kuai zi, ren mai tong, tai chong mai sheng, yue si yi si xia, gu rou zi … ." ("qi comes from heaven comes quickly, the ren mai unblocks, the tai chong is strong, within a month have a baby …"). The *Su wen-gu kong lun* said, "ren mai wei bing, nu zi dai xia jia zhu" ("if the illness from the ren mai, then women leuccorrhagia and blockages in the abdomen"). Wang Shu he in the *Mai jing* wrote, "ren mai ye, dong, ku shao fu yao qi xia yin heng gu, yin zhong qie tong" ("ren mai, moving, not comfortable in the lesser abdomen goes down from the umbilicus to around heng gu point, private parts painful"); "chong mai ye, dong, ku shao fu tong, shang qiang xin, you jia shan, jue yun, yi shi niao …". ("chong mai, moving, lesser abdomen painful, attacks the heart, has a jia (blockage) hernia, dead baby, and cannot control the urine …"). Xu Ling tai said, "Fan zi fu ren, xian ming chong, ren zhi mai" ("If treat women's illness, first treat chong and ren channels", then he also said, "chong ren mai jie qi bao zhong, shang xun bei li, wei jing luo zhi hai. Ci jie xue zhi suo chong sheng, tai zhi suo you ji, ming yu chong ren zhi gu, ze ben yuan tong xu, er hou suo sheng zhi bing, qian tian wan xu, ke yi zhi qi suo cong qi" ("chong ren channels all start from the bao, go around to the back, is the sea of the jing luo. Blood comes these jing luo, the baby is connected by these jing luo. If know what is chong ren, then you know the illness source and then all the illnesses whether there are many you still know where they come from") (*Yi luo liu shu*). Lu Zong hou said, "dai xia yi dai wei bing er de ming" ("leuccohrragia, it is named from the illness of the dai") etc. From the women's disease including the body passing the baby, period, and dai, the mechanism of illness emphases the importance of the connection of the chong-ren-dai channels, and the classification of all the illnesses which come from the illnesses caused by the chong-ren-dai channels' unable to adjust very well. These illnesses, in the mechanism of illnesses, has a good connection with the liver-spleen-heart-kidney and bao gong etc. each zang fu and each jing mai. All these are controlled by and lead by the chong-ren-dai in the qi jing, so the ren-chong-dai illness characteristics include together illness change of the zang fu and the jing mai. At the same time, this also gets a clearer system of women's illness which includes zang fu, jing mai and their mechanisms of illness. It has an important meaning for the differential treatment of illness.

(ii) Practical use meaning of the qi jing theories in the medicine treatment area

How to give medicine to treat qi jing illnesses? It mainly uses some medicines with the same approximate actions as the jing mai. Like tonify if weak in the case of the ren-du two mai as in the use of *gui lu er xian jiao (lu jiao, gui ban, ren shen, gou qi, ao cheng jiao,* then take with jiu (wine). *Lu* has the strongest yang qi, suitable for making the du mai unblock, *gui* totally gets the most yin qi, good at making the ren mai unblocked. *Ren shen* tonifies the qi, increases the yang, *gou qi* supports the yin and helps the jing, so it is suitable to tonify the ren-du mai). From the range major treatment analysis, if after an illness and weak, urinary dripping, lou xia, impotency, seminal emission, premature ejaculation, leuccorrhagia, lou tai etc. illness in the internal medicine. From the zang fu differential analysis, it mainly belongs to liver and kidney weak yin deficiency, spleen and kidney yang deficiency, and spleen and lungs both deficiency. And from the medicine classification, *lu jiao* goes to kidney and liver, *gui ban* into the spleen and liver, *ren shen* into the spleen and lung, and *gou qi* into the spleen and liver. It presents good connection between the ren-du two mai and with the liver-spleen and kidney-lung.

We also can see that medicines have related special characteristics in the treatment of qi jing illness. Many doctors in olden days summarized their experience in this area, like in the *De pai ben cao* which records the medicines which go into the qi jing: *ba ji* goes to the chong mai, *bie jia* goes on the chong mai, *gui ban* unblocks the ren mai, *chuan duan, long gu* treats the dai mai becomes ill, *bai guo* unblocks the du mai, *hu gu* enters the yin yang two qiao, *gui zhi* travels the yang wei etc. etc. Zhu Xiao nan did a summary of dai medicines from his practical experience: raises the dai mai: *sheng ma, wu wei zi*, fixing and supporting the dai mai: *long gu, mu li, wu zei gu, chun bai pi*. Stops the dai mai pain: *bai shao, gan cao*. Warms the dai mai's cold: *ai ye, gan jiang*. Cleans out the dai mai's damp-heat: *huang qin, huang bai, bai zhi tan, che qian zi*. Tonifies the dai mai's yin: *dang gui, shou di*. Zhu also summarized the medicines and prescriptions of the wei mai like eg. the major medicines of the yang wei are *huang qi, bai shao, gui zhi*; combined with *dang gui, chuan chiong* which governs the yin wei etc. etc. (see Shang hai zhong yi xue yuan pian *Ke lian lun wen hui pian* 1963 (6).

Zhu also summarized the gui jing medicines re chong, ren. In the book *Chong ren tou tao (Zhong yi za zhi* 1962 August p. 1):

1. Into chong mai medicines:
    (1) Tonifies the chong mai's qi: wu zhu you (*Ben cao gang mu* Yin Wang ancient discussion); ba ji tian (*Ben cao gang mu*); gou qi zi, gan cao, lu xian (*De pei ben cao*); lu rong (*Nu ke yao zhi*); zi he che, cong rong, zi shi ying, du zhong (*Lin zhen zhi nan*).
    (2) Tonifies the chong mai's blood: dang gui, bie jia, dan shen & chuan chiong (*De pei ben cao*).
    (3) Lowers the chong mai's adversity: mu xiang, bing lang (*De pei ben cao*).
    (4) Consolidates the chong mai: shan yao, lian zi (*Fu qing zhu nu ke*).

2. Into ren mai medicines:
    (1) Tonifies the ren mai's qi: lu rong (*Nu ke yao zhi*); fu pen zi (*Lin zhen zhi nan*); zi he che (*Xing xuan yi an ji lu*).
    (2) Tonifies the ren mai's blood: gui ban, dan shen (*De pei ben cao*).
    (3) Consolidates the ren mai: bai guo (*Fu qing zhu nu ke*).

Zhu and other research doctors did a lot of research in practice and experiments with animals, they indicate their obviously tonifying effects on the chong ren. They will recover and increase gonad hormones, so they can adjust the period, help the bao gong raise up, and recover normal sexual activity. This also confirms that the chong-ren controls the blood and that the bao tai qi jing theories are correct. The research re the qi jing medicines is valuable in the practical treatment of illness. It not only makes the qi jing theories more perfect, it adds more content to the jing luo theory and also confirms the practical treatment indicated meaning of the qi jing theories in the medicine treatment area. Qi jing theories have a widely-researched future in the use of medicine and direct practical treatment. It makes, when treating illness, use different ways and adopt different roles in the range of treatment with medicine. Also, this continuously adds and extends further investigation into qi jing theories and allows us to do deep research into chinese medicine. In turn, this gives very big benefit to medicine theories in general.

(iii) The practical treatment meaning of qi jing theory in acupuncture treatment method.

Direct theories, doctrinal reasons, and differential methods of acupuncture are the same with chinese medicine treatment methods. However, in individual practice, methods of treatment also have differences. The basis of acupuncture is the points, ie. whether it is suitable or not to give acupuncture on certain points has a relationship with a particular conclusion and with particular related results. In the qi jing ba mai, the distribution of the ren, du two mai have their own points, but the ren, du two mai have major treatment ranges. These treatment ranges together include matching illnesses which are controlled by the jing luo of the ren, du two mai, thereby extending the use range of the points. Example, ya men pt. (GV.15) has an action on treating dumbness, but in the olden days literature there was no record that dumb illness belonged to the du mai illnesses. In an example of the illness, the yang wei has "bu neng yan" ("cannot speak") illness and ya men is the meeting point of the yang wei and the du mai. This indicates that qi jing theories is one of direct theories of acupuncture treatment and follows the rule of selecting points according to suitability in practical use. Re practical methods for deciding which points to use, olden days doctors also give examples based on qi jing theories like the "ba mai jiao hui xue" ("the eight channel meeting points") ie. the illness of the chong mai use gong sun (SP4), the illness of the yin wei use nei guan (P6), the illness of the du mai use hou xi (SI3), the illness of the yang qiao use shen mai (UB62), the illness of the dai mai use zu lin qi (GB41), the illness of the yang wei use wai guan TH5), the illness of the ren mai use lie que (Lu 7), and the illness of the yin qiao use zhao hai (K6). These ba mai meeting points are examples of using shu points of the twelve jing mai to treat qi jing illnesses, they also indicate the important meaning in the acupuncture practical usage of the meeting points of the jing mai. Based on this, combine the olden theories and philosophy and get "ling gui ba fa" and "fei teng ba fa". "Ling gui ba fa" and "fei teng ba fa", these two methods are based on the 8 channels 8 points, using decided-upon points for opening the points on time. These two types of measures to decide and use points have been confirmed by long time treatment experience. The indicating meaning of the qi jing theories in the acupuncture practical use is confirmed.

CHAPTER 3

··

Jing bie, luo mai, jing jin, pi bu

1. The twelve jing bie

(1) The characteristics of the jing bie

The "jing bie" is the twelve mai which is separate from the circle line of the whole body. It goes into the body, ie. is another branch. However, it has differences with the normal jing mai, so it is called the "bie xing zhi zheng jing", simply called the "jing bie". Its major characteristics are:

1. Get off and combine, goes out and comes in (li he chu ru): the jing bie of the yang jing, after starting from the ben jing bie, goes ahead into the chest abdomen internal viscera. Most of them go out from the neck, and combine with the yang jing of the twelve jing, they are the starting-off points. The jing bie of the yin jing after starting from ben jing mai, go and circle at the body internal viscera, and meet or is parallel with the jing bie of the yang jing. They present the surface and the internal, and don't come back to the ben jing. However, they combine with the yang jing which is presented as surface and internal within it. This type of yin jing jing bie, which starts from the ben jing mai bie, is called "li". The phenomena of yin jing into the yang jing is called "he". The phenomena of the yang jing grasping and entering the yang jing is called "chu". While, after the yang jing jing bie circulates in the body, then it is called "ru".

2. "liu he":

(1) The jing bie of the foot tai yang and the foot shao yin:

a. The jing bie of the foot tai yang: after coming out of the hollow of the knee parts of the foot tai yang jing mai, it goes out. Its one branch extends and distributes to the buttocks and di (sacrum) 5 cun under and goes to the anus. Belonging to the urinary bladder, and spreading its luo on the kidney, it then goes along the back bone to the place of the heart and

102

spreads out. Another line directly goes from the back bone to the neck, and it still belongs to the foot tai yang jing jing mai.

b. The jing bie of the foot shao yin: after starting from the hollow of the knee of the foot shao yin jing mai, then goes and meets the foot tai yang jing bie. Then goes up to the kidney organ, and from the fourteenth vertebrae goes out and belongs to the du mai. Also, the jing bie which goes directly up and connects with the tongue root, then goes out on the neck, and belongs to the foot tai yang jing jing mai.

(2) The jing bie of the foot yang ming and the foot tai yin:

a. The jing bie of the foot foot yang ming: after starting from the thigh part of the foot yang ming jing mai, into the abdomen, belongs to the stomach, spreads its luo on the spleen, goes up passed the heart, and then goes up along the oesophagus (shi guan) out to the mouth. Extended to the nose bone and the eye socket (yan kuang), it also has a connection with the eye system, and belongs to the foot yang ming jing mai.

b. The jing bie of the foot tai yin: from the thigh part of the foot tai yin jing mai, then meets the yang ming jing bie, goes up to connect with the throat parts, and to the tongue.

(3) The jing bie of the foot shao yang and the foot jue yin:

a. The jing bie of the foot shao yang: after starting from the thigh bone of the foot shao yang jing mai, around the thigh joint into the edge of the hair of the private parts (yin bu mao ji), meets the foot jue yin jing bie. From here gets another branch and goes between the ribs, into the chest and abdomen, belongs to the gall bladder and spreads its luo onto the liver. It then goes towards the heart, and goes up along the oesophagus and out the lower jaw, by the mouth, spreads on the face, and connects with the eye system. In the external corner of the place of the eye, belongs to the foot shao yang jing jing mai.

b. The jing bie of the foot jue yin: from the foot fu of the foot jue yin jing mai, starts to go up and reaches the edge of the hair of the private parts. It meets the jing bie of the foot shao yang and goes together.

(4) The jing bie of the hand tai yang and the hand shao yin:

a. The jing bie of the hand tai yang: after starting from the shoulder joint part of the hand tai yang jing mai, it goes into the armpit, goes toward the heart, and then goes down to connect with the small intestine.

b. The jing bie of the hand shao yin: after starting from the 2 tendons of the armpit (ye wo) of the hand shao yin jing mai, goes into the chest, belongs to the heart, then goes up towards the throat. It goes out but shallowly at the face, and meets the hand tai yang jing jing mai at the internal corner of the eye.

(5) The jing bie of the hand yang ming and the hand tai yin:

a. The jing bie of the hand yang ming: after starting from the hand of the hand yang ming jing mai, it goes along the arm and the elbow ru parts, and distributes on the chest and the breast etc. parts. Another branch goes from the shoulder ru parts, starting by going into the back neck bone, going down towards the large intestines, and going up belonging to the lung. And then going along the throat, goes out at the clavicular fossa (que pen), and belonging to the hand yang ming jing mai.

b. The jing bie of the hand tai yin: after starting from the armpit parts of the hand tai yin jing mai, it goes behind the shao yin, into the chest, goes to the lung organ, and distributes at the large intestine. It then goes up and out at the clavicular fossa, along the throat, and belongs to the hand yang ming jing jing mai.

(6) The jing bie of the hand shao yang and the hand jue yin:

a. The jing bie of the hand shao yang: after starting from the top of the head parts of the hand shao yang jing mai, it goes into the clavicular fossa, goes down to reach triple heater and then distributes in the chest.

b. The jing bie of the hand jue yin: after starting from the armpit lower 3 cun parts of the hand jue yin jing mai, it goes into the chest, and belongs to the triple heater. It then goes along the throat, and goes out but shallowly on the back of the ear. In the gastric bone parts, it belongs to the hand shao yang jing jing mai.

In the twelve jing bie, whether there is yin jing jing bie or yang jing jing bie, in the beginning each starts from the ben jing jing mai. And at last combines on the 6 lines yang jing; it also mixes with the yang jing jing mai. All this contributes to the 6 he connection of the jing bie.

"Liu he" can be simply summarized as follows:

(1) The foot tai yang and foot shao yin meet, in the lower part, on the back of the knee. In the upper parts, they meet on the neck.
(2) The foot shao yang and foot jue yin meet at the edge of the pubic hair.
(3) The foot yang ming and the foot tai yin meet at the thigh bone together.
(4) The hand tai yang and the hand shao yin meet together at the eye internal corner.
(5) The hand shao yang and the hand jue yin meet together at the gastric (wan) bone.
(6) The hand yang ming and the hand tai yin meet together at the throat.

The road of the jing bie circulation, on the elbow and knee upper parts, zang fu, and body, even neck, obviously present surface and internal connection of yin yang both jing with each other. This indicates yin yang surface and internal both jing, not only start from major jing mai, and connect in the zang fu and at the end of the four limbs but also in the body have a go-out and go-into, separate and combining of jing bie (this makes up the "6 he" connection). Its distribution and connection, is more complex than the four limbs, so it emphasizes the connection between the surface and internal jing, and the zang fu.

3. There are no illness symptoms recorded for jing bie, because the jing bie come from original jing mai, most of the symptoms are included in the jing mai symptoms.

4. The circulation parts of the jing bie have some places where the jing mai circulation does not go. In the 6 yin jing mai, apart from the foot jue yin jing mai which can go up to reach the top of the head, the hand shao yin jing mai goes up and connects with eye system. The other four yin jing mai only reach the throat. However, the 6 yin jing bie, after reaching the head, face, neck, and throat, all meet together with the 6 yang jing bie and go into the 6 yang jing mai. So, the 6 yang jing mai in the head and face, already received the 6 yin jing bie qi and blood; this is the reason why the 6 yin jing also have an action on the head and face. Therefore, if the yang jing have an illness, you can treat the yin jing related to the yang jing like surface and internal. This confirms the connection of yin and yang, and surface and internal.

(2)   The function and practical meaning of the twelve jing bie.

The twelve jing bie are in fact, branches of the twelve jing mai, but this branch mai distribution has some special characteristics. And, in addition, its mai qi distribution range is wide, as it constructs another composition of the jing luo system. Analysis of its function and practical use value from the detailed distribution of the jing bie, are major paths as follows:

1.   increase the surface and internal belonging-to luo connection of the twelve jing mai: the distribution and circulation of the twelve jing mai has surface jing and internal jing - they help each other. The yang jing control the surface, belongs to the bowels luo (connecting to) the organs. The yin jing control the internal, belongs to the organs luo (connecting to) the bowels. The twelve jing bie increase these connections. The "6 he" connection makes the connection of surface and internal, which is the twelve jing jing mai distribution in the yin jing and the yang jing of the legs, get another important connection. After the jing bie goes into the chest and abdomen internal organs, most of the jing bie circulate in the zang-fu which its jing mai belong to. Especially, the yang jing jing bie all connect with the organs and bowels which have a connection with it; this makes the connection of surface and internal, ie. both jing, in the internal parts are very good. It also makes the organs and bowels in the internal body help each other very well. However, this surface and internal mixing together connection, is the cross connection of the twelve jing mai itself. The zang fu belong to the luo, and along with the distribution of the luo mai etc. factors, there are a lot of other factors, but the twelve jing bie increase this connection. This has an important meaning in the theory and practical use. In the acupuncture practical use, its important to direct the theory regarding how to get the point (how to decide which point to use). For instance, "tou xiang xun lie que" of the four total points ("head, neck look for lie que (Lu7)"). Another instance, the lung has a fever with recurring evil, then use he gu (LI4), and qu chi (LI11). A further instance, spleen deficiency makes the transport and digestion abnormal and then presents with abdominal distended, and diarrhoea etc. symptoms, use zu san li (St36). Stomach qi develops gas pain, use gong sun (SP4) etc. All these are based on the theory of surface and internal xu luo (belonging to luo). It also provides theories for the zang xiang xue shou (zang xiang system), and the zang fu differentiation. Additionally, it gives the theory to the connection and the change between zang fu change and regards illness mechanisms.

2. It emphasizes the importance of jing mai in the head and face parts: of the twelve jing mai circling on the head and face, are mainly yang jing. By way of their connection with the circle distribution and the "liu he" connection, the yin jing qi and blood also goes up to the head. In this way, and in addition to a variety of jing mai connections in the qi jing area, it makes the jing qi of the human body connect with the head, brain and face, and wu guan (5 sense organs) parts. So, the *Ling shu-xie qi zang fu bing xin* said: "shi er jing mai, san bai liu shi wu luo, qi xue qi jie shang yu mian er zou kong qiao" ("the twelve jing mai and the three hundred and sixty five luo qi and blood all go up to the face and go from the face and go to the empty qiao (openings)"). This indicates that the head, face, and empty openings are important parts of the jing qi and meet together. There are many new developments in acupuncture methods in recent times. For example, ear acupuncture used for treating all body, four limbs and internal organ illnesses; as well as acupuncture anaesthesia. Another example, is face acupuncture and nose acupuncture, also used for anaesthesia. All these indicate the importance of face parts jing mai and their shu points, they can treat a wide range of illnesses. Its theory's basis is that there is a connection in each part of the head via the jing luo system, and the jing bie which circle it and meet together. It is the factor which makes the jing qi come together on the head and face parts. It has a practical meaning in chinese medicine ie. each branch explains zang xiang (the condition of the organs shows externally ultimately) theory. For example, "xin kai qiao yu shi" ("the heart has its opening on the tongue"), "shen kai qiao yu er" ("the kidney has its opening in the ear"), "gan kai qiao yu mu" ("the liver has its opening in lungs have their opening on the nose"), "pi kai qiao yu kou" ("the spleen has its opening onto the mouth"), and "qi hua zai chen" ("all present on the lips"). It also explains the internal connection between the head and face illnesses and zang fu jing mai.

3. Making the distribution and connection of the twelve jing mai more precise: by way of the circling and distribution of the twelve jing bie and the jing mai of the legs and the internal organs each part have more connection. Some parts and organs in which the twelve jing mai mai qi do not distribute, the jing bie causes them to get a connection. In this way, it increases the connective roads, making each part of the human body have a good connection. For example, in practical use, chinese medicine, whether internal medicine or other medicines, re some diagnoses and treatment processes, are all important especially between the heart and kidney 2 jing. In the

twelve jing mai, although we have an explanation about the circulation of the foot shao yin kidney jing, its jing mai is "luo yu xin" ("luo at the heart"), but the hand shao yin jing jing mai doesn't distribute to the kidney. In the foot tai yang jing bie, its circulation not only is on the urinary bladder but also spreads and luo ("san luo") on the kidney, then spreads on the heart. This has more of a connection between the heart and the kidney. Another example, in chinese medicine people always think that the stomach has quite a big effect on the heart, like "wei bu he ze wo bu an" ("if the stomach is not good, then you cannot sleep very well") (*Su wen-ni tiao lun*). So, in the internal medicine practice, it always uses medicine that harmonizes the stomach to fix the heart. This is the normal use and treatment process in chinese medicine. But in the twelve jing mai, the foot yang ming stomach jing doesn't distribute to the heart, and the hand shao yin heart jing also doesn't circulate on the stomach bowel. However, the distribution and circulation of the foot yang ming jing bie, belonging to the stomach, spreads on the spleen and then connects with the heart. They make the connection between the heart and the stomach, in this way, as a serious basis for chinese medicine when it comes to harmonizing the stomach and calming the heart spirit. A further example presents itself, when treating leucorrhagia illness in women's medicine, chinese medicine concentrates on adjusting the deficiency and excess of the kidney qi, but in the twelve jing mai circulation of the foot shao yin kidney jing, it doesn't have a direct connection to the dai mai. However, the distribution of the foot shao yin jing bie indicates that it comes from the du mai, so makes for connection between the kidney and the dai mai. In addition, the circulation of the jing bie in the surface of the body, increases the connection of some parts, like the foot tai yang jing bie circulates on the anus, and therefore it increases the connection of the foot tai yang jing mai and this part. In the foot tai yang urinary bladder jing points like cheng shan point (UB57) etc. has the function to treat haemorrhoids. This has a connection with the distribution road of the jing bie.

Summarizing the above, although the jing luo theories' main body is the twelve jing mai, it still relies on the twelve jing bie and other parts and has a very complex connection. In this way, it can have an action re the jing luo system of the human body. This also emphasizes that jing luo theories must combine with zang xiang theories, heping each other. By doing this, chinese medicine has a near-perfect meaning.

2. The luo mai.

(i) The distribution and function of the luo mai

The luo mai are the branch mai which go slant-wise (xie xing) from the jing mai. Most of them distribute on the surface of the body. There are fifteen lines, and there is one line in each of the twelve jing mai. Add the ren mai, and du mai luo, and the da luo (big luo) of the spleen, they are normally altogether called the "fifteen bie luo", simply the "fifteen luo". They are a major body in all the luo mai: while there are branches from the quite big luo mai, normally called the luo mai, there are smaller branches called the "sun luo". The luo floating on the skin, that can be seen with the eyes, are called the "fou (floating) luo". They also can be called the "xue luo". Regarding the fou (floating luo) which are equivalent to small blood tubes, therefore they are the "xi xiao xue guan". The branches of the luo mai which start the quite big luo mai, their mai qi slowly becomes small ie. from the line state extending and spreading to the area state. In this way, they have a perfect connection with every part of the body. The detailed distribution and function of the luo mai are as follows:

1. The distribution of the fifteen luo mai:

(1) The hand tai yin luo mai: its starting point is lie que (Lu 7) point. From the jian bei of the wrist, goes on the hand yang ming. Then goes parallel with the hand tai yin jing mai, directly into the middle of the hand, then distributes on yu ji (Lu10) point.

(2) The hand shao yin luo mai: its starting point is tong li (H5) point. From the back of the hand 1 cun, part goes to the hand tai yang jing. Also, goes up from the wrist 1 cun, along the jing mai going into the heart, connects with the tongue origin part (ben bu), and goes up to belong to the eye system.

(3) The hand jue yin (heart governor) luo mai: its starting point is nei guan (P6) point, 2 cun from the wrist. Distributes between the 2 tendons, along the jing mai and then goes up, connects with the pericardium, luo on the heart system.

(4) The hand yang ming luo mai: its starting point is pian li (LI6) point, 3 cun from the wrist. It goes with the hand tai yin jing, while another branch goes up to jian yu (LI15), goes up passed the qu chi, pian luo on the teeth parts. There is also a branch into the ear parts, meets with the zong mai parts.

(5) The hand tai yang luo mai: its starting point is zhi zheng (SI7)point, from the wrist 5 cun. It goes internally on the hand shao yin jing: a bie zhi (a branch channel) goes up passed the elbow parts, luo on the jian yu parts.

(6)   The hand shao yang luo mai: its starting point is wai guan (TH5) point 2 cun from the wrist, goes up from the external arm into the chest, meets with the hand jue yin jing.

(7)   The foot yang ming luo mai: its starting point is feng long (ST40) point, 8 cun from the external ankle, goes to the foot tai yin jing. There is a branch along the external jing bone which goes up, luo's (connects) on the head and neck parts and meets with the yang jing zhi qi (ie. qi of the yang jing), and then goes down and luo's on the throat part.

(8)   The foot tai yang luo mai: its starting point is fei yang (UB58) point, 7 cun from the external ankle, which goes on the foot shao yin.

(9)   The foot shao yang luo mai: its starting point is guang ming (GB37) point, 5 cun from the external ankle. It goes on the foot jue yin jing, and goes down to spread on the top of the foot (zu fu).

(10)   The foot tai yin luo mai: its starting point is gong sun (SP4) point, in the big toe original joint back 1 cun. Partly, it goes on the foot yang ming jing, while another branch goes into the abdomen and connects with the intestines and stomach.

(11)   The foot shao yin luo mai: its starting point is da zhong (K4) point, in the internal ankle, back around the foot heel. It goes on the foot tai yang jing, while another branch goes up with the jing mai under the pericardium (xin bao), and goes through on the back bone parts.

(12)   The foot jue yin luo mai: its starting point is li gou (Liv.5) point, 5 cun from the internal ankle. It goes on the foot shao yang jing, its branch goes passed the jing bone, to go out to the testes part and the reproductive organs (shen zhi.qi).

(13)   The ren luo mai: its starting part is jian tu (ie. wei yi) part, then goes down to jiu wei (CV15) point, and spreads on the whole abdomen.

(14)   The du luo mai: its starting point is chang qiang (GV1). From there, it goes along the back bone two sides on to the neck, spreads on top of the head; spreads and extends to around the shoulder (jian jia) part, and goes from right and left on the foot tai yang jing, into all the back bone.

(15)   The big luo of the spleen: its starting point is da bao (SP21) point. From yan ye lower 3 cun part, spreads on the chest and ribs parts, includes all the blood in the body.

As mentioned above, each bie luo starting part has a point. The fifteen luo mai normally use this point as a presentation. These points are called "luo points". Luo points have the function to treat each respective line illness. Now to summarize, the fifteen luo points are listed in table 7:

Table 7

Hand 3 Yin	Hand Tai Yin's Bie	—	Lie Que	(LU7)
	Hand Shao Yin's Bie	—	Tong Li	(H5)
	Hand Jue Yin's Bie	—	Nei Guan	(P6)
Hand 3 Yang	Hand Yang Ming's Bie	—	Pian Li	(LI5)
	Hand Shao Yang's Bie	—	Wai Guan	(TH5)
	Hand Tai Yang's Bie	—	Zhi Zheng	(SI7)
Foot 3 Yang	Foot Yang Ming's Bie	—	Feng Long	(ST40)
	Foot Tai Yang's Bie	—	Fei Yang	(UB58)
	Foot Shao Yang's Bie	—	Guang Ming	(GB37)
Foot 3 Yin	Foot Tai Yin's Bie	—	Gong Sun	(SP4)
	Foot Shao Yin's Bie	—	Da Zhong	(K4)
	Foot Jue Yin's Bie	—	Li Gou	(LIV5)
Front & Back Chest & Ribs	Ren Channel's Bie	—	Wei Yi	(CV15)
	Du Channel's Bie	—	Chang Qiang	(DU1)
	Spleen's Big Luo	—	Da Bao	(SP21)

Explanation: in the twelve jing, the foot tai yin spleen jing has one branch luo mai. Why is there another big luo of the spleen? This is because the stomach is the origin basis of qi and blood. The spleen is only a single organ, which mainly treats the middle jiao (heater), and cannot treat another organ. It also transports jing ye (saliva and fluids) for the stomach, so it has 2 luo mai.

Some books classify the big luo of the stomach as the main luo, and call it the "16 luo". Which is correct? This is a good question. The "big luo of the stomach" is presented in the book *Su wen-ping ren qi xiang lun*: "wei zhi da luo ming yue xu li, quan ge luo fei, qu yu zuo ru xia, qi dong ying biao, mai zong qi ye" ("the big luo of the stomach is called xu li, spreads on the lung, goes out under the left breast, its movement is suitable to wear clothing, the mai relates to the zong qi". The *Su wen-ping ren xiang lun* chapter mainly describes the mai qi and indicates that the breathing has a connective change with the four seasons. As well as emphasizing the "wei qi wei ben" ("the stomach qi belongs to the source") theories and the idea of "wei zhi da luo" ("the stomach belongs to the big luo") sentence explanation, these mainly indicate that the stomach qi is the zong qi of the mai. The meaning of "da luo" here perhaps means the stomach qi goes up the line. Compared to the *Ling shu-jing mai* pian description of the fifteen luo mai. It explains in its luo mai description and symptoms, whether consistently or mainly, there are differences so here we don't clarify whether "wei zhi da luo".

2. The function of the fifteen luo mai

One of the functions of the fifteen luo mai is the relationship between the surface and the internal jing in the twelve jing. Its connective methods are not the same as the "6 he" of the jing bie - it emphasizes the body function of the yang jing, and also emphasizes the connection of internal parts. The luo mai are the yin jing luo mai and they go to the yang jing, the yang jing luo mai also goes to the yin jing, therefore the luo mai of the yin and yang jing connect with each other, although the luo mai go into the chest and connect with the internal organs. It doesn't have a fixing connection with the su luo, but it mainly connects and distributes on the surface and internal jing in the limbs.

The second function of the fifteen luo mai is that the fifteen luo mai have the function of controlling all the body's luo mai. The fifteen bie luo are the main part of the luo mai. They control the normal luo mai, the sun luo, the fou mai, and the blood luo (xue luo) etc.

Another function of the luo mai is that they have the function to transform and protect the qi and blood, so that they give benefit to the whole body's organs. Because of the luo mai distribution, ie. "zhi er heng zhe" ("a lot of branches cross"), a lot of small distributions and the network of the whole body, then have a wide connection with all the body's organs. So the yin wei, and the qi and blood which circulate in the jing mai, can distribute to the whole body by way of the sun luo and give nutrition to all the organs/tissues, and then maintain the normal activities of the body. Therefore, the luo mai are an important connection road to make the jing mai enable diffusion and spread on all the body's organs/tissues. The luo mai and the jing mai are connected with each other, ie. the jing mai shows the "line" distribution while the luo mai shows the network type "area" spread distribution. In this way, it not only makes the human body become an each-organ-connecting-with-each-other body, but also makes all the body connect and help each other.

(ii). Practical meaning and symptoms of the luo mai

The symptoms of the luo mai are quite simple in olden times records. From these symptoms, it gives us some idea about the function of the luo mai and then allows us to understand their related illnesses. Now, we will describe the following from the *Ling shu-jing mai* chapter:

1. The bing hou (symptoms) of the hand tai yin luo mai:
    excess condition: hand and wrist parts hot,
    deficiency condition: breath short, bedwetting, frequent urination.
2. The bing hou of the hand shao yin luo mai:
    excess condition: the chest feels full and distended,
    deficiency condition: cannot speak.
3. The bing hou of the hand jue yin luo mai:
    excess condition: heart pain,
    deficiency condition: upset (fan xin).
4. The bing hou of the hand yang ming luo mai:
    excess condition: tooth pain, deafness,
    deficiency condition: feels cold in the teeth, chest feels blocked inside,
5. The bing hou of the hand tai yang luo mai:
    excess condition: bone joints loose, elbow and arm cannot use (loss of function),
    deficiency condition: wart on the skin which looks a small spot on the skin which afterwards itches.
6. The bing hou of the hand shao yang luo mai:
    excess condition: elbow parts spasm (contraction),
    deficiency condition: elbow and arm loose and cannot bend.
7. The bing hou of the foot yang ming luo mai:
    excess condition: dian illness, kuang illness (madness),
    deficiency condition: legs and feet wasting and thin and not strong, cannot bend, when the luo qi goes jue ni (the wrong way) then hou bi (throat blocked) will happen, suddenly loss of voice.
8. The bing hou of the foot tai yang luo mai:
    excess condition: blocked nose, headache, back pain,
    deficiency condition: clear watery runny nose, blood from nose.
9. The bing hou of the foot shao yang luo mai:
    excess condition: qi goes the wrong way (ni) then loss of consciousness (ie. faints),
    deficiency condition: foot muscle wasting and not strong, cannot stand up after sitting.
10. The bing hou of the foot tai yin luo mai:
    jue qi goes up and then will have cholera (huo luan) and then vomiting.
    excess condition: very painful in intestines,

deficiency condition: distention of the abdomen caused by the accumulation of gas and fluid due to the dysfunction of the liver and spleen (tympanitis).

11. The bing hou of the foot shao yin luo mai:
    excess condition: urine long bi,
    deficiency condition: waist pain.

12. The bing hou of the foot jue yin luo mai
    if illness qi goes up then testes swelling, suddenly gets a hernia.
    excess condition: strong (qiang) yin (very rigid penis erection),
    deficiency condition: private parts very itchy.

13. The bing hou of the ren luo mai:
    excess condition: skin on the abdomen painful,
    deficiency condition: skin on the abdomen itchy.

14. The bing hou of the du luo mai:
    excess condition: back straight and not flexible,
    deficiency condition: head heavy and dizziness.

15. The bing hou of the spleen big luo:
    excess condition: painful in the whole body,
    deficiency condition: the joints in all four limbs not strong (no force).

The luo mai symptoms shown in the *Nei jing* are not many, but they give people some good ideas. One of which, is that each luo mai described different symptoms about excess conditions and deficiency conditions, and explained the importance of excess conditions and deficiency conditions in different treatment. Another one is that it lists the symptoms of luo mai "qi ni" ("qi adverse") about the foot yang ming, the foot tai yin, the foot shao yin, and the foot jue yin etc. It also emphasizes the importance about jing luo "qi xue tiao he" ("qi and blood help balance each other") in the physiological and illness mechanism. Both of them have great importance re practical use and theories.

From the analysis from the luo mai surface and the internal jing connection, the luo mai symptoms should include surface and internal 2 jing symptoms. But, there are many symptoms which have been discussed in the twelve jing symptoms, so the previous luo mai symptoms just provide some examples. In practice, one should concentrate on using theories, and not become limited by the symptoms mentioned above. Example, the foot yang ming luo point feng long (ST40), can treat throat bi, craziness (dian kuang), going up to high places and singing a song (ben gao er ge), take off all the clothing and run around, abdomen painful etc. foot yang ming symptoms. It can also treat face swelling, four limbs swelling (shui bi), upset, heart painful, chest painful like someone beating you, body heavy, vomiting etc. foot tai yin symptoms. It can furthermore treat beng lou (metrorrhagia and menorrhagia), irregular periods, all caused by the "pi neng tong xue" ("spleen unable to control the blood") etc. illness. Because "zi wei du chu yang ming" ("if want to treat the wasting illness just take the yang ming"); also, suitable for limbs and feet not strong (or weak), and skin parts muscle wasting etc. illness. Because the lung and stomach mai qi connect with each other, it also treats cough illness. All of this can be proven in practice. This indicates that the luo mai theories have an indicated meaning and practical use value in acupuncture practice.

Re the luo mai theories and in the name of practical use, there are still the "acupuncture floating luo" ("zhen ci fou luo"), the "xue luo" ("blood luo"), and the "sun luo". All these methods treat illness. Example, the book *Ling shu-za bing* chapter: " ....yao ji qiang, qu zu tai yang guo zhong xue luo" (" ....if the waist and spine are straight and hard, then take the foot tai yang hollow of the knee xue luo"). The *Ling shu-jing mai* chapter, " ....ci luo mai zhe, bi zhen qi jie shang shen xue zhe" ("if want to use acupuncture on the luo mai, must insert in the joints by way of the blood"). Re water distended illness (shui zhang yi), "xian xie qi zhang zhi xue luo, hou tiao qi jing" ("first discharge its distention, via the xue luo, and then adjust its jing"), Following the *Ling shu-shui zhang,* it is found that this insertion-of-the-luo method has some new developments particularly in recent years. For example, after inserting at the luo, use huo guan (glass cupping), so that removal of the blockages at the luo mai can be undertaken to allow qi and blood can go through and get a good result with this illness.

In addition, by observing the colour change on the surface luo mai, and judging which illness is at fault, this is the area to decidedly use luo mai theories. Like, the *Ling shu-jing mai* chapter: "fan zhen luo mai, mai se qing, ze han, qie tong; chi zhe you re" ("when diagnose luo mai, if the mai colour is blue/green (qing), then there will be cold, and moreover pain; if the colour is red there will be heat"). And, "han duo ze ning qi, ning qi ze qing hei; re duo ze niao ze ze huang chi" ("more cold then stagnancy, stagnancy there will be blue/green and black; if more hot then will be shiny (glossy), if more niao ze (?) then there will be yellow and red") (*Su wen-jing luo lun*). This is the practical use for luo diagnosis then. About the theories surrounding luo diagnoses, the *jing mai* chapter also indicates: "fan ci shi wu luo zhe, shi ze bi jian, xu ze bi xia" ("if belong to the fifteen luo, then excess will present outside, if deficiency then will be lower down"). In the excess illness of the luo mai, blood congestion and qi blockage of the luo mai on the surface of the body, will present as luo mai blocked blood. Otherwise, when the qi and blood are not enough, because the luo mai are deficient, it is not easy to see the luo mai. From the above mentioned, the luo mai diagnosis theories and practical experience can be seen as a reference for the clinical use.

In summary of the above, the luo mai theories and symptoms have some direct meaning for chinese medicine on every subject. They are one of the compositions which make up many areas in jing luo science. It is worthy of further study.

3.   The jing jin

(i)   The characteristics, distribution and function of the twelve jing jin

The twelve jing jin are the jing luo system's adjusting parts of the body's external. Because their circulation -distribution symptoms and function etc. concentrate on the jing rou (tendons and muscles), so they are called the "jing jin".

The circulation characteristics of the jing jin are just on the four limbs and the body, including the chest and abdomen. They don't go into the internal organs. They emphasize the jing luo system's control function of the surface of the body. They also, along with the twelve jing mai, present internal and external; the twelve jing bie emphasize the internal organ circulation methods, they are all different.

The jing jin distribution characteristics can be summarized as "jie ju san luo". "Jie" means a combination of the words "jing jin", they are mainly on joint and muscle parts. "Ju" also means a combination of the word "jing jin", they are mainly on the ji jian (muscle) parts. "San" means the spread of jing jin, they are on the muscle wu li parts. "Luo" is the connection function of jing jin, it limits/controls the four limbs and one hundred bones, is beneficial to the joints.

The circle and distribution rule of the jing jin are: all start from the ends of the four limbs, and circle and meet on the wrists, elbows, armpits, shoulders, ankle bones, knees, and condyles etc. joints and then distribute on the chest and back. Finally, on the head and body.

Now, we will explain each jing jin's detailed distribution as follows:

1.   The foot tai yang jing jin: starts from the small toe, goes up, stored on the external ankle, slanting up, stored on the knee; it goes down externally to the ankle and stores on the heel, goes up and stores on the back of the knee; its branch on the outside side of the calf muscle then goes up to the inside side of the back of the knee while another one goes up parallel and stores on the buttocks. Then goes up to the back bone and then to the back of the neck, its branch goes into the root of the tongue. And another goes directly and

stores on the zhen bone, and then goes up to the top of the head and goes down from the forehead and stores on the nose; while a branch is the "mu shang wang" ("net on the eyes"), goes down and stores by the nose. Another branch from the armpit external side, stores on the shoulder yu, another branch goes into the armpit and goes out to the que pen (supraclavicular fossa) and stores on the wan bone; a branch goes out from the que pen, slanting up by the nose.

2. The foot shao yang jing jin: starts from the second small toe, goes up and stores on the external ankle, goes up by the external side of the knee, a branch starts from the external condyle above the tibia bone then goes up to the thigh, front part of which stores on the fu tu, the back part stores on the jue di: directly goes up to the parts of the rib and then goes through to the front side of the armpit which then connects with the breast parts and stores on the que pen. Its direct jing jin then goes from the armpit, goes up and spreads and goes through the que pen and goes out from the front side of the foot tai yang, and along the back of the ear, goes up to the corner of the forehead, meets on the top of the head and goes up to the cheek and stores by the nose. A branch stores on the external corner of the eye.

3. The foot yang ming jing jin: starts from the foot 3 toes, ie. in the middle three toes, sores on the foot fu, slanting goes up distributes on the external bu bone, and stores on the external side of the knee, goes up directly and stores on the pi xu, then goes up to the ribs and connects to the back bone. Its direct part stores on the knee, a branch spreads on the external pu bone and then meets on the foot shao yang; from the knee goes up directly along the fu tu, goes up stores on the pi parts, meets together on the private parts, goes up to distribute on the abdomen and stores on the que pen; extends to the neck and goes up to the mouth and meets by the nose, stores under the nose, meets on the foot tai yang, is the "mu shang wan" ("net covering the eyes"). A branch from the cheek stores in the front of the ear.

4. The foot tai yin jing jin: starts from the internal side big toe, goes up stops on the internal ankle; directly goes to the parts and stops on the pu knee in the knee, goes up from the internal side and stores on the pi, meets on the private parts; then goes up to the abdomen stores on the umbilicus, circles in the abdomen, stores on the ribs parts, spreads on the chest; its internal part adjusts on the back bone.

5. The foot jue yin jing jin: starts from the surface of the big toe, goes up and stores on the front of the internal ankle, along the internal side of the jing, goes

up and stores on the internal pu bone, along the internal side stores on the private parts, connects with every jing jin.

6. The foot shao yin jing jin: starts under the small toe, slanting goes under the internal ankle with the jing of the foot tai yin and stops on the heel, meets with the jing of the foot tai yang, goes up stores on the internal pu bone, goes up along the internal side, stores on the private parts with the jing of the foot tai yin. A branch goes along the back bone up to the back of the neck and stores on the zhen bone and meets with the jing of the foot tai yang.

7. The hand tai yang jing jin: starts on the small finger goes up stores on the back of the wrist, goes up along the internal side of the front of the arm, stores on the back of the ru bone, extends and stores under the armpit; its branch goes to the back of the armpit, goes up around the shoulder blade and the scapula, along the neck, goes out to the front of the jin of the foot tai yang, stores on the wan bone of the back of the ear; one branch jing starts from the back of the ear and goes into the ear; its direct part goes out of the ear and goes down to store on the chin and then goes up to connect with the external corner of the eye. Another branch jing from the cheek goes to the chu yu (teeth) parts along the front of the ear, connects with the external corner of the eye, forehead, and stores on the corner of the head.

8. The hand shao yang jin jing: starts from the end of the ring finger goes out and stores on the back of the wrist, goes up along the front of the arm to store on the point of the elbow, along the external side of the arm goes out to the shoulder and then to the neck and meets the hand tai yang; its branch goes in and connects with the base of the tongue after going down to the corner of the cheek; another branch jing goes up from the qu ya parts along the front of the ear reaching the external corner of the eye and goes up past the forehead to store on the corner of the head.

9. The hand yang ming jing jin: starts from the end of the index finger to go to storing on the back of the wrist, then goes along the front arm to store on the external elbow, then along the arm to store on the shoulder. Its branch goes around the shoulder and goes to the back bone; directly goes to the parts along the shoulder goes up to the neck; a branch stores by the nose directly goes out on the front of the hand tai yang, and goes up to the left corner of the forehead and spreads on the head part and goes down to the right side cheek part.

10. The hand tai yin jing jin: starts from the big finger and along the finger stores on the back edge of the thumb muscle (yu ji), along the cun mouth external side goes up to the forearm to stop in the elbow; then goes up along the internal

side of the arm and goes into the armpit, goes out on the que pen and stores on the front of shoulder, stores on the que pen on the upper parts, while the lower parts store on the chest spreads on the guan ge, and meets under the ge (diaphram) and to the ribs.

11. The hand jue yin jing jin: starts from the middle finger goes with the jin of the hand tai yin stores on the internal side of the elbow, along the internal side of the front arm to store on the armpit, goes up along the ribs front and back sides and spreads here, its branch goes under the armpit, spreads on the chest, stores on the guan ge parts.

12. The hand shao yin: starts from the internal side of the small finger, stores on the rei bone in the back of the hand, goes up stores on the internal side of the elbow, goes up into the armpit parts, meets the hand tai yin on the breast parts, stores on the chest, along the chest ge, goes down to connect with the umbilicus.

The above is from the records of the *Ling shu-jing jin*. Its sequence are: the foot three yang, the foot three yin, the hand three yang, and the hand three yin. This is very useful, it indicates not only they are part of connection re the whole body circulation and the yin and yang, surface and internal aspects among the jing, but there is a connection with the three yang jing. This is the composition of the "si jue":

1. The foot three yang jing jin: meet on the face cheek parts
2. The foot three yin jing jin: meet on the "yin qi" (private parts)
3. The hand three yang jing jin: meet on the "jiao" (one side of the head)
4. The hand three yin jing jin: meet on the chest ge parts (feng).

The methods of distribution of the jing jin, not only are different from the twelve jing mai, which transport with the yin yang shou zhu and then become the circulation parts, but also are different from the twelve jing bie, which separate and combine with the surface and internal 2 jing. The jing jin consists of the jing rou system in the jing luo system with its special connection, spread and distibution methods.

One of the jing jin's functions is its connection to the hundred bones and therefore its maintainence of the function of all of the body. The human body has differences between hard and soft, and tendons and tissues. Hard tendons all distribute near the limbs, neck and back bone, are strong and have force, and can connect the four limbs and hundred bones. Soft tendons distribute on the chest, abdomen, head and face, soft and thin, this is their function to connect with each other. If it is the tendons of the hand and feet three yang they go on external, and people have more hardness; if it is the tendons of the hand and feet three yin then they go internal, and they are more soft. The twelve jing tendons include tissue, muscle, and tendon membrane etc. functions, and consists of the connection parts shallow and surface in the jing luo system.

Another function of the jing jin is that it protects the organs in each part of the whole body. The *Ling shu-jing mai* chapter said, "gu wei gan, mai wei ying, jing wei gan, rou wei chang" ("bones become gan, the vessels ying nutritive level, jing is the framework, muscles/tissues are the walls"). "Jing wei gan" actually means the muscles connect with the bones, and can bend and stretch, presenting strong and forceful. "Rou wei chang" means the muscles, (includes the fat under the skin), distribute on the surface of the body and four limbs shallow parts. Then becomes important external tissues which avoid organ injury and avoid external evil.

The twelve jing jin belong to the twelve jing mai, they depend on the jing qi of the twelve jing mai, so they circle and distribute mostly the same as the twelve jing mai. However, the jing jin also have some circle parts, and excess jing mai circling. On the other hand, the jing jin function actively still relies on the jing luo qi and blood. This indicates to us when we study, we should consider the internal connection between jing jin and jing mai jing qi, which combine jing jin and jing mai. In this way, we can get the perfect knowledge about jing jin function.

(ii).   The symptoms and practical meaning of the jing jin

1.   The bing hou (symptoms) of the foot tai yang jing jin: the small toe pulls/tugs strongly (chu qiang), foot heel swelling and painful, joint contraction heavy, back strong and reverse bending, neck hard, armpit feels like something pulling under it, shoulder cannot raise, que pen part painful, and cannot turn left or right.

2.   The bing hou of the foot shao yang jing jin: the 4th toe tugs/pulls strongly, pulling external knee tendon, the knee cannot bend or straighten, the back of the knee hollow tendon is heavy (ji), the front pulls the thigh, the back pulls the sacrum, goes up the ribs, painful pulling of the que pen breast part and neck part, tendons tense, from left to right the right eye cannot open, goes up past the right corner of the head, and goes parallel with the qiao mai, left luo on right side, so an injury is on the left corner and then right foot cannot use, it is called as "wei jing xiang jiao" ("net tendons cross").

3.   The bing hou of the foot yang ming jing jin: the middle toe pulls/tugs strongly, the small leg (calf) tendon twists, the tendons and muscles in the feet parts

jump/shake/vibrate and are hard, the fu tu tendons are twisted, the thigh front is swollen and distended, hernia, the tendons and muscles in the abdomen are heavy, pulling of the que pen and face, the mouth slanted suddenly, the tendons pulled and tense then the eye cannot close; belong to heat then the tendons are loose and the eye cannot open. The tendons in the cheek are cold requiring treatment in the cheek, ie. put in the corner of the mouth; if there is heat then the tendons are loose and cannot contract/draw back, it can also make the corner of the mouth slanting.

4. The bing hou of the foot tai yin jing jin: the big toe pulls/tugs strongly, the internal ankle painful, twisted tendons with pain, pulled bone in the knee and painful, bottom of the internal side of the thigh pulled and painful, private parts painful, connect to the umbilicus and then the 2 sides of the ribs painful, 2 sides of the chest pulled, and internal back bone painful.

5. The bing hou of the foot jue yin jing jin: the big toe pulls/tugs strongly, the front of the internal ankle is painful, there is a pulling in the knee which is also painful, the internal side of the buttocks are painful and then has twisted tendons, the private part's function is at a loss, if you have more sex then the yin (testes etc.) contracts, if injured by the cold then the yin contracts, if injured by the heat then the yin private parts become loose and cannot contract.

6. The bing hou of the foot shao yin jing jin: the bottom of the feet has twisted tendons, the parts it passes and stores at are painful and have twisted tendons. When the symptoms of this jing jin happens then one suffers from epilepsy illness, shaking and convulsions (jing feng). If the Illness involves the external the head is not able to lower or bend (ie. nod), trismus. If the illness involves the internal then cannot lie down with the face up. So in the case of yang illness, then the waist adverse (opisthotonos), cannot bow one's head or lower, if yin illness cannot look up.

7. The bing hou of the hand tai yang jing jin: the small finger spasmed strong and painful, the internal elbow rei bone back edge painful, along the side of the arm connecting to the armpit, the armpit and the back of the armpit painful, and around the shoulder connecting to the neck painful. Tinnitus and painful (in the ear), pain goes down transfers to the chin, myopia (short-sighted). If the neck tendons are tense, then tendon fistula (scrofula); if the neck parts are struck by the cold and heat evil then neck swelling.

8. The bing hou of the hand shao yang jing jin: the parts it passes through are strong and spasmed, twisted tendons, or the tongue parts are curled up and shrunken (juan suo).

9. The bing hou of the hand yang ming jing jin: the parts it passes through are strong and spasmed, pain and twisted tendons, the shoulder cannot raise, neck cannot turn left or right,

10. The bing hou of the hand tai yin jing jin: the parts it passes through are strong and spasmed, twisted tendons, pain, extreme cases even becoming "xi ben" (a form of accumulation), the ribs parts tense, vomiting blood.

11. The bing hou of the hand xin zhu (jue yin) jing jin: the parts it passes through are strong and spasmed, twisted tendons, goes ahead to the chest parts then has pain in the chest and get xi ben illness.

12. The bing hou of the hand shao yin jing jin: the tendons tense and contracted inside, there is a hardness hidden under the heart, and produces a "fu liang" (another form of accumulation) illness; there are tendon illnesses on the upper limbs, the elbow parts will have pulling and are tense like when you catch fish with a net, along the parts this jing jin passes and relates to the tendons, tendons and muscles make for pain.

The twelve jing jin belong to the twelve jing mai and are covered under the same as the jing mai. However, they have many parts that have illness, ie. already excess parts of the jing mai circulation like the hand yang ming jing mai stops at ying xiang (LI20) but he gu (LI4), yang xi (LI5) etc. all can treat illnesses of the head parts. The reason is that its jing jing go on the head and face parts and can "shang zuo jiao, luo tou, xia you han" ("goes to the left corner, spreads to the head, and goes down to the right cheek"). This indicates the range of the twelve jing treatment. There are many things that the jing jin circulation can result in and are not caused by the jing mai's jing bie circulation. In analysing the jing jin system, they mainly present as illnesses which are about the movement function areas ie. like pulling, and spasming/contracting of the tendon mai, twisted tendons, vibrating/shaking, stiff overly strong joints, and bending and stretching not well. These symptoms are in addition to some of the tendon and muscle illnesses which are not described by the jing mai before. So, the symptoms of the jing jin, add to the content re the movement functions in the jing luo system.

The symptoms of the jing jin are the symptoms of the tendon and muscle system in the jing mai; and the jing jin's function and activity relies on the jing luo's qi and blood from the zang fu. So, the body surface tendons and muscle illness are connected with the jing mai, and internal organs. From the analysis of the jing jin systems in the whole or greater view, we can understand the usage value of the jing jin symptoms in practical use.

According to the theories of jing jin in the systematic technigue areas, there are fen ci (parts piercing) (muscle piercing), hui ci (section piercing), (muscle membrane piercing), guan piercing (joint piercing, muscle membrane), etc. in content (*Su wen-bi lun*).

In acupuncture treatment, if the jing jin has an illness which results from cold evil, it mainly presents as a tense illness. We can use fan needling piercing technique. And after inserting the needles, we can use fire at the right temperature at the end of each needle to remove cold evil. One can also use moxa in place of fire or warm needling. Warm needling treatment has some good results in treating frozen shoulder, and the ratio of efficacy is more than 90% (see *Wen zhen liao fa*). Besides bi illness, the after-effects of stroke, and tenosynovitis etc. have good results from this type of treatment. Re the hot illness, the tendons and muscles are loose and cannot contract, so use the hand techniques like shu ci yi chu (quickly pierce or insert then the illness goes out) to discharge the yang evil. All this is of practical use in jing jin theories.

Because there is a mechanism of illness connection between the jing jin, the internal organs and the jing luo in practical treatment, for injury by the internal use of medicine which can cause muscle atrophy, spasm and shrinkage (ie. infantile paralysis) one can circulate the blood and remove stagnation, unblock the jing and circulate the luo. This example, also has a good connection with jing jin theories. At the present, the treatment of infantile paralysis after-effects causing tan huan and wei suo, have resulted in new developments in jing jin theories and practical usage. Analysis from the function of the muscle, to name one such example in point, has meant the understanding of "zhu dai yin" ("the main problem controls another problem"), and "shang dai xia ("the upper is more important/carries the low"). These are both important in treating some illness caused by ma bi (numb arthritis) muscle contraction, pulled by another muscle, then resulting in some abnormal shape. This analyses the imbalanced condition of the muscle force and then increases the treatment results further.

The above explains the practical usage value of jing jin symptoms and their theories. We also need to know that the twelve jing jin hou have also been classified under the movement/activity system muscle illness and therefore I will make this summary of the matter. This is actually a summary from olden times. People believed that re the muscle or tendon, the jing mo (tendon membrane) includes the soft tissue, the moveable organs and part of the function of the nerves. So, the twelve jing jin bing hou practical meaning extends the range of the illnesses and, in fact, lists them. It has important meaning to the Jing luo theories, development and practical use.

4.   The pi bu (skin parts)

(i)   The meaning and function of the twelve skin parts

The skin parts are the distribution of the jing luo system in the skin. They have two meanings: one refers to the whole, another refers to the parts. With regards to the whole area understanding, the skin parts are the most shallow parts of the skin that present on the external of the human body and are the parts which directly contact with the atmosphere and has a sensitivity to the external weather. They have an adjusting function to all these changes and then protect the human body from evils.

The skin parts have this function mainly based on the "zheng qi" of the human body, especially re the function of the wei qi. The wei qi is distributed on all the skin, like the *Su wen-bi lun* said: the wei qi "xun yu pi fu zhi zheng" ("the wei qi goes around the skin"), and "chong pi fu" ("all around the skin"). And the *Ling shu-ben zang* said: "xian xing pi fu" ("first goes around the skin"). And furthermore, the *Ling shu-jing mai* etc. also stated, that if the wei qi was comfortable and then the "pi fu tiao rou, chou li zhi mi yi" ("the soft skin is very good, like young people, very fine"), in other words evil cannot invade internally.

The skin parts also have a good connection with the lungs like the *Su wen-ke lun* said, "pi mao zhe fei zhi he ye" ("the skin has a problem then you have a problem with the lungs"). So, if lung qi deficiency and people will get a common cold easily. In chinese medicine external illness theories, whether the Shang han theories or the Wen bing theories, it is equally called a surface illness. The major meaning is that illness change caused by evil attack the skin parts is because of evil going inside the parts. The Shang han theories, when they discuss the external intake, first feel they show at the tai yang jing system group; if the illness evil on the surface doesn't disappear, it will go into the shao yang jing or the yang ming jing. These theories prove that it is the wei qi around the skin parts which is responsible. If the wei qi loses its protective action then "pi fu xian shou xie qi" ("the skin will firstly be attacked by evil qi"). So, in the Wen bing theories, although it is called "wen bing shang shou, shou xian fan fei" ("if warm evil attacks, first attack the lungs") (Ye Xiang yan *Wai gan wen re pian*) (below is the same), it indicates that the "fei zhu qi wei wei" ("the lungs control the qi but the qi belongs to the wei qi"). It also indicates: "fei zhu qi, ze he pi mao, gu yun zai biao" ("the lungs control the qi, the qi has a connection with the skin and body hair, so this qi is on the surface"). So, the Wen bing theories differential emphasizes the wei, qi, ying, and xue groups/parts. All this, is the knowledge of olden people on the whole of the skin.

The meaning re parts of the skin is that the distribution range of the twelve jing mai is in the surface of the human body surface. The *Su wen-pi bu lun* said: "pi bu yi jing mai wei qi" ("the skin parts are based on the jing mai"), because they have twelve jing mai so the skin is also divided into twelve parts; the skin parts are the jing mai on the skin. However, the skin parts are different from the jing mai and also different from the luo mai. They have a good connection with the luo mai especially with the fou luo. The *Su wen-pi bu lun* said: "fan shi er jing luo mai zhe, pi zhi bu ye" ("if the twelve jing mai illness this includes the skin parts illness"). The skin parts, as a differential of the human body surface of the jing luo, is different to the to the jing luo. Its difference from the jing luo is that the jing luo is presented as a line distribution; the luo mai is presented as a net distribution; but the skin parts emphasize the classification of "mian" ("area"). Its range mostly belongs to the position of jing luo distribution but it has a little bit wider use to the jing luo. Chinese medicine theories consider the parts illness of the jing luo mainly to have a connection with the skin parts which they relate to. Like the *Su wen-pi bu lun* said, "xie ke yu pi, ze cou li li kai, kai ze xie ru ke yu luo mai, luo mai man, ze zhu yu jing mai, luo mai man, ze ru she yu zang fu ye. Gu pi zhe you fen bu, bu yi er sheng da bing ye" ("if evil guest in the skin, then the cou li (the pores) stay open, the cou li open then the evil qi goes into the luo mai, the luo mai full then it goes into the jing mai, the jing mai full then it goes into the zang fu organs. So, if the skin has a parts problem then maybe have a big illness"). This indicates that it cannot be divided into different skin parts of the jing mai and its luo mai's jing mai parts and their illnesses. The jing luo zang fu illness has a good connection with the skin parts that the evil has come in. Like the *Ling shu-xie qi zang fu bing xin* said, "chu yang zhi hui, ci zai yu mian. (Xie) zhong ren ye, … zhong yu mian, ze xia yang ming. Zhong yu xiang, ze xia tai yang. Zhong yu jia, ze xia shao yang" ("every yang meets on the surface (or face), if evil attacks the people on the face, then goes to the yang ming. If evil attacks on the neck, then goes to the tai yang. If attacks the cheeks, then goes to the shao yang"). So, skin and jing mai, and zang fu illnesses connect with each other. This indicates different connections between the whole and the parts. It further presents chinese medicine theories about the view of the whole body.

(ii).   The practical use of the twelve skin parts theory

The twelve skin parts have a tight connection on the physiology along with the 5 zang 6 fu, the twelve jing mai, and the qi blood ying wei. It also has a tight connection with the mechanism of illness. In the *Ling shu-jing mai* chapter "shi dong" and "suo sheng bing" etc. have many illnesses presented as problems with the skin parts. Like, The foot yang ming jing jin qi excess, it must be hot before the illness happens. On the other hand, if deficiency there must be cold before illness. And, also in the case of the hand yang ming jing qi excess, then where the mai passes it will be hot and swollen. While, if deficiency then there will be cold and inability to recover. The *Su wen-ci re lun pian* said, "gan re bing zhe zuo jia xian chi, xin re bing zhe yan xian chi, pi re bing zhe bi xian chi, fei re bing zhe you jia xian chi, shen re bing, yi xian chi" ("those with liver heat illness then the left jaw/cheek is red first, those with heart heat illness then the visage is red first, those with spleen heat illness then the nose is red first, those with lung heat illness then the right jaw/cheek is red first, kidney heat illness the cheeks are red first"). The *Ling shu-lun yi zhen chi* chapter: "shou suo du re zhe yao yi xia re", zhou qian du re zhe ying qian re, zhou hou du re zhe jian bei re, bi zhong du re zhe yao fu re … yu shang bai rou you qing xue mai zhe, wei zhong you han" ("those who are solely hot in the hands under the waist is hot, those solely hot in front of the elbows the pectorals/breasts are hot, those solely hot behind the elbows the shoulders and back are hot, those solely hot in the arms the waist and abdomen are hot … .on the white flesh of yu ji (Lu10) have blue/green blood vessels, then the stomach has cold"). Also: those whose chi(cubit pulse) skin is slippery and shiny, is due to wind. Those whose chi skin is course/uneven, have wind bi (arthritis), Those whose chi skin is rough like fish scales, wither … All these illnesses are the effects of skin illnesses, but show that the skin parts have a tight connection with the 5 zang and 6 fu.

Based on these theories, diagnosis in external medicine judges the source of illness, in the jing mai and the internal organs, resulting in ulcers that occur on the skin parts. For example, like the bin ulcer (ju) which belongs to the foot shao yang jing; the dui kou ulcer which belongs to the du mai, and especially to the foot tai yang urinary bladder jing; the fu tu ulcer which belongs to the foot yang ming stomach jing; the waist ulcer which belongs to the foot shao yin kidney jing etc.. In visual diagnosis, checking the colour change on the skin and fou luo is one of the types of colour diagnoses (se zhen). At present, green/blue and black normally means pain illness, if dark black colour it normally means bi illness, if yellow and red colour it normally means a hot illness, if pale and white colour it normally means a deficiency and cold illness etc.. In addition, and at present, skin colour diagnosis also observes the papules on the skin (mainly on the back). Check the reflection of the hardness state on the skin, the sensitivity differences, and the electricity conduct changes on the skin etc. all of which are references in the diagnoses of illness and its new developments re skin parts theories in this type of diagnosis.

In the treatment areas, there are olden insertion methods like "ban ci" and "mao ci" that insert shallowly in the skin (*Ling shu-guan zhen* chapter). The present insertion methods, that is called skin needling, is a development of them. The practical use of skin needling has a connection with jing luo parts from examination to selection of points. Another example, like internal skin insertion methods such as "pi nei zhen fa" ("skin internal needling technique"), "chao zhi fa". ("treating the haemorrhoid technique"), and "fu tie fa" are all based on the same mechanism. The moxa used in acupuncture treatment methods is also an action from area of skin parts. Besides ultraviolet ray light put on the points, there is the jing luo magnetic treatment. They are all based on jing luo theories. The latter uses magnetic change needles action on special jing luo points on the surface of the body or "yi tong wei shu" ("if pain use shu points") (magnetic source use is not the same, there is chi tu (red earth) - Co (cobalt) Hg magnetic combined metals plant to produce constant magnetism and magnetic unit from 600 - 2000 GC; there is Samarian (Sm) - cobalt and carium (Ca) - cobalt permanent magnetic body, magnetic body, magnetism strength from 1,300 - 2,500 GC etc., on the methods there is external application methods and circulation of magnetism methods etc.). Although its mechanism is quite complex, its direct theories and jing luo theory - especially the theory about skin parts have a tight connection.

To summarize the previous, skin parts theories have a wide use in acupuncture treatment on every illness, along with the development and creation of treatment methods on the surface of the body. Skin parts theories increase one's depth and breadth to understanding. Summarized in one sentence, jing luo theories have a rich content but still need development and study, this needs further research in the future.

PART 2

THE PRACTICAL USE OF
THE JING LUO THEORIES

CHAPTER 1

....

Jing luo theories indicate direct meaning and practical use of acupuncture treatment methods.

The criteria and development of acupuncture treatment methods is the basis in forming jing luo theories. Jing luo theory also directs the practical use of acupuncture from theory directly to acupuncture treatment methods. Following only proven jing luo theories about the direct meaning of acupuncture methods from the selection of points prescription and hand techniques.

Section 1
Acupuncture selection of points methods is the practical use of jing luo theories.

Acupuncture treatment is the same with other aspects of chinese medicine. You must base it on yin and yang, the wu xing, and ying wei qi xue etc. fundamental theories. In other words, there is a need to use observation, smell, enquiring, and translation/interpretation/correspondence main methods and differential treatment. However, as far as treatment methods go, acupuncture treatment methods have special characteristics.

Acupuncture treatment directly uses xue (acupuncture) points, by the conduction and reaction of the jing luo in adjusting ying wei qi and blood and the zang fu function of the human body. By way of recovery of the related and dynamic balance of yin and yang in the body so as to get a good result. In this view, jing luo and points are the fundamentals of acupuncture treatment.

Re the main range and common characteristics of points, we have a preliminary description in the jing luo theories section. However, illness change and symptoms are very complex. In practical usage, it needs to imply related and special characteristics of points flexibly, under the direction of the jing luo theories to give a suitable prescription of points to get the satisfactory treatment results. So, whether some acupuncture point formulas are suitable or not is the key point of seeing whether treatments will be good or not.

Acupuncture point formulae rules have been described deeply in the *Nei jing*. After continuous development, it has formed quite a perfect theory. For example, according to the sources of illness can get the points ie.: "bing zai shang zhe xia qu zhi; bing zai xia; zhe gao qu zhe; bing zai tou zhe qu zhi zu; bing zai yao zhe qu zhi guo" ("if the illness is on the upper parts then take from the lower parts; if the illness is in the lower then take from the higher parts; if the illness is on the head then take the points from the feet; if the illness happens in the waist then take the point from the back of the knee") (*Ling shu-zheng zhi* chapter). Because of "xie qi yu jing, zuo sheng ze you bing, you sheng ze zuo bing" ("evil is on the jing, left side excess then right side illness, if right side excess then left side illness"). And so, there is also "bing zai zuo zhe qu zhi you, bing zai you zhe qu zhi zuo" ("if illness is on the left then get a point from the right, if illness is on the right then get a point from the left") rule to get points.

When describing the connection of "te ding xue" ("special points") and internal organs and jing luo illness change, the *Ling shu-xuan qi yi ri fen wei si shi* chapter said, "bing zai zang zhe, qu zhi jing; bing bian yu se zhe, qu zhi ying; bing shi jian shi zhe zhi, qu zhi shu, bing bian yan zhe, qu zhi jing; jing man er xue zhe, bing zai wei; ji yi yin shi bu jie de bing zhe, qu zhi yu he" ("those illness at the zang, select its well point; those illness change re colour, select its spring point; those illness sometimes there and sometimes not, select its stream point; those illness change re voice, select its river point; those whose channels are full and have bleeding, illness at stomach; and those whose drinks and foods don't digest to the point of being an illness, select its sea points"). The *Nan jing - liu shi ba nan* added the explanation, "jing zhu xin xia man, ying zhu shen re, shu zhu ti zhong jie tong, jing zhu chuan ke han re, he zhi ni qi er xie" ("the well points govern under the centre is stuffy, the spring points govern body heat, the stream points govern the body heavy and the joints painful, the river points govern asthma coughing and cold-hot, the sea points govern adverse qi and diarrhoea"). The *Ling shu-xie qi zang fu bing xing* chapter said, "ying shu zhi wai jing, he zhi nei fu" ("the spring and the stream points treat the external channels, the sea points treat the internal bowels"). The *Ling shu-jiu zhen shi er yuan* chapter said, "wu zang you yi ye, ying chu shi er yuan. Shi er yuan ge you suo chu. Ming zhi qi yuan, guan qi ying, er zhi wu zang zhi hai yi" ("if the wu zang have an illness, it comes from the twelve yuan; the twelve yuan come from different parts. If we know their yuan (source) and observe their reflection, we can know the illness of the 5 zang") etc. All these descriptions indicate some use rule of the "tie ding shu xue".

According to the mechanism that points out that not only are they the reflected points of the zang fu jing luo illness change but also they are the stimulating points of treatment. In practical use, they are the selected point routes and methods ie. "yi tong wei shu". Like the *Qian jin fang* said, "ren you bing tong, ji leng nian qi shang, rou li dang qi qu, bu wen kong xue, ji de bian kuai huo tong qu, ji yan 'ah shi', jiu ci jie yan" ("if people have an illness then press his upper part, if get the suitable parts can get the pain parts or comfortable parts without requiring points, this is called 'ah shi', using this method, everybody gets this experience"). This selecting points route has been developed by countless people so its treatment range has been extended in the areas of practical treatment and illness diagnosis.

The above acupuncture formulae points rules are all directed by the jing luo theories because the jing luo are distributed and circling according to fixed parts. So, the select points rule is essentially "jing mai suo guo, zhu zhi suo ji" ("if on the jing mai parts then treat those parts and you will get good results"). Because the jing luo circulation has crossings and a complex distribution phenomenon, so there is also a flexible selection-of-points rule. Re some special formulae points method for selecting xue points, they are all the practical use of jing qi theories or qi jing, luo mai, jing bie and jing jin theories originally from the jing luo theories.

Now, we will list the use of the acupuncture fifteen select points methods and then further describe the acupuncture practical use of jing luo theories:

1.   The three parts select points method.

The "three parts" means parts like neighboring or remote parts:

a.   The parts select points method: the major target is to get the points from the illness-take-place parts, in the surface of the muscles of the four limbs. One needs to use the select points rule of "yi tong wei shu". Like when important organs or some illness change occurs, and you cannot get the regular points, you can select points next to the place. Regarding this select points method, there are quite good results on pain or chronic illness like stomach pain ie.. zhong wan (CV12), while in the case of abdomen pain, tian shu (ST25) etc.

b.   Neighbouring select points method: in the next illness parts, (there are related positions with illness parts jing luo) select suitable shu points to increase treatment result. One can use this method in a mixed use with other methods. Like, for example, nose illness take shang xing (GV23), wrist pain get wai guan (TH5), ankle joint illness change get jue gu (GB39) etc.

c.   Remote parts selection method: this also called "along-the-jing-to-get-the-points method". In other words, along the jing mai distribution road, at the other end of the jing mai circulation road to get the shu points method. This method is a very fundamental selection method in acupuncture practical use. It is suitable for every illness, like eye illness use guang ming (GB37); ear illness use zhong zhu (TH3); tooth-ache use he gu (LI4) etc. Ren and du 2 mai xue (points) can treat mainly parts and its next neighbouring illnesses i.e. can also have a treatment function on the whole body. To name some cases in point, da zhui (GV14) can treat common cold, white bood cells reduced and less condition, bronchitis, schizophrenia (jing shen fen lie zheng), malaria and malaria like illnesses, hepatitis etc.; guan yuan (CV4) can treat functional uterus bleeding, seminal emmission, impotency, urinary tract infection, nephritis, and all body deficiency etc. This is a very important technique when getting the points.

The three parts select points method is usually partly in mixed use in practice. For example, stomach pain: re parts one needs zhong wan (CV12), re neighboring one needs zhang men (Liv.13), and remote route one needs zu san li (ST36) and gong sun (SP4). They can also be used individually according to the illnesses and be used flexibly.

2.   Shu mu select points method.

The "shu xue" (back main points) are the parts which are transformed by the zang fu jing qi. There are 5 zang shu and 6 fu shu, and they all distribute in the foot tai yang urinary bladder jing (channels) of the back. Because they are on the back so they are also called the "bei shu". The "mu xue" are the parts in which zang fu meet together. There are 5 zang and 6 fu mu and they distribute in the chest and abdomen parts. As the shu and mu points have a tight connection with the zang fu, so when the 5 zang and 6 fu have an illness change, the shu mu select points method can be used. Flexible use of the shu mu points, cannot only treat the illness of the zang fu, but also can treat the illness which has a related illness mechanism in the internal organs indirectly. Just like liver opens onto the eyes, take the liver shu in order to treat eye illness. The kidney opens onto the ear, so take the kidney shu in order to treat kidney deficiency deafness. According to the practice rule, when take the shu mu select points for zang fu illness, normally still use the remote select points method of "zang bing qu shu, fu bing qu he" ("if zang illness take the shu, if fu illness take the he"). In the back shu points, it not only includes the shu points of the 5 zang and the 6 fu, but also includes other organs' shu points in the chest and abdomen eg. gao huang shu (UB43), ge shu (UB17), qi hai shu (UB24), guan yuan shu (UB26), zhong lu shu (UB29), and bai huan shu (UB30). One also can select points flexibly according to the illness. Normally, use shu mu select points methods such as:

(1) Gan shu (UB18) matched/married with qi men (Liv14) (liver mu). Main treatment: liver illness, ribs painful, vomiting out sour liquids, jaundice, sometimes hot sometimes cold etc.

(2) Xin shu (UB15) matched with ji que (CV14) (heart mu). Main treatment: heart pain, palpitations, convulsions, epilepsy (dian jian), insomnia etc.

(3) Fei shu (UB13) matched with zhong fu (Lu1) (lung mu): Main treatment: lung illness, cough, asthma, coughing blood etc,

(4) Pi shu (UB20) matched with zhang men (Liv.13) (spleen mu): Main treatment: spleen illness, abdomen distended, edema (shui zhong), rib pain, intestinal noises, diarrhoea, jaundice etc.

(5) Shen shu (UB23) matched with jing men (GB25) (kidney mu): Main treatment: seminal emmission, leucorrhoea, kidney deficiency, waist pain etc.

(6) Dan shu (UB19) matched with ri yue (GB24) (gall bladder mu): Main treatment: distended and full, ribs painful, vomiting, jaundice etc.

(7) Xiao chang shu (UB27) matched with guan yuan (CV4) (small intestine mu): Main treatment: urine long bi, bedwetting, diabetes (xiao ke) etc.

(8) Da chang shu (UB25) matched with tian shu (ST25) (large intestine mu): Main treatment: constipation or diarrhoea, abdomen distended, edema etc.

(9) Pang guang shu (UB28) matches with zhong ji (CV3) (urinary bladder mu): Main treatment: urine blocked or too much (ie. high frequency) urination, bedwetting, the 5 lin (urinary disturbances) etc.

(10) Wei shu matched with zhong wan (stomach mu): Main treatment: stomach painful, vomiting, indigestion etc.

(11) San jiao shu (UB22) matched with shi men (CV5) (triple heater mu): Main treatment: edema, urine is not good (bu li). (Can't use on women).

(12) Jue yin shu (UB14) matched with tan zhong (CV17) (pericardium mu): Main treatment: chest pressure uncomfortable, difficult to breath etc.

3.   Front and back select points method.

This treatment is from each part of the body, front and back shu points. Its basic theory is mainly that one should use the special function of the qi jing ren du 2 mai; or the surface and internal connection of the twelve jing mai, to select points.

(i)   Head parts: ren zhong (GV26) matched with feng fu (GV16), treats sudden zu zhong (?). Qian ding (GV21) matched with hou ding (GV19) treats headache. Ya men (GV15) matched with lian quan (CV23) to treat yin ya (can't speak loudly). Tian zhu (UB10) matches with ying xiang (LI20), to treat blocked nose.

(ii)   Chest and back parts: tan zhong (CV17) matched with ge shu (UB17), to treat chest pressure and uncomfortable. Shen zhu (GV12) matched with tian tu (CV22), to treat cough and asthma.

(iii)   Abdomen and waist parts: guan yuan (CV4) matched with ming men (GV4), to treat seminal emmission and impotency. Gui lai (St29) matched with ci liao UB32), to treat irregular menstruation.

(iv)   Four limbs parts: san yin jiao (SP6) matched with hou xi (SI3), to treat five fingers numbness. Nei guan (P6) matched with zhi gou (TH6), to treat chest and ribs distended and full, qu ze (P3) matched with tian jing (TH11) or qu ze (P3) matched with shao hai (H3), to treat elbow joint painful. Bi guan (St31) matched with cheng fu (UB36), to treat buttock joint (gu guan jie) painful. Qu quan (Liv.8) matched with xi yang guan (GB33), to treat knee joint painful. Ran gu (K2) matched with jin men (UB63), to treat very strong numbness in the hands and feet.

4.   The twelve jing surface and internal select point method.

According to the relationship of surface and internal, in the zang fu jing luo, to select points, this is a common case in acupuncture practice. Like, tai yuan (Lu9) (lung channel) matched with he gu (LI4) (large intestines channel) to treat common cold caused by external wind-cold, zu san li (St36) (stomach channel) matched with gong sun (SP4) (spleen channel) to treat gastritis, and stomach painful. Yin xi (H6) (heart channel) matched with hou xi (SI3) (small intestines channel) to treat night sweating (dao han). Cheng shan (UB57) (urinary bladder channel) matched with fu liu (K7) (kidney channel) to treat haemorrhoids with blood, abdomen painful, and diarrhoea. Da ling (P7) (pericardium channel) matched with yang chi (TH4) (triple heater channel) to treat wrist joint pain. Feng chi (GB20) (gall bladder channel) matched with xing jing (Liv.2) (liver channel) to treat glaucoma.

5. Yin yang select points method (also called zhu ke (host guest) select points method.

   a. The shu points of the yin jing and the shu points of the yin jing are matched. Like, gong sun (SP4) is matched with nei guan (P6), to treat abdomen painful. Shen men (H7) is matched with san yin jiao (SP6), to treat insomnia, seminal emmission.
   b. The shu points of the yang jing are matched with the shu points of other yang jing. Like, qu chi (LI11) is matched with zu san li (St36) to treat stomach and intestines illness, fever illness. Zhi gou (TH6) is matched with yang ling quan (GB34) to treat the ribs painful. and liver and gall bladder illnesses.
   c. The shu points of the yin jing are matched with the shu points of the yang jing. Like, zu san li (St36) is matched with nei guan (P6) to treat stomach wan (gastric cavity) is distended and painful. He gu (LI4) is matched with fu liu (K7) to treat common cold caused by the external and then has a hot body, without sweating.

6. Yuan luo select points method (also called zhu ke (host guest) select points method).

The "yuan xue" are the twelve yuan points which are the twelve jing mai distributed on the hands and feet, wrist, and ankle parts. The *Nei jing* said: "fan ci shi er yuan zhe, zhu zhi wu zang liu fu zhi you yi zhe ye" ("all the twelve yuan points treat illness of the 5 zang and 6 fu"), "wu zang you yi, dang qu zhi shi er yuan" ("if the 5 zang have an illness should take the twelve yuan points").

The "luo xue" are the fifteen luo points of the fifteen luo distributed on the four limbs, abdomen and sacrum etc. They have a connection function re yin yang surface and internal jing of the twelve jing mai.

Yuan luo match each other, and connect internal and external, upper and lower parts. They can treat both internal organs and surface of the body illness.

Although the yuan luo select points method belongs to surface and internal match range, it is not readily matched as surface and internal 2 jing, but instead mainly considers the jing mai yuan points that cause the illness. Regarding other concerns, are the luo points of the jing mai that presents surface and internal. This is a correct and limited select points method to select the points (ie. the yang jing has yuan points, the yin jing hasn't yuan points in the "wu xing shu" and instead is replaced with shu points so the 6 yin jing are shu yuan together as one).

A detailed use in practice is described as follows:

a. Tai yuan (Lu9) matched with pian li (LI6): Main treatment: cough, panting and wheezing, swelling (fu zhong) in the upper parts (points presented as a yuan point (zhu or host) matched with a luo point (ke or guest), the same follows).

b. He gu (LI4) matched with lie que (Lu7): Main treatment: externally caused common cold and cough, headache or left side headache.

c. Chong yang (St42) matched with gong sun (SP4): Main treatment: stomach painful and vomiting, intestinal sounds, and abdomen painful.

d. Tai bai (SP3) matched with feng long (St40): Main treatment: chest and abdomen distended and stuffy, phlem fluid (tan yin) cough.

e. Shen men (H7) matched with zhi gou (TH6): Main treatment: violent palpitations, fright and palpitations, epilepsy, eyes dizzy (mu xuan).

f. Wan gu (SI4) matched with tong li (H5): Main treatment: head and neck hard and painful, tongue is not flexible so cannot speak.

g. Jing gu (UB64) matched with da zhong (K4): Main treatment: waist and back painful, eye illnesses, feet painful.

h. Tai xi (K3) matched with fei yang (UB58): Main treatment: headache and throat swelling, cough, eyes dizzy.

i. Da ling (P7) matched with wai guan (TH5): Main treatment: chest and ribs painful, upset, and vomiting blood.

j. Yang chi (TH4) matched with nei guan (P6): Main treatment: chest and ribs distended and painful, headache, and fever.

k. Qiu xu (GB40) matched with li gou (Liv. 5): Main treatment: lesser abdomen hernia painful, ribs distended and painful.

l. Tai chong (Liv.3) matched with guang ming (GB37): Main treatment: gall bladder and liver fire too hot, red eyes swelling and painful.

7. Jie jing pei xue select points method.

This method's special characteristics are to select points alternatively on the same jing mai to make the jing qi go through and make sensitive the needle connection. It is usually used for four limbs contraction and bi illness.

If treatment for four limbs wei bi (flaccid paralysis and pain): jian you (LI15), bi nao (LI14), qu chi (LI11), he gu (LI4); jian niu (TH14), nao hui (TH13), tian jing (TH10), wai guan (TH5).

If treatment of lower limbs wei bi: huan tiao (GB30), yang ling quan (GB34), xuan zhong (GB39), zu lin qi (GB41); bi guan (St31), yin shi (St33), zu san li (St36), xian gu (St43).

If treatment of waist and back pain: shen shu (UB23), da chang shu (UB25), wei zhong (UB40), kun lun (UB60).

8.   Huan zhou select points method.

Get the points from around the illness change parts in order to make every jing qi and blood go through around the illness change parts. This method is mainly used for four limbs bi pain or for injury (contusions, bruises) etc.:

If treat wrist joint painful: yang chi (TH4), yang xi (LI5), da ling (P7), yang gu (SI5).

If treat the elbow joint pain: qu chi (LI11), shao hai (H3), tian jing (TH10), xiao hai (SI8).

If treat the shoulder joint pain: jian jing (GB21), jian san zhen (triple shoulder points).

If treat the hip joint pain: bi guan (St31), cheng fu (UB36), huan tiao (GB30), yin lian (Liv. 11).

If treat the knee joint pain: both xi yan (St35 + Ex. Pt.), qu quan (Liv.8), wei zhong (UB40), xi yang guan (GB33).

If treat ankle joint pain: jie xi (St 41), shang qiu (SP5), kun lun (UB60), qiu xu (GB40).

9.   Xi hui select points method.

"Xi" has the meaning of "between" and "go through without anything stopping it". Xi points mainly distribute between tendons and bones so it is called xi. They are one of the special shu points. There is altogether twelve jing and 2 directions (er wei), 2 openings (er qiao), together sixteen points. They are key points to treat acute illness and pain in the practical treatment. "Hui xue" are mainly the points from the zang fu, qi and blood, tendons, mai, bones, and marrow 8 things. The *Nan jing-si shi wu nan* said, "re bing zai nei zhe, qu yu hui zhi qi xue ye" ("if hot disease inside then take the meeting qi points"). In practical use, they are not limited to hot diseases, they are also used in internal illnesses. If an illness belongs to one area we can use related meeting points. Now, we will describe the meeting points and xi points as follows:

(1) Xi points

Lung jing - kong zui (LU6): main treatment of coughing adversely with spitting of blood, headache, throat swelling.

Heart jing - yin xi (H6): main treatment of heart pain, vomiting blood, night sweating.

Liver jing - zhong du (Liv.6): main treatment of beng lou, hernia pain, lesser abdomen very painful.

Spleen jing - di ji (SP8): main treatment of waist and ribs distended and painful, urine blocked, suddenly edema, irregular periods.

Kidney jing - shui quan (K5): main treatment of heart and chest stuffy and painful, feet heels swelling and painful.

Pericardium jing - xi men (P4): main treatment of heart and abdomen painful, vomiting blood, nose bleeding.

Above are the yin jing xi points.

Large intestines jing - wen liu (LI7): main treatment of headache, face swelling, face and tongue swelling and pain, throat painful, malignant boil.

Small intestines jing - yang lao (SI6): main treatment of hands and shoulders swelling pain, cannot see clearly.

Gall bladder jing - wai qiu (GB36): main treatment of head and neck painful and hard, chest and ribs distended and painful.

Stomach jing - liang qiu (St34): main treatment of stomach pain, breast swelling and painful, knee swelling and pain.

Urinary bladder jing - jin men (UB63): main treatment of childrens' jing feng (convusions), epilepsy, deafness.

Triple heater jing - hui zong (TH7): main treatment of hand and shoulder are sore and numb, ribs painful.

Above are the yang jing xi points.

Yang qiao - fu yang (UB59): controls left and right yang in the body.

Yin qiao - jiao xin (K8): controls left and right yin in the body.

Yang wei - yang jiao (GB35): controls the surface of the body.

Yin wei - zhu bin (K9): controls the internal of the body.

Above are the qi jing xi points.

(2)   Ba hui points (8 hui points).

> Fu (bowels) hui - zhong wan (CV12): mainly treats 6 fu illness.
> Zang (viscera) hui - zhang men (Liv.13): mainly treats 5 zang illness.
> Jin (tendon) hui - yang ling quan (GB34): mainly treats tendon illness.
> Sui (marrow) hui - jie gu (GB39): mainly treats marrow illness.
> Xue (blood) hui - ge shu (UB17): mainly treats blood illness.
> Gu (bone) hui - da zhu (UB11): mainly treats bone illness.
> Mai (vessel) hui - tai yuan (LU9): maily treats vessel illness.
> Qi (qi -energy) hui - tan zhong (CV17): mainly treats qi illness.

Xi points and hui points are all key points out of all the jing points. In practical use, they are used together to help each other, like the stomach jing xi point liang qiu (St34) matched with the fu hui zhong wan (CV12) to treat stomach pain and vomiting sour liquid etc. When making a diagnosis, you can use them flexibly according to differentiation and zang fu jing mai.

10.   Ben jing select points method.

This select points method is the method for illness change of internal organs using shu points treatment of the ben (original) jing.

The *Nan jing-liu shi jiu nan* said: "bu xu bu shi, yi jing qu zhi zhe, shi zheng jing zi sheng bing, bu zhong ta xie ye, dang zi qu qi jing" ("if people don't have deficiency and are not excess and then should take the jing. That is for the initial illness, get the zhu jing, ie. if not attacked by other evils, should take its jing. This indicates the use range of the ben jing select points method. In practical use, we should be concerned with special characteristics of the points position and compare the twelve jing symptoms (bing hou). Now, we will give examples as follows:

(1)   Lung illness: coughing and panting, coughing blood, Take tai yuan (LU9), lie que (LU7), yu ji (LU10), chi ze (LU5), zhong fu (LU1).

(2)   Heart illness: palpitations, violent palpitations, insomnia, epilepsy. Take shen men (H7), tong li (H5), ling dao (H4).

(3)   Spleen illness: diarrhoea, abdomen full, abdomen pain. Take gong sun (SP4), san yin jiao (SP6), da heng (SP15), fu ai (SP16).

(4)   Kidney illness: seminal emmission, bed wetting, impotency, edema. Take fu liu (K7), zhao hai (K6), tai xi (K3), ran gu (K2).

(5)   Liver illness: rib pain, hernia. Take tai chong (Liv.3), da dun (Liv.1), qi men (Liv.14), zhang men (Liv.13).

(6) Pericardium illness: heart pain, upset, vomiting blood, epilepsy. Take lao gong (P8), da ling (P7), nei guan (P6), jian shi (P7).

(7) Stomach illness: vomiting, hiccoughs, stomach wan painful, indigestion. Take shang ju shu (St37), zu san li (ST36), nei ting (St44), liang men (St21).

(8) Urinary bladder illness: urine can't go through, the 5 lin, Take pang guang shu (UB28), shen shu (UB23), qi hai shu (UB24), wei yang (UB39).

(9) Gall bladder illness: ribs painful, jaundice, Take ri yue (GB24), jing men (GB25), yuan ye (GB22), yang ling quan (GB34).

(10) Triple heater illness: sweating out and cheeks panful, goitre block. Take wai guan (TH5), zhi gou (TH6), tian jing (TH10).

(11) Large intestines illness: nose bleeding, throat painful, abdominal noises, abdominal pain. Take qu chi (LI11), wen liu (LI7), xia lian (LI8), he gu (LI4).

(12) Small intestines illness: jaw painful, cheeks swelling, urine won't flow. Take shao ze (SI1), hou xi (SI3), yang lao (SI6), xiao hai (SI8).

(13) Ren mai illness: 7 hernias, leucorrhagia, abdominal mass/lump illness. Take qu gu (CV2), zhong ji (CV3), guan yuan (CV4), qi hai (CV6).

(14) Du mai illness: epilepsy, tetanus, Take da zhui (GV14), jing suo (GV8), ming men (GV4), yao yang guan (GV3).

The ben jing select points method and indirect jing select points method are very similar; both the ben jing select points method uses pei xue (matching points) and the indirect jing select points method use pei xue. The indirect jing select points method emphasizes treating the illness change of the four limbs jing luo. The ben jing select points method, by comparison, emphasizes the zang fu internal illness change. In the practical use, you can use them flexibly but should have emphasis on some parts.

11. End of limbs select points method.

This method uses the shu points on the upper and lower limbs which are similar. It is suitable for zang fu illness and all body illness:

Si wang points - wei zhong (UB40) matched with qu ze (P3), mainly treats high fever, chest and abdomen very painful, four limbs spasmed.

Si guan points - he gu (LI4) matched with tai chong (Liv.3), mainly treats body hot, headache, palpitations, convulsions (tic).

Lao gong (P8) matched with yang ling quan (GB34), mainly treats epilepsy and mania condition (kuang zheng).

Ba xie matched with ba feng, mainly treats 4 limbs swelling (fou zhong), hands and feet numbness.

Hands twelve jing matched with feet twelve jing, mainly treats the 5 centres upset and hot, high fever and loss of consciousness (fainting, muddled-headedness ie. hun mi).

Shi xuan matched with qi duan (GV28 or Ex.pt.), mainly treats cholera vomiting and diarrhoea, upset, rash and collapse from fright (jing jue).

12.   Upper and lower select points method.

This method is according to the *Nan jing*, "bing zai shang zhe qu zhi, bing zai xia zhe gao qu zhi" ("if the disease is in the upper take the lower points, if the disease is on the lower parts take the upper points"). According to this rule to select points:

  a.   Upper illness, take the lower points method:
If upper parts have an illness change, take the lower parts to treat, like: gan feng tou teng (liver wind headache), take yong quan (K1), xing jian (Liv. 2); eye illnesses and swelling painful, take tai chong (Liv.3), guang ming (GB37); stomach and abdomen illnesses, take zu san li (St36) matched with nei ting (St44); zu san li (St36) matched with gong sun (SP4). For waist and back illness, take wei zhong (UB40) matched with kun lun (UB60); wei zhong (UB40) matched with cheng shan (UB57).

  b.   Lower parts, take upper parts method:
If lower parts have illness change, use upper parts to treat, like blocked nose and nose bleeding, take shang xin (GV23), tong tian (UB7); lower limbs tan huan (paralysis), take yao yang guang (GV3), in-between the 12th vertebrae and ci liao (UB32).

  c.   Upper and lower parts methods used together:
Normally, according to the jing mai circulation, select the points from the upper ends and the lower ends of the jing mai ie. take the head and the tail, like a back out-of-joint and painful, take ren zhong (GV26) matched with chang qiang (GV1). Prolapse of the anus and internal haemorrhoids, take bai hui (GV20) matched with chang qiang (GV1), Ben tun (adverse rising of accumulated qi usually from the kidneys) qi adverse, take tian tu (CV22) matched with qi hai (CV6).

13. Wu xing shu (5 elements points) select points method.

"Wu xing shu" means the sixty-six special shu points which are the jing, ying, shu, yuan, jing, and he under the four limbs and at the elbow and knee joints in the twelve jing mai. Its meaning is: "suo chu wei jing, suo liu wei ying, suo zhu wei shu, suo xing wei jing, suo ru wei he" ("out is well points, stay is spring points, put into/inject is stream points, go is river points, and come in/enter is sea points"). Because every point matches with the wu xing, so it is called the "wu xing shu". This select points method is according to the 5 elements and the creation and destruction theories. Select the shu points one by one; then combine the selecting points rule of "xu ze bu qi mu, shi ze xie qi zi" ("deficiency then tonify its mother, excess sedate its son"). Example: lung excess illness, cough and panting and chest fullness then sedate the he (sea) point chi ze (water) of the ben (original) jing. Because the lung belongs to jin (gold/metal), and chi ze (LU5) belongs to water, metal can create water, this is the method of excess then sedate the son. Another example, lung deficiency illness, a lot of sweating, and less qi then tonify the shu point tai yuan (LU9) (earth) of the original (ben) jing. Because tai yuan belongs to earth, earth can create gold/metal, earth is the mother of gold, this is the meaning of deficiency then tonify the mother. Every jing, tonify and sedate/reduce, can do like this method. When take the points then can read the Table 8 and the Table 9.

Table 8 The Twelve Jing Jing Ying Shu Jing He Chart

Heavenly Stems	Jing Bie	Mother Point	Point Bie	5 Elements Mutually Create	Son Point	Point Bie	5 Elements Mutually Create
Jia Wood	Gall Bladder Channel	Xia Xi (GB43)	Ying Water	Water Creates Wood	Yang Fu (GB38)	Jing Fire	Wood Creates Fire
Yi Wood	Liver Channel	Qu Quan (LIV8)	He Water	Water Creates Wood	Xing Jian (LIV2)	Ying Fire	Wood Creates Fire
Bing Fire	Small Intestines Channel	Hou Xi (SI3)	Shu Wood	Wood Creates Fire	Xiao Hai (SI8)	He Earth	Fire Creates Earth
Ding Fire	Heart Channel	Shao Chong (H9)	Jing Wood	Wood Creates Fire	Shen Men (H7)	Shu Earth	Fire Creates Earth
Wu Earth	Stomach Channel	Jie Xi (ST41)	Jing Fire	Fire Creates Earth	Li Dui (ST45)	Jing Metal	Earth Creates Metal
Ji Earth	Spleen channel	Da Du (SP2)	Ying Fire	Fire Creates Earth	Shang Liu (SP5)	Jing Metal	Earth Creates Metal

Geng Metal	Large Intestines Channel	Qu Chi (LI11)	He Earth	Earth Creates Metal	Er Jian (LI2)	Ying Water	Metal Creates Water
Xin Metal	Lung Channel	Tai Yuan (LU9)	Shu Earth	Earth Creates Metal	Chi Ze (LU5)	He Water	Metal Creates Water
Ren Water	Urinary Bladder Channel	Zhi Yin (UB67)	Jing Metal	Metal creates Water	Shu Gu (UB65)	Shu Wood	Water creates Wood
Gui Water	Kidney Channel	Fu Liu (K7)	Jing Metal	Metal Creates Water	Yong Quan (K1)	Jing Wood	Water Creates Wood
Bing Mutual Fire	Triple Heater Channel	Zhong Zhu (TH3)	Shu Wood	Wood Creates Fire	Tian Jing (TH10)	He Earth	Fire Creates Earth
Ding Mutual Fire	Pericardium Channel	Zhong Chong (P9)	Jing Wood	Wood Creates Fire	Da Ling (P7)	Shu Earth	Fire Creates Earth

	YIN CHANNELS					YANG CHANNELS						
POINT NAME JING BIE	JING WOOD	YING FIRE	SHU EARTH	JING METAL	HE WATER	POINT NAME JING BIE	JING METAL	YING WATER	SHU WOOD	SOURCE	JING FIRE	HE EARTH
LUNGS (METAL)	SHAO SHANG (LU.11)	YUJI (LU.10)	TAI YUAN (LU.9)	JING QU (LU.8)	CHE ZI (LU.5)	LARGE INTESTINE (METAL)	SHANG YANG (LI.1)	ER JIAN (LI.2)	SAN JIAN (LI.3)	HE GU (LI.4)	YANG XI (LI.5)	QU CHI (LI.11)
SPLEEN (EARTH)	YIN BAI (SP.1)	DA DU (SP.2)	TAI BAI (SP.3)	SHANG QIU (SP.5)	YIN LING QUAN (SP.9)	STOMACH (EARTH)	LI DUI (ST.45)	NEI TING (ST.44)	XIAN GU (ST.43)	CHONG YANG (ST.42)	JIE XI (ST.41)	ZU SAN LI (ST.36)
HEART (FIRE)	SHAO CHONG (H.9)	SHAO FU (H.8)	SHEN MEN (H.7)	LING DAO (H.4)	SHAO HAI (H.3)	SMALL INTESTINE (FIRE)	SHAO ZE (SI.1)	QIAN GU (SI.2)	HOU XI (SI.3)	WAN GU (SI.4)	YANG GU (SI.5)	XIAO HAI (SI.8)
KIDNEYS (WATER)	YONG QUAN (K.1)	RAN GU (K.2)	TAI XI (K.3)	FU LIU (K.7)	YIN GU (K.10)	URINARY BLADDER (WATER)	ZHI YIN (UB.67)	TONG GU (UB.66)	SHU GU (UB.65)	JING GU (UB.64)	KUN LUN (UB.60)	WEI ZHONG (UB.40)
PERI-CARDIUM (MUTUALFIRE)	ZHONG CHONG (P.9)	LAO GONG (P.8)	DA LING (P.7)	JIAN SHI (P.5)	QU ZE (P.3)	TRIPLE HEATER (MUTUAL FIRE)	GUAN CHONG (TH.1)	YE MEN (TH.2)	ZHONG ZHU (TH.3)	YANG CHI (TH.4)	ZHI GOU (TH.6)	TIAN JING (TH.10)
LIVER (WOOD)	DA DUN (LIV.1)	XING JIAN (LIV.2)	TAI CHONG (LIV.3)	ZHONG FENG (LIV.4)	QU QUAN (LIV.8)	GALL BLADDER (WOOD)	QIAO YIN (GB.44)	XIA XI (GB.43)	LIN QI (GB.41)	QIU XU (GB.40)	YANG FU (GB.38)	YANG LING QUAN (GB.34)

TABLE 9

When using this selecting points method, we should pay attention in that if a point does not belong to the 5 shu points range, then we cannot use "zi mu bu xie fa" ("son and mother tonify and sedate technique"). Also, when select points with zi mu bu xie fa, it should be based on the illness, condition of the needle, ie. whether tonifying or sedating, whether using son and mother points of the original jing, whether using son and mother jing, or whether using son and mother points of the son and mother jing. If deficiency, then notify its mother, if excess then sedate its son according to the select points method and the treatment rule. When one needs to tonify and sedate from amongst the jing points, still have the other rules "xie jin dang xie ying" ("when sedate the well points should sedate the spring points"), and "bu jing dang bu he" ("tonify the well points should tonify the sea points"). This alternative method of tonifying and sedating well points (because the well points are on the fingers and toes, and are very sensitive) can be used for bi jue ji zheng (blockage collapse sudden/acute conditions. We can prick-and-bleed quickly and easily, but it is not suitable for the complete hand technique involved in tonifying and sedating. Eg. if meet the heart jing and need to tonify shao chong point (H9) and change to tonify shao hai (H3); or if meet the pericardium jing and need to tonify zhong chong (P9) and change to tonify qu ze (P3); or if meet the pang guang jing and need to tonify zhi yin (UB67) and change to tonify wei zhong (UB40) etc. Because the he (mother) can create jing (son), tonifying he is equal to tonifying jing. This is the meaning of if deficiency, then tonify its mother. If meet the spleen jing and need to sedate yin bai (SP1) can change to sedate da dun (SP2); or if you meet the stomach jing and need to sedate li dui (St.45) can change to sedate nei ting (St.44) etc. because the jing (mother) can create the ying (son). Sedating the ying is equal to sedating the jing. This is the meaning of if excess then sedate the son.

The 5 elements shu select points method is also based on the *Nan jing-liu shi ba nan* which said, "jing zhu xin xia man, ying zhu shen re, su zhu ti zhong jie tong, jing zhu chuan ke han re, he zhu ni qi er xie, ci wu zang liu fu jing ying shu jing he suo sheng bing ye" ("the well points control under the heart full, the spring points control the body hot, the stream points control the body heavy and the joints painful, the river points control panting and coughing and going cold-hot, and the sea points control qi adverse and diarrhoea, these are all the 5 viscera and the 6 bowels well, spring, stream, river, and sea points." In this each point treatment range, given the individual needs of the original jing illness change, choose points flexibly. If the illness patients pulses are floating, and panting and coughing and going cold-hot, and the chest is full, from the differential view it should be the lung channel illness; if the patient can be seen as having under the heart is full, use the lung channel's well point shao shang (LU11); if the body is hot, use the lung channel's spring point you ji (LU10); if the body is heavy and has joint pain, use the lung channel's stream point tai yuan (LU9); if there is panting and coughing, and going cold-hot, use the lung channel's river point jing qu (LU8); if there is adverse qi and diarrhoea, use the lung channel's sea point chi ze (LU5). If the patient's pulse is floating and moderate (huan), the abdomen is distended stuffy, the food doesn't digest, the body is heavy, and the joints painful, likes to sleep, when dong qi is at the umbilicus, press and there is little pain then from a differential view, this is the foot tai yin spleen jing illness; if full under the heart, use well point yin bai (SP1) of the spleen jing; if the body is hot, use spring point da du (SP2) of the spleen jing; if the body is heavy and the joints painful, use the stream point tai bai (SP3) of the spleen jing; if panting and coughing, and cold-hot, use the river point shang qiu (SP5) of the spleen jing; if adverse qi and diarrhoea, use the sea point yin ling quan (SP9) of the spleen jing.

14. Hard and soft select points method (another name is husband and wife select points method).

In the Chinese Old books, there is a rule which is called wu men (5 doors) and shi bian (10 bian) which uses the tian gan (heavenly stems) as part of acupuncture treatment theories. The words 5 door has two explanations: one is the mother and son which are distributed as the jing, ying, shu, jing, and he. Another is that, what makes the tian gan change and what makes the 5 types match, is called husband and wife points.

The twelve jing na jia (or tian gan) method (fa) includes jia (gallbladder), yi (liver), bing (small intestines), ding (heart), wu (stomach), ji (spleen), geng (large intestines), xin (lungs), ren (urinary bladder), gui (kidney); triple heater also belongs to ren, pericardium luo together becomes gui. Zhang Jing yue changed the last two phrases: the triple heater yang home (fu) must return to bing, the bao luo (pericardium) is from yin day's fire sign.

The twelve jing na zi (di zhi) fa: lung yin, da (chang) mao, stomach chen palace, spleen si, heart wu, small (intestines) wei inside, shen pang (guang), you kidney, pericardium wu, hai (san) jiao, zi gall bladder, chou liver through.

The 5 yun transport jia and ji together transform (hua) earth (tu), yi and geng together transform metal/gold, bing and xin together transform water, ding and ren together transform wood, wu and gui transform fire.

Tian gan has yin and yang differences, yang is as husband, yin as is wife. According to the ten tian gan, which match each other, there are jing points. This is where husband and wife points come from. In the treatment area, select this type of husband and wife points. There are two practical methods:

A. Jia yi matched together: this means that when inserting into the points that belong to the gall bladder jing, add one point from the spleen jing. Like, for example, yin ling quan (spleen) matched with yang ling quan (gall bladder), "chu xi zhong zhi nan ao" ("use these points can remove the pain of knee swelling") (*Yu long fu*). Shang qiu (spleen) matched with qiu xu (gall bladder), "jiao tong kan zhui" ("all this can remove feet painful") (*Yu long fu*). Yi and geng matched together, this means when take the points of the liver jing, they are matched with the points of the large intestines. Like, he gu (LI4) matched with tai chong (ben jing), shou lian jian ji tong nan ren, he gu zhen shi yao tai chong" ("when the hand leading edge and shoulder and spine are very painful, use he gu and tai chong") (*Shi xuan fu*); wen liu (LI7) (large intestines) matched with qi men (Liv. 14) (liver jing), "xiang qiang shang han, wen liu qi men er zhu zhi" ("if the neck is hard and attack by cold, use wen liu (LI7) and qi men (Liv.3)") (*Bai zheng fu*). Bing and xin matched together, this means points of the small intestines jing matched with points of the lung jing like hou xi (SI3) (small intestines jing) matched with lie que (LU7) (lung jing), "hou xi pei lie que, zhi xiong xiang you tong" ("use hou xi (SI3) and lie que (LU7) together to treat pain in the chest and the neck") (*Qian jin fang*). Ding and ren matched together, ie. points of the pericardium jing matched with the points of the urinary bladder jing. Like wei yang (UB39) (urinary bladder jing) matched with tian chi (P1) (pericardium jing), "wei yang tian chi, ye zhong zhen er shu san" ("use wei yang (UB39) and tian chi (P1) together can release the swelling in the armpit") (*Bai zheng fu*). Wu and gui matched together, it means points of the stomach jing matched with points of the kidney jing. Like, yin gu (K10) (kidney jing) matched with zu san li (St.36) (stomach jing), "zhong xie huo luan, xuan yin gu san li zhi chen" ("attacked by evil and cholera, use yin gu (K10) and zu san li (St.36)") (*Bai zhen fu*).

2. Another commonly used method relating to husband and wife selecting points method, use jia and yi matched together as example:

   (1) Take the gall bladder jing points to treat spleen illness. Like the patient whose abdomen is distended and eats little, feels the body is very heavy and tired, and the face and the eyes and the body present yellow, the skin is itchy, very thirsty and bitter, have a fever, stools like slurry, urine is not very good and red colour, pulse is ru shu (soft and rapid), tongue surface is yellow and sticky. From the differentiation

view, it is a case of damp-heat warms the spleen. According to the husband and wife select points method, jia yi are matched together, so take the gall bladder jing ri yue (GB24) and yang fu (GB28) points.

(2) Take the spleen jing points to treat gall bladder illness. Like the patient whose eyes are dizzy (mu xuan), has deafness, bitter in the mouth, vomiting some bitter fluid, chest full and ribs painful, sometimes hot and sometimes cold, easily angry, cannot sleep very well at night, pulse bowstring and rapid and excess (xuan suo shi), tongue coating yellow tongue body red. From the differential view, it is a case of gall bladder jing excess heat. When do the treatment, take da du (SP2) and da bao (SP21) points of the spleen jing, which in other words is jia ji matched together, ie. husband and wife select points method.

Others, ie. every jing, is based on the tian gan matched together. Can select points as mentioned above for some illnesses. It is not necessary to describe in detail.

The 5 elements increase together (sheng) and also are destroyed together (ke). In the creation and destruction relations there are many changes. Hard and soft matched together select points method is based on the olden doctors' yin yang 5 elements theories. In regard to some practical use experience, we should combine and select acupuncture points and then change to get this select points method. Re the 5 elements create (sheng) and destroy (ke), metal can destroy wood however as it is geng it belongs to yang hard's metal, yi belongs to yin soft's wood, but cannot arrive at mutually destroy, and moreover there is a hard soft mutual exchange, therefore yi and geng, on the other hand, are of the same nature and can mutually combine. Again, they are apart of hard and soft points technique and have their basis in their origin's physiology. The 5 element points are paired to the source (yuan) physiology, and also overall, yi uses geng as hard, geng uses yin as soft, so use yin channel Jing (well) points belong at yi wood, yang jing (well) points belong at geng metal, and therefore have the treatment effect of yin and yang paired together with yin yang mutual conclusions, hard and soft mutually have the source origin cause. It gives each point a physiological cause, raising separation from combining.

15.   The eight mai meetings selecting points method.

The qi jing ba mai are not all going and circulating on the four limbs. However, from the cross and meet relations of the twelve jing mai, these are the points connecting with the qi jing on the four limbs. The ba mai's course-and-meet points amounting to a total of 8 points out of the qi jing ba mai which also connect with the four limbs. Using these 8 points upper and lower together to treat the qi jing and other illnesses, this select points method is additionally called the ba mai zhao hui (cross and meet) select points method.

What the Eight Mai cross and meet points method mainly treats can be seen in the table below, table 10:

CHANNEL NAME	POINT NAME	CONTROLLING CURE SUMMARY
CHONG YIN WEI	GONG SUN (SP4) NEI GUAN (P6)	Combines at chest, heart and stomach
DAI YANG WEI	LIN QI (GB41) WAI GUAN (TH5)	Combines at eye canthus, ear back, shoulder, throat, cheek (jaws)
DU YANG QIAO	HOUXI (SI 3) SHEN MAI (UB62)	Combines at eye inner canthus, throat, neck, ear, shoulder, elbow
REN YIN QIAO	LIE QUE (LU7) ZHAO HAI (K6)	Combines at lung system, larynx and pharynx, chest and diaphragm

TABLE 10

Out of the ba mai zhao hui points there are two select points methods, ie. they have come from the ba hui zhao hui points method. One is Ling gui ba fa (Qi jing na gua fa), and the other is Fei teng ba fa.

Ling gui ba fa is mainly based on the 8 points of the qi jing ba mai and then use the ba gua, jiu gong (9 palaces) and the tian gan and di zhi etc., selecting points according to the time methods.

Ling gui ba fa is based on the ba gua, and makes the kan gua (1) match with shen mai (UB62), the qian gua (6) match with gong sun (SP4), the dui gua (7) match with hou xi (SI3), the kun gua (2) match with zhao hai (K6) (the central palace kun 5 should select K6), the li gua (9) match with lie que (LU7), the xun gua (4) match with lin qi (GB41), the zhen gua (3) match with wai guan (TH5), and the gen gua (8) match with nei guan (P6). After that, based on yin yang, tian gan and di zhi can be used to select point times. This ba fa composition, not only includes the ba mai, the ba points and the ba gua but also have the gan zhi numbers which are the basis for ba fa select points. The numbers of gan zhi has the dai day (modern day) and dai hours (modern hours) two types. Dai (substituted) days count tian gan in which jia ji are 10, yi geng are 9, ding ren are 8, wu gui bing and xin are 7. Di zhi counts chen xu chou and wei as 10, shen you as 9, yin mao as 8, and si wu hai zi as 7. Modern day hours then counts tian gan so that jia ji becomes 9, yi geng becomes 8, bing xin becomes 7, ding ren becomes 6, and wu gui becomes 5. While regarding the di zhi, zi wu becomes 9, chou wei becomes 8, yin shen becomes 7, mao you becomes 6, chen xu becomes 5, and si hai becomes 4. This is where gan zhi modern numbers come from. It is based on the 5 elements produced numbers and gan zhi yin yang production. Ling gui ba fa calculates points with them.

Use method: use the gan zhi number of the day and hour. Add together, to get the sum of four numbers, and then according to the yang day divide by 9, yin days divide by 6. Delete the sum of the gan zhi and then the residue is the shu point you should compare with the ba gua numbers ie. this is the shu point that at that time should open.

If the sum can be divided completely, yang day is 9 re calculation it is suitable to open point, on the other hand, if it is a Yin day then calculate as 6, it is suitable to open point gong sun (Sp 4).

Fei teng ba fa is also based on the ba mai ba points. It is a selecting points method according to the time but this method only wants to know the tian gan of that day each time, then can get the points. We don't need to use yang 9, yin 6, 10 change open and close calculation. For instance, jia zi day according to zi jian yuan (zi returns to the source) methods, zi shi (time period/hour), it is suitable to become jia zi shi (time period/hour), can take gong sun (SP4); and chou shi should be yi chou time period, can take shen mai (UB62); bing yin time period, can take nei guan (P6) ... and so on. Select points with this method ie. 6 jia and 6 ren, 6 yi and 6 gui, 6 bing, 6 ding in-between ... times. Then, we select open points the same.

Re Ling gui ba fa selecting points use, it follows the select points principle that is based on time select points, fixing time select points, and major and assisting points combination. They are similar to zi wu liu zhu method. However, the use of zi wu liu zhu has yang days and yang times (hours) to select points, and yin days and yin times (hours) selecting points rule. While, in the ba fa, there is no such rule. The twelve shi chen (time periods) in any day can calculate shu points according to the equation to process acupuncture. This is the difference with the old selecting points method.

Zi wu liu zhu method also use jing, ying, shu, jing, and he from the twelve jing to make up the sixty-six points it uses. And combined with the tian gan, di zhi, and the sixty jia zi etc., it uses particular times to open points along with a variety of assistant points (Ling gui ba fa and zi wu liu zhu according to the ancient books one opens points without using this principle).

The above outlines the use of fifteen point selection methods.

Section 2
Acupuncture hand methods. Practial use of jing qi theories

In acupuncture practice, use the correct differential and sensitive points but if the hand technique (shou fa) is not suitable, you cannot get the expected result; sometimes you even get adverse results. All acupuncture doctors think acupuncture hand techniques are very important, they warn that "zhen jiu bu lin shou fu liu min" ("acupuncture is not good if use of hand techniques is not good"). So acupuncture hand techniques is an important key to get the good results in practical usage.

Acupuncture hand techniques must be under the "de qi" (qi zi), basis, to get the good results. The *Ling shu - jiu zhen shi er yuan* indicates, "si zi er qi bu zi, wu wen qi su qi zi er qi zi, nai qi zi, wu fu zhen." ("when use acupuncture and qi doesn't come don't ask the number, when use acupuncture and qi comes then it's gone don't use needle again." "wei chi zi yuo, qi zi er you xio. Xiao zi xin, yao feng zi qui zhen, xin hu you jian chang dian, qi zi dao bi yi." "the major point of using acupuncture is to get the qi and then get the results, just like wind blows the clouds and then you can see the sky and this is the key problem of acupuncture"). All this indicates that "de qi" is the key problem to use acupuncture hand techniques. (De qi) at present is called "zhen gan" or "jing luo gan chuang zian ziang" ("field and transfer phenomenon"). In modern day, a lot of acupuncture practice, acupuncture anaesthesia and other experiments all present "de qi" is one of the most important aspects in getting acupuncture results and for acupuncture anaesthesia (zhen ma ma zhen) to be successful.

By observation and measurement in the jing luo field and retransfer phenomena, in jing luo sensitive people, these further confirm the existence of the jing luo; it also explains the importance and usefulness of jing luo theory.

According to the *Ling shu -jing mai* chapter, "sheng zi xie zi xu zi bu zi ri zi ci zi, han zi liu zi, xian xia zi jiu zi, bu sheng bu xu, yi jin qu xi" ("if excess then should sedate /relax/discharge it, if weak then should tontify /add, if hot then have an illness, if cold then it will keep, then if hollow down then use moxa if not excess or not deficient then use the channel (jing) to get it.")rule. Acupuncture hand techniques mainly are divided into bu fa, xie fa, ping bu ping xie fa. In acupuncture practice, should follow bu xie rule correctly. The *Ling shu-xie qi zang fu bing xin* chapter indicate, "bu xie fa xi bing yi jia" (use "bu or xie" – if use wrong one then the illness will become bad), this tells the people that it is very important to use bu xie methods.

Now describe acupuncture bu xie hand techniques about "shao shan huo" and "tou tian liang", then analyse the indicated meaning re jing qi theories about the acupuncture hand techniques:

1.   Literature record

"shao shan huo" and "tou tian liang" are types of big bu and big xie hand techniques. From their operation methods and function, their development is based on the *Ling shu - zhen jiu shi er yuan* chapter about bu xie theories and the *Su wen - zhen jiu* chapter, "ci xu zhu shi zi zen xie re ye, ... man er xie zi zi, zhun xia kan ye "("you insert in cases of deficiency then get the excess, is hot under the needle, if full then discharge is cold under the needle").

In the olden times literature, people who described cold hot and bu xie were the early people in the Jin like Dou mi. His book *Zhen jiu zi nan* indicated "fu bin huo re zi, zi zi yi han ye. He ru? Xu qi han zi, xian chi ru rang zi fan, hou de qi tuo xie zi yin zi fen, fu lin bin ren gi qi ru er tian qi qu, jin an sheng chen zi xi su zu, qi bin ren zi jiu qing bing yi" ("people get an illness, then get a fever, treat with cold if with cold first and insert into the yang zi fen and then get the qi put inside into the yin zi fen. This results in the earth qi coming in and the sky qi coming out from the patient. Just follow these methods then the patient will feel clear.")

"Fu bing er han xi, zi zi yi re ye he ru xu qi re xi, xiang qi ru yin zi hun, huo de qi xu yin zhu zi yang zi fen, fu lin bing ren tian qi ru er di qi qu, ye an shen shu zi zi qu zu, qi bing ren zi jiu he huan yi" ("people feel very cold then treat with hot, if people need hot then first insert into the yin zi fen and then get the qi along the needle to the yang zi fen, then the sky qi comes in and earth qi goes out, it also follows that this method used several times then the patient will feel better.")

Su feng's book *Zhen jiu da chuan* indicates "shao shan huo" and "tou tian liang" two terms. After that, it becomes two methods of big bu and big xie in acupuncture. There are detailed records Yang zhu Zhou's book *Zhen jiu da chen*.

2.   Which one is suitable

When you judge the illness, should tell the difference between deficiency and excess, cold and hot; according to the illness, use correct methods then will get the good results, avoid sometimes deficiency, sometimes excess.

(1)   Shao shan huo

It can bu yang, remove cold (chu han), suitable for all deficiency cold illness, and there is a "zhu yang" ("increase the yang") function. It can treat long term tan huan (hemiplegia), very difficult ma han bi (numb and cold), wind cold malaria, four limbs very cold, cannot sleep caused by heart and kidney doesn't cross (co operate), kidney deficiency type waist sore, seminal emission, premature ejaculation, impotency, and amenorrhoea caused by heart and spleen not strong enough (bu zu), liver and kidney both deficiency cause cannot see clearly, stomach ptosis and ptosis in the internal organs, prolapse of the uterus, stomach pain caused by deficiency and cold, abdomen pain, indigestion and qi deficiency constipation, cold diarrhoea, five o clock diarrhoea, stroke (tuo) illness, vital gate fire diminishing, high blood pressure coming from deficiency and common cold from external cold wind.

(2) Tou tian liang

It can xie yang (ie. remove heat), is suitable for all the really hot illnesses, it has zhi yin (treat the yin function), it can treat wind-phlegm type wind stroke, throat wind, dian kuang (depression and craziness), malaria, only hot by itself, ie the muscles become hot and bones very dry, diarrhoea, lower-down the evil, remove the heat, mutual fire excess too strong, stomach excess types fever pain, abdomen pain, constipation, excess type high blood pressure, bi illness, one side wind too strong people (pian feng), heat in the blood chamber then amenorrhoea, in hot days get diarrhoea, red dysentery, wind heat toothache, fire eyes, all inflammation illnesses (throat inflammation, teeth root inflammation, middle ear inflammation tonsillitis etc), external medicine afterwards damage, bi condition, and external wind heat.

3. Xun Zhi Xie Wei

Shao shan huo and Tou tian liang are kinds of hand techniques of combined tonifying and sedating, it should be operated on separately. The amount of excitation is quite strong. When you choose the point position, you must choose the point which is quite far from the internal organs, blood vessels, tendons (jing jin), or abundant muscled places, and quite sensitive places, then it is easy to make an operation and get success. However, re the points for operation, it is not suitable to take too many points. Usually take one or two points. The correct location of the points is very important.

For example problems in the head, feng chi (GB20), tai yang (Extra), bai hui (GV20), (although these are travsverse needling points they can be used). In upper limbs, jian yu (LI 15), qu chi (LI 11), chi ze (Lu 5), wai guan (TH 5), nei guan (P6), he gu (LI 4). In abdomen part, zhong wan (CV 12), tian shu (St 25), qi hai (CV6), guan yuan (CV4). In the back and waist parts, da zhui (GV14), jian zhong shu (SI 15), jian zhen (SI 9), shen shu (UB23), da chang shu (UB 25). In the lower limbs parts, huan tiao (GB 30), feng shi (GB 31), yang ling quan (GB34), zu san li (St 36), wei zhong (UB 40), cheng shan (UB 57), san yin jiao (Sp 6), xuan zhong (GB 39).

For those muscles small and thin, for example 12 jing - well points, shi xuan points, the shi wang points, etc and chest part, head - face parts, must use transverse needle point positions, and those shu points near the zang fu, the nine orifices, heart area, lung area or liver, gall bladder, kidney, urinary bladder, ears, eyes … etc areas, all are not suitable to use this kind of hand technique.

When taking points, for those disease conditions of the four limbs, head and face, should take the local points or the near points as the majors points, combining the follow-the -channels taking method. For those diseases of the back and waist, chest and abdomen, and organs and bowels, should follow the channels and take the points. Use the local points or near points as assistants.

4.   Hand Techniques and Operation

(1)   Shao shan huo

1.   Travelling/walking down yin techniques; use left hand to hold correctly the point position, the right hand holding the needle insert into the point. Let the needle go down three times sequentially, the first enters the tian (heaven) part under the skin, the next comes to the ren (person) part, the next goes through the ren part, then goes further to the di (earth) part. At the end, from the earth part, directly take the needle out of the skin. The first is shallow, then deep, the needle force is making an emphasis in the deeper part, slow insert and quick take out. Down yin technique.

Note (1) After needle body enters the point inside, from the shallow part moderately slight twirling insert to the deep part. Again, from the deep part, very quickly twirling and pull/retract to the shallow part, up and down, go and come, use according to follow the balance by degrees, can make it excess (shi) by tonifying. The needle tip enters moderately, from shallow to deep part, guides the yang heat, overcomes the yin cold, that is called jiang (down) yin.

2.   When twirling the needle, from the basis of sore (suan), numb (ma), distended (zhang), heavy (zhong) sensations, let the finger force go down, twisting the needle in the left direction, each time 180 – 360 degrees, that means the

holding-needle right hand, one's thumb is going forward, then the index finger is going backwards, repeat is to operate, then can produce the feeling of heat.

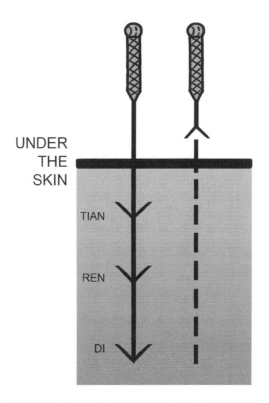

FIGURE 2: REDUCE YIN TECH.

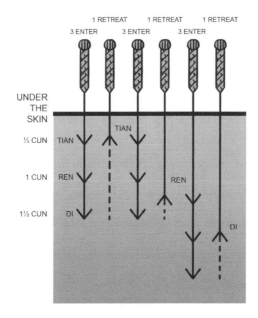

FIGURE 3: 9 ENTER 3 RETREAT

3. Slow pull and tense pressing, the meaning of tense (jin) here means heavy, the meaning of slow (man) means light. When entering the needles at the tian, person, and earth parts, for pressing and inserting the needles, should use a heavy insertion or light pulling.

4. Travelling nine yang shu (number). *Zhou yi* - dan shu (simple numbers), qi shu (old number), is yang - 9 number becomes old yang (lao yang), the 7 number becomes young yang (shao yang). Entering needle at tian, ren and di parts, when twirling (or pulling-inserting), the needle end going down should press in section, making the force at the end of the needle, each part twirling (or pulling-inserting) 3 times, 3 times 3 is 9, this becomes 9 yang number (also can at each part, operate 9 yang number), can make a stop for a while then repeat the operation. Pressing (An)- according to the practical experience, the 9 and 6 numbers are not exactly required, for the normal patient you can use 3 times 3 is 9 technique. For those patients who are not very sensitive (ie more insensitive) you can operate the 9 yang number in each level. If the patient is very sensitive he can't bear the 9 and 6 numbers, then you can operate 3 or 2 numbers. Has the same effect.

5. Follow and saving – the following of the travelling of channel qi and then tonify its qi, like the three yin channels of the hand and the three yang channels of the foot. From upper to lower, after needling then twirling insertion, letting the sensations of soreness, numbness, distendedness, heaviness travel downwards same as going down the path of the channel qi.

6. Travel - vibrate - scrape technique (zhen gua shu) - first use the thumb and the index finger of the left hand to fix the needle body, again use the thumb of the right hand to vibrate or scrape the handle of the needle so it goes down below. The vibrating and scraping is done 30 to 60 times then can produce the feeling of heat.

7. Entering the needle when the patient is breathing out and pull out the needle when the patient breathes in.

8. After needling and when come out, immediately use a finger (or a cotton ball) press and knead the needle hole.

Indications - when the needle comes out, if you want to tonify, then you should quickly press and knead the needle hole so the true qi can remain inside. That is, letting the true qi remain inside, not letting the arriving yang qi get out. So closing the needle hole can retain the true qi, that's the reply/response of guiding yang to the internal/inside for tonification.

(2) Tou tian liang

1. Travel and raise up yang technique: holding the needle method is exactly the same as shao shan huo. So make the needle insertion go directly into the earth part, then three times, as separated steps, pull out the needle from the ren part and the heaven part out to beyond the outside of the skin. First deep, later shallow, the needle force is emphasised on the surface (biao) level, quick insert inside, slow withdrawal.

    Raising up yang technique (Figure 4) or nine retreat three enter technique (Figure 5).

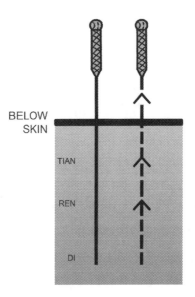

FIGURE 4: RAISE YANG TECH.

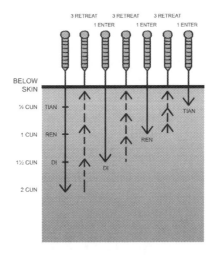

FIGURE 5: 9 RETREAT 3 ENTER TECH.

Indications:

> (1) Use fingers quickly and rapidly, insert from the shallow part into the deeper part. Again moderately, slowly twirl the needle and pull out from the deep part to the shallow part, up and down, back and forth, according to the use of qi to judge the needle movement, can make it deficient (xu), is sedation (xie). That is to say, quick and rapid needling, and moderate and slow withdrawal, layer by layer, guiding evil qi out and spreading (fa san), is sedation.
>
> (2) Because it is required that yin qi come forth, it must happen after yang evil is extracted, ie. yin overcomes yang. So that one can achieve this purpose it is required from yin (inside) guide yang (outside), let the strong qi fire (qi huo) be guided from the earth part to the heaven part and spread outwards, then the yang is gone and the yin will come, that is why it's called raising out the yang.

2. When twirling the needle based on the sour, numb, distended and heavy sensations, make the finger force more upwards, twirling the needle to the right hand direction each time 90-180 degrees C, that is with the right hand holding the needle, the needling hand (ci shou) use one's thumb to twirl backwards. The index finger twirls forward, then repeat this operation and you will produce the feeling of coolness.

3. Tensely pull out, slowly press. When we treat with needle at earth, person (ren), and heaven parts we should use heavy withdrawal and light insertion.

4. Travelling 6 yin number. *Zhou yi Yi jing:* even numbers are yin, the number 6 is lao (old) yin, the number 8 is shao (young) yin. When withdrawing and twirling the needle at earth, person, and heaven parts, pull up the needle end, make the force at the needle body, twirling (or withdrawing inserting) two times each level. Two times three equals six. Then this is a 6 yin number (can also at each level operate the 6 yin number), can stop for a while, then repeat the operation.

5. Welcome and grab it. Follow the opposite direction of channel travelling paths; for example, like the hand 3 yang channels and the foot 3 yin channels, are from lower to upper, therefore when twirling and inserting after needling, make the sour, numb, distended, and heavy sensations travel down lower, just opposite to the oncoming paths of the channel qi.

6. Travel, vibrate and scrape technique. Using the thumb of the left hand, fix the needle body first, then use the index finger (or the thumb) of the right hand to

vibrate and scrape the needle handle upwards, doing this operation 30 to 60 times, this can produce the feeling of coolness.

7.   Inserting the needle when the patient is breathing in, withdrawing the needle when breathing out.

8.   When pulling out the needle, shake the needle so that the needle hole is enlarged, don't press and seal the hole after withdrawing the needle.

Note: when withdrawing the needle, you should shake and enlarge the hole if you want to sedate (xie fa), don't press, knead the hole, so you spread the evil qi. Opening the needle hole is for the yang evil to go out efficiently, and makes a lot of yi qi come in. This is equal to the principle of guiding yin and expelling out and therefore is sedating.

Indications: according to the number 8, re operating procedures of shao shan huo and tou tian liang hand techniques, this is to adjust qi carrying out the procedure under the guidance of channels and collaterals theory. For example, with travel down yin technique and raising up yang technique and slow pull up (man ti) and tense pressing (jin an) and tense pulling (jin ti) and slow pressing (man an), the purpose is to adjust qi on the deep and shallow levels. For twirling hand techniques, re travel 9 yang number or 6 yin number, and for shaking and scraping techniques, the purpose is to circulate the qi and make the qi go faster (qiu qi). Following and saving, and welcoming and catching, the purpose is to adjust qi. Re controlling the travelling direction of the channel qi, and re entering and pulling out the needle following the patient's breathing, the purpose is in cooperating with and controlling the flow direction of the channel qi. After the needle comes, out press and knead, or not pressing and kneading the needle hole according to whether you wish to save the qi or let the qi go out.

From the above analysis, we can see that the purpose of needling hand techniques is mainly to adjust the qi, but adjusting qi of course cannot be separated from channel qi theory, that's why the needling technique is a specific application of channel qi theory.

As described above, acupuncture combined point prescription and needling hand technique are most key questions in acupuncture practice. The above describes and verifies that channels and collaterals theory has great importance for the key introduction to needling and hand techniques. This illustrates the theoretical value and meaningfulness of channel and collateral theory.

CHAPTER 2
Channel and Collateral Treatment Introduction

Introduction

The channel and collateral treatment takes the position of response re the channels and collaterals theory as basic starting point. Using the channel and collateral theory and chinese medicine theory as an introduction to bian zheng (diagnosis of the patient's condition) and its practice, at any possible point position, inject some kinds of drugs and apply certain hand techniques to achieve specific treatment purpose.

The characteristics of channel and collateral treatment is not only to pay attention to hand technique in the acupuncture treatment but to emphasise the influence of different needling sensations during treatment. Also, one should consider the application of drugs and how they can influence the patient's body. Re the operation procedure, it can be of some advantage to inject small amounts of drugs on a point position, or to use water injection treatment (shui zhen) technique or block therapy (feng bi Liao fa), but when treating it is also important to emphasise differential diagnosis and relative skills in applying channel and collateral theory and traditional chinese medicine theory.

The program of differential diagnosis and practical treatment of the channel and collaterals is that after having a general knowledge of the patient's condition you can proceed. Mainly using touch diagnosis to check the unusual changes in the patient's channels and collaterals (ie at the channel points)- that is the channel response according to the positive feedback and after checking out the fourteen channels with reference to the four diagnoses (si zhen) and using the channel and collateral theory and Chinese medicine theory to proceed with analysis and synthesis. On the basis of differential daignosis combined points prescriptions, selecting certain drugs and applying certain drugs and applying certain hand techniques pertaining to predictive needling, results may be used to achieve the purpose of treatment.

Re the channels and collaterals treatment has a wide effect on appropriate conditions it can not only be used for some acute diseases but also be used for some unknown and relatively complex disease conditions. It can not only be used for treatment but can also be used to further investigate and analyse disease conditions and further discover the solution to disease and sickness.

Section 1
Diagnostic Techniques

The Characteristics of Yang Type Responses

1. The positive responses of surface level channel points: if the colour, shape and temperature are different from normal, then it belongs to positive responses, and then can further investigate the positive response matters.
2. Positive response matters: under the skin or in the muscle level, if you touch or feel a round shape, thin flat shape, cone shape, oval shape, block shape or string-bean like air balls (qi pao), this will indicate a positive response matter. Different shapes of positive response objects are related to different area functions so therefore it is related to different diseases. For example, the cone shape, and the large bar shape indicate a patient suffering an acute disease, ie. an excess (shi) condition in chinese medicine. Thin round shapes and thin bar shape are usually found in chronic disease, which is a deficiency (xu) condition in chinese medicine. If fei shu point (UB 13) has a cone shape or block sections this usually indicates pneumonia (acute type), that's an excess (shi) condition. If there is a bar section at the same location that indicates chronic trachiitis: if the patients has a thin flat oval shaped block section that usually means lung T.B.
3. Channel points pressing pain: if the relevant channel points have obvious pressing pain or sensitivity, then this belongs to a positive reaction.

The Technique of Looking for Positive Reaction Techniques

So to find out the positive reaction material requires one to use touch diagnosis using the finger or thumb belly. There are four kinds of touch diagnosis;

1. Sliding technique (hua dong); using the finger or thumb belly, lightly use a sliding movement along the channel and collateral lines, it is easy to find out from this the positive reaction objects on the surface of the channel points.
2. Pressing-rubbing technique (an rou fa): so if the practitioner uses a little bit heavier pressure and uses more force when doing the sliding movement

technique, it is easy to find out the positive reaction objects in the muscle and under the skin.

3. Moving-pressing technique (yi ya): using a heavy force, also using the end point of the finger belly to test/examine/explore the positive reaction objects at the deeper layers.

4. Pushing movement technique (tui dong fa); using the finger belly of the thumb

Moving along the channel and collateral lines then pushing and examining at the same time. This method is suitable for xi (cleft) points and yao di bu (waist vertebrae parts) touch diagnosis.

The Examination Sequence for Touch Diagnosis

1. The first travelling line (xing xian) of the back part: out from the spinal vertebrae both sides 0.5 cun, equal to or similar to the Hua tuo jia ji points.

2. The second travelling line of the back part out from the spinal vertebrae both sides 1.5 cun, includes the 12 channels zhang-fu points.
   For the above two travelling lines, which start from the upper and end at the lower, we can use sliding movement technique and pressing- rubbing technique.

3. The third travelling line of the back part; also out from the spine both sides 3 cun, channel points indications are similar to their relevant back shu points.
   So we can do the touch diagnosis from lower to upper using the pressing, rubbing, or moving pressing techniques.

4. Mu points: the mu points of the 12 points are all located on the chest, and abdomen parts. We can use moving-pressing techniques for these points.

5. Xi (cleft) points: the xi point of the 12 regular channels (including the four xi points of the Extraordinary channels, means the total becomes 16 points) all located on the four limbs, can follow the channel and collateral travelling lines of each channel using the pushing-movement technique to find out the positive reaction object. Pushing movement tracks should be accurate, and the fingers should be stable and the force should be smooth and balanced.

6. The related shu points and special points; here we can emphasise the yuan (source) points and the special points to find out the positive reaction objects.

Following the above sequence, and applying the sliding movement, moving-pressing, pressing-rubbing and pushing movement etc technique at the shu points parts or in the neighbourhood of the shu points we can find out the positive reaction objects, the skin tension, and the degree of pressing pain, and therefore lead to the treatment of channel points.

Section 2
Treatment Techniques

Operation Method

1. Firstly, the practitioner should tell the patient that after treatment he/she will have some normal reactions, eg, soreness (suan), distendedness (zhang), sunken heaviness (chen zhong), tiredness without force (pi fi wu li).

2. Each time you choose the point position related to the disease, you must carry out normal skin sterilisation, then hold as if holding a pen. The syringe size should be 2-5 ml, and the needle head 4-5 ½ size. On each point, the practitioner should inject 0.2-0.5ml of medicinal fluid. On some of the head and face parts shu points or on some of the four limbs shu points, it is not suitable to do point injection. Here you can combine with needling treatment.

3. Do the injection one time each day or every second day, seven days or fourteen days make one course. Take 4-7 day rest between two courses.

4. Hand technique and needle sensation; according to the different characteristics of different diseases, the practitioner should use different hand techniques to obtain different needle sensations. This will have a close relationship with the treatment effect.

There are four normal kinds of hand techniques and needle sensations.

(1) Repeated Type: when the needle touchs the positive reaction object, there will be a feeling like soreness (suan), numbness (ma), or distendedness (zhang). When injecting the medicine, if the patient reports one of these sensations this will indicate that the treatment effect, particularly for common disease, will be very good.
Obtaining method: the practitioner must choose the positive point, and needling should activate and inject the medicine at a medium speed.

(2) Line Shape Type: that is when the practitioner injects the medicinal liquids, the patient should have a line shape type sensation. It is suitable for chronic deficiency weakness (xu ruo) patients.

Obtaining method: the practitioner should use smaller hypodermic needle and the medicine density should be less, and the insertion method should be slow.

(3) Pen Type: that is the needle sensation conduction track is strong and big and gives a pen type sensation conduction. It is suitable for the patient with a strong body.

Obtaining method: the practitioner should select a hyodermic needle which is big and has a high density medicine. The speed of insertion of the medicine is quick.

(4) Wide Band shape Feeling: the sensation conduction should be like a wide band shape, radiating outwards. It is suitable for excess heat (shi re) conditions.

Obtaining method: the practitioner should use big needling and a high density medicine and very quick insertion of the medicine.

Medicine Selection

Having the following conditions or situations will allow us to use channel point injection medicines:

(1) must be easy to absorb, without side effects
(2) must have certain excitations
(3) must pay attention to the actions of the medicines and their reasons for use.

With regards to practical treatment the first two practical conditions are most important. Using one medicine can treat various kinds of disease. Sometimes mixing a few related disease medicines can increase the effects.

The most commonly used channel point injection medicines are:

(1) vitamin C
(2) vitamin B1
(3) vitamin B12
(4) Chinese medicine injection liquids, dang gui solution, chuan wu, hong hua solutions, deng zai xi xin solution, chai hu solution, ban lan gen solution.
(5) brain tissue liquid, placenta tissue liquid

Section 3
Common Disease Treatment

The suitable diseases for using the channels and collaterals treatment technique is basically the same as acupuncture. Therefore, all the diseases that acupuncture can treat, it can treat; so the point position of the channels and collaterals treatment technique is the positive reaction objects. If you cannot touch the positive reaction objects, you can introduce the channel points to do treatment. However, the practitioner should always maintain using the principle of don't lose it's channel, otherwise lose it's point.

1.   Common cold

Diagnostic channel points: da zhui (GV14), one side or both sides, where the muscle membrane is raised up or tense, feng men (UB 12) one side or both sides, where there is muscle belly tension or where there are blockage sections.

Treatment technique: enter the needles 5 - 8 fen, injecting the mmedicine fast obtaining the pen type needling sensation.

2.   Tonsillitis, pharyngitis

Diagnostic channel points: 7th cervical vertebra one side or both sides, where ever there are round or oval shaped blockages.

Treatment technique: select a 5 fen - 1 cun needle, use injection solution. If acute type, add qu chi (LI 11) (one side or both sides), you ji (LU10).

3.   Bronchitis

Diagnostic channel points: fei shu (UB 13) one side or both sides, in acute types you will see oval shaped blockages; in chronic types you will see round shaped or thin flat shaped blockages.

Treatment technique: select 3-5 fen needles, use injection solution. The needle sensation should feel like it is radiating to the front of the chest.

Acute type patients add qu chi (LI 11); chronic type patients add kong zui (Lu 6) (one side or both sides), if bronchial asthma add tanzhong (CV 17).

4.   Pneumonia

Diagnostic channel points: fei shu (UB 13) one side or both sides, where there are diamond or oval shaped blockages; for those acute type patients often you will find oval shaped blockages at the fei re xue (Ex.pt.); da zhui one side or both sides, where the muscle belly raises up. There should be a sensation of pressure or pain.

Treatment technique: combine one side or both sides zu chi (LI 11), kong zui (LU 6), use injection solution.

5. Lung Tuberculosis

Diagnostic channel points: jie he xue (Ex.pt.), fei shu xue(UB 13), the side the disease occurs, you should be able to feel round shaped blockages, while at xhong fu (Lu 1) there will be the sensation of pressure pain.

Treatment technique: select a 5-8 fen needle, inject the medicine at a medium speed. Sometimes there will be a line shape type radiation towards the chest.

6. Tuberculosis of the lymph nodes.

Diagnostic channel points: jie he xue (Ex.pt.), one side has round shaped blockages, cervical lymph nodes or below the jaw lymph nodes are swollen big and hard.

Treatment technique: select a 5-8 fen needle, needle into the blockages or the swollen large lymph nodes. Slowly inject the solution.

7. Stomach pain, gastritis, stomach and duodenal ulcers

Diagnostic treatment channel points; pi shu (UB 20), wei shu (UB 21), wei cang (UB 45) one side or both sides, however most patients will show shaped or thin shaped blockages or cylindrical sections on the right side. With regards to ulcers, you will feel round shaped blockages at the ulcer point accompanied with the sensation of pressing pain.

Treatment technique: select a 8 fen - 1 cun needle and inject medicine. Combine with jiu wei (CV 15)

8. Vomiting, hiccoughs

Diagnosis treatment of channel points; add wei cang (UB 50), you should see block sections and bar slabs for those hiccoughs, block sections can generally be touched at ge shu (UB 17).

Treatment technique: insert the needle 5-8 fen, inject the medicine using pressure pushing. The needle sensation should feel like it is radiating towards the front of the body. You may combine with jiu wei (CV 15), shou san li (LI 10), left side or right side.

9.   Constipation, diarrhoea

Diagnosis and treatment channel points, on the left side or right side wen liu (LI 7), pi shu (UB 20), da chang su (UB 25), you will find blockage sections or sensitive pressing pain.

Treatment technique: insert the needle 8 fen to 1 cun, then inject the medicine.

10.   Hepatitis

Diagnosis and treatment channel points; on the left side or right side, at gan shu (UB 18), gan re point (Ex.pt.) and on right qi men (Liv 14), zhong du (Liv 6), you can generally feel blockage sections or sensitive pressing pain.

Treatment technique: insert 5-8 fen, injecting the medicine at medium speed. The needle sensation should radiate towards the liver region. You can combine with gan yan point (Ex.pt.).

11.   Waist and leg pain

Diagnosis and treatment of channel points: on the right side or the left side of the waist - sacral vertebra or on both sides, you generally find sensitive pressure painful spots, or round shapes, or string bean shaped blockage sections. In the neighbourhood of bai huan shu (UB 30), you can also usually find round shaped blockage sections. With regards to sciatica, at dan shu (UB 19) (illness side), there should be round shaped or thin flat shaped blockage sections or sensitive pressing pain.

Treatment technique: can combine with zu san li (St 36), yang ling quan (GB 34). Inserting the needle 8 fen - 1 cun, use strong pressure to inject the medicine. The needle sensation should feel like it is radiating towards the leg.

12.   Chest pain.

Diagnosis and treatment of channel points opposite positions to the part of the chest pain at the back, like fei shu (UB 13), du shu (UB 16) having block sections or sensitive pressing pain. The centre position of the chest has pain and hui zhong (TH 7) has pressing pain.

Treatment technique: enter the needle 5-8 fen medicine injection. Using pressure inject the medicine at medium speed. Needle sensation radiating towards the front of the chest.

13.   Shoulder and upper arm pain

Diagnosis and treatment of channel points; jian wai shu (SI 14), jian tong dian (Ex.pt.), round shaped block sections or sensitive pressing pain.

Treatment technique: enter the needle 5-8 fen medicine injection. Injecting the medicine at medium speed. The needling sensation should radiate towards the shoulder and the arm.

14.   Torticollis (Wry neck)

Diagnosis and treatment of channel points; between tian zhu (UB 10) and tian rong (SI 17) there should be sensitive pressing pain points.

Treatment technique: entering needle 5 fen. Combine with xuan zhong (GB 39) (left side or right side), using medicine injections and injecting the medicine at medium speed.

15.   Sinusitis, upper jaw sinus cavity inflammation, epistaxis (nose bleeding)

Diagnosis and treatment of channel points: both sides of the sixth cervical vertebrae, round shape block sections. Fei shu (UB 15) having flat slab block sections.

Treatment technique: entering needle 3-5 fen. Using medicine injection, inject the medicine at a moderate to slow speed. The needle sensation should feel like a mild form of conduction going towards the upper or head parts. Allergic type sinusitis, combined with zi tian zu chi (Ex. Pt.) (located below LI 11 - 1 cun). Nose bleeding, combine with right or left side jian jing (GB 21) (when inserting the needle 3-5 fen, you should be careful not to needle too deep).

16.   Oral cavity inflammation, oral cavity pappy (ie. ulcerated)

Diagnosis and treatment of channel points: at chen jiang point (CV 24) you should find block sections or pressing pain.

Treatment technique: insert the needle 3 fen, using medicine injections, you can combine with chen jiang (CV 24), pi shu (UB 20), left side or right side qu chi (LI 11).

17.   Middle ear inflammation, otis mastoidea

Diagnosis and treatment of channel points: at yi feng (TH 17), there should be pressing pain or block sections. Shen shu (UB 23) is a positive point.

Treatment technique: insert the needle 8 fen - 1 cun. Using medicine injection, combine with qu chi (LI 11) (disease side).

18. Conjunctivitis (syndesmitis)

Diagnosis and treatment of channel points: at fei shu (UB 15), pi shu (UB 20), gan shu (UB 18) you should find positive reaction points.
Treatment technique: insert needle 5-8 fen, using medicine injection.

19. Nebula, keratoleukoma (leukoma).

Diagnosis and treatment of channel points; at gan shu (UB 18) and on one side or both sides of the fourth cervical vertebrae, you should find round shaped block sections or flat blockage sections.
Treatment technique: insert needle 5-8 fen, using medicine injection.

20. Optic atrophy, retinitis

Diagnosis and treatment of channel points: at gan shu (UB 18) and shen shu (UB 23) you should find flat slab or round shaped block sections, and under feng shi (GB 20) you may find slab or round shaped block sections.
Treatment technique: insert needle 5-8 fen, entering from the slab block section under feng chi towards the opposite side eyes direction. Use placenta tissue liquid, or vitamin B1.

21. Neurasthenia

Diagnosis and treatment of channel points: at jue yin shu (UB 14), you can usually find round shaped or oval shaped block sections. xin shu (UB 15), gan shu (UB18), left side or right side having positive reactions.
Treatment technique: insert needle 3-5 fen, medicine injection. If the patient has gastro intestinal disorder or irregularity, add liang qiu (St 34) or zu san li (St 36), (left side or right side).

22. Headache, nervous type headache

Diagnosis and treatment of channel points: under feng chi (GB 20) or at tian zhu (UB 10), you should find round shaped block sections.

Treatment technique: insert needle 3-5 fen, medicine injection. Can combine with lie qie (LU 7).

23. Facial nerve paralysis (palsey)

Diagnosis and treatment of channel points: on the diseased side qian zhen point (Ex. Pt.) you should find round shaped block sections. Wen liu point (LI 7) may also have oval shaped block sections.

Treatment technique: insert needle 3-5 fen, medicine injection. Can also combine with disease side yin xiang point (LI 20).

24. Nephritis

Diagnosis and treatment of channel points: at shen shu (UB 23) and at shen re point (Ex.pt.), in acute cases oval shaped or diamond shaped block sections can usually be seen. For those chronic cases, one may see flat slab shapes or thin bar chains.

Treatment technique: insert needle 8 fen - 1 cun, medicine injection.

25. Bed wetting

Diagnosis and treatment of channel points: shen shu (UB 23), pang guang shu (UB 28), and zhong shu (GV 7), all should have both sides round shaped block sections or pressing pain.

Treatment technique: insert needle 8 fen - 1 fen, medicine injection. Using pressure inject the medicine so that a needle feelings radiates towards the front. Can combine with zhong ji (CV 3), shui fen (CV 9).

26. Irregular mensuration, adenitis

Diagnosis and treatment of channel points: at pi shu (UB 20) or gan shu (UB 18), and at guan yuan shu (UB 26), local area you should find some round shaped tubercules or pressing pain. Insert needle 8 fen - 1 cun, medicine injection. Inject medicine at a medium speed with a needle sensation radiating downwards or upwards. Can combine with san yin jiao (Sp 6).

27. Urticaria, pruritus, eczema

Diagnosis and treatment of channel points: at da zhui (GV 14), fei shu (UB 13), ge shu (UB 17), qu chi (Li 11) have nodes or pressure pain.

Treatment technique: Insert 3 – 5 fen inject in herbal solution. Those lower limbs a lot add xue hai (Sp 10), those upper half body add jiu wei (CV 15); Pruritus condition add left side or right side da zhu (UB 11); eczema combine san yin jiao (Sp 6). Skin itching a lot condition add left side or right side da zhu point (UB11); eczema combined with san yin jiao (Sp6).

28. Psoriasis, neuro - dermatitis

Diagnosis and treatment of channel points: at da zhui (GV 14), left side or right side should show positive reactions. At the seventh thoracic vertebrae or the eighth thoracic vertebrae, either on the left side or right side, you should also be able to find bar sections or positive reactions.

Treatment technique: insert the needle 5-8 fen, medicine injection. Can be combined with qu chi (LI 11).

29. High blood pressure

Diagnosis and treatment of channel points: at xue ya dian (Ex.pt.), on the left side, one should find round shaped block sections, while at tian zong (SI 11) there may also be sensitive pressing pain. Gan shu point (UB 18) additionally, may have positive reactions.

Treatment technique: insert needle 3-5 fen, medicine injection. Can combine with ze tian qu chi [under qu chi (LI 11) 1 cun].

30. Anemia

Diagnosis and treatment of channel points: at ge shu (UB 17) and at pi shu (UB 20), the muscles often tend to become soft and relaxed or sunken or one may see small bar sections.

Treatment technique: insert needle 3-5 fen, medicine injection.

31. Nervous (alarmed, flustered), palpitations

Diagnosis and treatment of channel points: at xin shu (UB15) (left side) one may often see round shaped block sections.

Treatment technique: insert needle 3-5 fen, medicine injection. Can combine with ju que (CV 14), yin xi (H 6).

32. Schizophrenia, depression and epilepsy (dian xian)

Diagnosis and treatment of channel points: at da zhui (GV 14), xin shu (CV 15) (left side), and yi shu (UB 49) (left side or right side), you should be able to feel positive reactions.

Treatment technique: insert the needle 3-5 fen. With regards to depression and epilepsy, you can combine with jiu wei (UB 15), and ya men (GV 15), medicine injection. On the other hand for schizophrenia you may combine with needling ren zhong (GV 26).

33. Haemorrhoids, prolapse of the anus

Diagnosis and treatment of channel points: at da chang shu (UB 25), and guan yuan shu (UB 26), you should find round shaped or thin flat shaped block sections.

Treatment technique: insert the needle 8 fen - 1 cun, medicine injection. For those haemorrhoid patients who have bleeding with the stools, can combine with ge shu (UB 17), kong zui (LU 6).

34. Hernia

Diagnosis and treatment of channel points; at xiao chang shu (UB 27), and guan yuan shu (UB 26), you should find round shaped block sections.

Treatment technique: insert the needle 5 - 8 fen, medicine injection. Can combine with qi men [Extra point beside guan yuan (CV 4) to the side (i.e. lateral) 3 cun].

35. Uterus prolapse

Diagnosis and treatment of channel points: at pi shu (UB 20), you will quite often find the muscle soft and relaxed or sunken or having a small bar section. Gan shu (UB 18) also usually has pressing pain or block sections.

Treatment technique: insert the needle 5 - 8 fen, medicine injection. Can combine with tan zhone (CV 17), qi men (Extra point, as above), san yin jia (SP 6), all of which should have positive reactions in their respective local areas.

36. Hair loss

Diagnosis and treatment of channel points: at du shu (UB 16) and shen shu (UB 23), there should be round shape block sections.

Treatment technique techniques: insert the needle 5 - 8 fen, medicine injection.

37. Stroke, after - effects

Diagnosis and treatment of channel points: for those with half body numbness or hemiplegic, use gan shu (UB 18), shen shu (UB 23), and jian tong dian (Extra pt.) all of which should have block sections or bar sections.

Treatment technique: inserting the needle 5 -8 fen, medicine injection. If the lower limbs are affected, can combine with yang ling quan (GB 34). For those patients whose tongue is stiff and cannot speak, can combines with xin shu (UB 15), and you can needle lian quan (CV 23); for those patients with high blood pressure, and dizziness, combine with xue ya dian (Extra pt.).

38. Whooping cough

Diagnosis and treatment of channel points: at fei shu (UB 13), (you should find block sections), tan zhong (CV 17).

Treatment technique: insert needle 5 - 8 fen, medicine injection. Can combine with ding chuan point (Extra pt.).

39. Thromboangitis obliterns (Buerger's disease)

Diagnosis and treatment of channel points: at xin shu (UB 15), pi shu (UB 20), ge shu (UB 17), and in front of the area around the inside of the ankle bone, you should find positive reaction points.

Treatment technique: insert needle 5 - 8 fen, medicine injection.

40. After effects of infantile paralysis

Treatment principle

1. Take the touch positive reaction points as the major treatment channel points. Normally at gan shu (UB 18), dan shu (UB 19), wei shu (UB 21), and shen shu (UB 23) you can touch bean chain shape, round shape, or bar section reaction objects.
2. Treatment course: from 1 - 5 years old, 7 times as a course. Over 6 years old, 10 - 15 times at a course, can stop 3 -5 days between the courses.
3. After the treatment has some effect, you should incorporate specific exercises to improve the effect. The channel and collateral treatment is usually used only on the disease side.
4. For each treatment use only one group of treatment points, or two groups in appropriate combination.

Divide into groups for treatment (according to the different conditions of the limbs and body)

1. Difficulty in raising the legs group (the main problem is the muscle is paralysed), take the zu yang ming stomach channel as the main treatment channel.

Points:

(1) Qi chong (St 30), fu tu (St 32), 1 cun above feng shi (GB 31), jie xi (St 41), needling pierce actual local points. jie xi (St 41), add
(2) Bi guan (St 31), ci liao (UB 32), zu san li (St 36),

2. Foot turned inside group (external side muscle group paralysis), take gall bladder channel, and urinary bladder channel as the main treatment channels.

Points:

(1) Feng shi (GB 31), zu san li (St 36), shen mai (UB 62), and zheng nei fuan (Ex.pt). Can needle shu gu (UB 65), or jing gu (UB 64).
(2) 2 cun above feng shi (GB 31), yang ling quan (GB 34), and xuan zhong (GB 39). Can needle shu gu (UB 65), kun lun (UB 60), jing gu (UB 64).

3. Foot turned out group (internal muscle group paralysis), take spleen channel as main treatment.

Points:

(1) Xue hai (Sp 10), di ji (Sp 8), and zheng wai fan (Ex.pt.). Can needle da du (Sp 2).
(2) Qi men (Liv 14), san yin jiao (Sp 6), and Zhao hai (K 6). Can needle yin bai (Sp 1).

4. Horse-foot (talipes equinus)

Points:

(1) Fu tu (St 32), zu san li (St 36), and ji xi (St 41). Can needle nei ting (St 44), and yin men (UB 51). At cheng shan (UB 57), can also inject an appropriate amount of 0.5 -1% procaine.

(2)   Bi guan (St 31), xia ju xu (St 37), zu xia qiu dian (Ex. Pt), qiu xu (GB 40), and shen mai (UB 62). Can needle xiang jian (Liv 2). At cheng shan (UB 57), and kun lun (UB 60), can inject appropriate amount of 0.5 - 1 % procaine.

5.   Shoulder external muscle group paralysis (internal sore type): jian wai shu (SI 14), da zhu (UB 11), dan shu (U B19), tian zong (SI 11), jian yu (LI 15), tai bi xue (Ex.pt.), bi shen (Ex.pt.), jian jia gu wai yuan, positive block section (jian tong dian). The above points according to the different conditions make combination in use.

6.   Hand fingers contracted (spastic), cannot take objects; jian wai shu (SI 14), qu chi (LI 11), yu ji (Lu 10), he gu (LI 4), hou xi (SI 3), lao gong (P 8), yang chi (TH8), si feng (Ex.pt.). The above points can appropriately select from.

41   Deafness, dumbness (aphasia)

(i)   Treatment principle

1.   Treatment principles is that for deafness, is to treat dumbness by training the patient to speak. So, deafness and dumbness should be combined in treatment. Using channel and collateral injection acupuncture treatment and speaking training. Combine these three measures as a treatment technique.
2.   Find and touch the positive points as major treatment points. Usually can touch thin flat shape block sections, round shape block sections, and sensitive pressing pain, at shen shu (UB 23), san jiao shu (UB 22).
3.   Each ten times as a course. Stop 3-5 days between the courses.

(ii)   Treatment technique

1.   Treatment as a group: according to the total degree of deafness and dumbness, half deaf and dumb, after treatment of the listening ability, recovery comes back, accordingly can divide the group for treatment.
2.   Major channel points: san jiao shu (UB 22), shen shu (UB23), hui zong (TH 7), yi feng (TH 17), tian gong (SI 19), wai guan (TH 5), ting ming (Ex. pt.), er men (TH 21), xia ting hui (tiang hui below 5 fen), long xue (Ex.pt.), zhong zhu (TH 3), etc. Alternative section - usually for deafness combine the disease side yi feng (TH 17). After having listening ability, add ya dian (Ex.pt.), ya men (GV 15), xian shu (UB 15), etc.

Needling shang lian quan (Ex.pt.), tou wei (St 8), external jin jiang yu ye (Ex. Pt.).

3. First time treat patient, use shu points using medicine injection. The other channel points combine with acupuncture. After two times treatment, for those points surrounding the ear, use a small amount of medicine injection. This will improve or maintain listening ability. Has some effect.

4. Should treat those combination diseases. For deafness combined with tinnitus, should combine with yi ming (TH 17), he gu (LI 4), zu san li (St 36), xia ting hui (Ex.pt.). For those with low intelligence combine with xin shu (UB 15), shen shu (UB 23), shen men (H 7), bai hui (GV 20). For those having digestive tract syndrome, combine with wei shu (UB 21), da chang shu (UB 25).

The above statement indicates or points out the practical diagnosis and treatment of main points in the channel and collateral treatment technique. So, channel and collateral treatment technique, as an acupuncture practical assistant to treatment techniques, has some practical value in use.

CHAPTER 3
....
Instruction Of Channel And Collateral Theory In Application Of Medicine (Yao)

Chinese medicine theory in instruction of practical application, mainly has si qi (four qi) and five wei (tastes), sheng jiang fou chen (raising, lowering, floating and sinking), and medicines gui jing (return to the channel). So the four qi is the conversion of medicine characteristics as the five tastes are the classification of the medicine tasks. Sheng jiang fou chen is the action of medicine on the human body; medicine gui jing is the specific action and result of medicine on the human body. Organ and bowels, channel and collaterals desire change. They all together make an integral medicine theory system and guides the practical application of medicine.

The following analysis is the relationship between the medicine theory and channel and collateral theory, and in the instruction meaning of channel and collateral theory in application of medicine.

Section 1
Relation between the four qi and the channel and collateral theory

Therefore, the so called qi is the medicines' characteristic. The four qi means the medicine is cold, hot, warm or cool ie. the four different kinds of medicine characteristics. Cool and cold, warm and hot, the only difference is in the field of medicine characteristics. However, cold, cool and warm and hot, are two kinds of different medicines which have the opposite properties. The four qi classification is mainly determined by the different reaction and treatment effects after the medicine acts on the human body. So the cold and cool medicines have clean out effects (qing re), remove fire (xie huo) and remove toxins (jei du), they are used for curing hot conditions. For example, shi gao (gypsum), zhi mu (anemarrhena), huang lian (coptis), zhi zi (cape jasmine fruit), yin hua (honeysuckle), lian qiao (forsythia) etc. Some herbs are warm/hot medicines for removing cold, warming the internal (wen li), assist yang (zhu yang) used for curing cold conditions. For example, fu zi (aconite), gan jiang (dried ginger), rougui (cinnamon), ai ye (artemesia), ba ji (morinda) etc.

Su wen zhi zhen ao da lun said "for those adverse/inverted try positive, for those correct, then try as negative. For those having heat, then cool, for those having cold, then heat them; for those deficiency, then tonify it, for those excess, sedate it". This is a correct/true treatment. The four qi points out the general rule of medicine application when applying the principal of true treatment (zhen zhi).

However, the medicine classification of the four qi is not very detailed. The correct procedure points out the rule applying medicine for specific disease conditions. The twelve channels disease forecasting and according to the channels and zang fu, through cold hot deficiency and excess conditions, make a predictive condition, allowing for an introduction to the four qi application. So, the 12 channels make for forecasting, this indicates that the medicine connects with the climate condition. Having a great inspiration for other doctors to treat disease according to the zang fu ben zhen (formation treatments) using four qi theory and according to the disease conditions using medicine. Such as Zhang yuan su, summarised zang-fu example, cold hot deficiency and excess medicine formulation/formulae (Table 11), according to warm cool, tonify sedate as the treatment principal.

According to zang fu jing luo and concluding using this medicine treatment, this indicates that the four qi, when it was created, had a clear reaction with the channel and collateral theory. The four qi theory application, only under the direction of channel collateral theory, can have application while in the product situation.

TABLE 11: Zang Fu External Internal Cold Hot Deficiency Excess Use Of Herbs

1. Lungs

Deficiency Excess

Reduce Excess

Sedate The Son: Zhe xie, ting li, sang pi, di gu pi.

Remove Dampness: Ban xin, bai fan, bai fu ling, yi ren, mu gua, chen pi.

Reduce Fire: Geng mi, shi gao, Han shui shi, zhi muscle, he zi.

Unblock Stagnancy: Zhi qiao, bo he, sheng jiang, mu xiang, xing ren, hou pou, za jiao, jie geng, su geng.

Tonify Deficiency

Tonify Mother: Gan cao, ren shen, sheng ma, huang qi, shan yao.

Moisten Dryness: Ge ke, e jiao, mai dong, chuan mu, bai he, tian hua fen, tian dong.

Consolidate Lungs: Wu mei, su qiao, wu wei zi, bai shao, wu bei zi

External Root

Clean Out Heat ----- Clean out root heat (Clean metal): Huang qin, zhi mu, mai dong, zhi zi, sha shen, zi wan, tian dong.

Remove Cold

Warm Root Cold (Warm Lungs):
Ding xiang, huo xiang, kuan dong hua, tan xiang, bai dou kou, yi zhi ren, sha ren, shu mi, bai bu.

Spread Root Cold (Remove Surface):
Ma huang, jiu bai, zi su.

		Sedate Excess	Sedate Heat:	Da huang, mang xiao, ge hua, qian niu, ba dou, yu li ren, shi gao.
			Sedate Qi:	Zhi qiao, mu xiang, chen pi, bing lang.
			Tonify Qi:	Za jiao.
	Deficienty Excess	Tonify Deficiency	Moisten Dryness:	Tao ren, ma ren, xing ren, di huang, ru xiang, song zi, dang gui, rou cong rong
2. Large Intestines			Dry Dampness:	Bai zhu, cang zhu, ban xia, liu huang.
			Raise Sunken:	Sheng ma, ge gen.
			Consolidate Collapse:	Long gu, bai e, he zi, su qiao, wu mei, bai fan, chi shi zhi, yu shi liang, shi liu pi.
	External Root	Clean Out Heat	Clean Out Root Heat:	Qin jiao, huai jiao, di huang, huang qin.

External Root — Clean Out Heat — Spread External Heat (Remove From Muscle): Shi Tao, Bai zhi, Sheng ma, Ge gen.

(Warm Interior): Gan

		Sedate Excess	Sedate Damp Heat:	Dai huang, mang xiao.
			Resolve Food & Drinks:	Ba dou, shen qu, zha rou, e gui, nao shi, yu jin, shan leng, qin fen.
	Deficiency Excess		Transport Damp Heat:	Cang zhu, bai zhu, ban xia, fu ling, chen pi, sheng jiang.
3. Stomach		Tonify Deficiency	Spread Cold Dampness:	Gan jiang, fu zi, cao guo, gong gui, ding xiang, rou guo, ren shen, huang qi.

External Root	Clean Out Root Heat (Lower Fire):	Shi gao, di huang, xi jiao, huang lian
	Remove External Heat (From Muscles):	Sheng ma, ga gen, dou chi.

		Sedate The Son:	He zi, fang feng, sang pi, ting li.
	Sedate Excess	Unblock Vomiting:	Dou chi, zhi zi, lou bu zi, chang shan, gua di, yu jin, ji zhi, luo lu, ku shen, chi xiao dou, yang tang, ku cha.
Deficiency Excess		Sedate Lower:	Dai huang, mang xiao, meng shi, da ji, xu sui zi, ge hua, gan sui.
		Tonify The Mother:	Gui xin, fu ling.
	Tonify Earth	Tonify The Qi:	Ren shen, huang qi, sheng ma, ge gen, gan cao, chen pi, huo xiang, yu zhu, sha ren, mu xiang, bian dou.
4. Spleen		Tonify The Blood:	Bai zhu, cang zhu, bai shao, jiao yi, da zao, gan jiang, mu gua, wu, me, feng mi.
	Remove Root Dampness	Dry Central Palace:	Bai zhu, cang zhu, chen pi, ban xia, nan xing, yu tou, cao dou kou, bai jie zi.
External Root		Clean The Bowels:	Mu tong, shi fu ling, zhu ling, huo xiang.
	Resolve External Damp ---------	Open the Ghost Door:	Ge gen, cang zhu, ma huang, du huo.

5. Small Intestines	Deficiency Excess	Sedate Excess Heat:	Qi Fen:	Mu tong, zhu ling, hua shi, qu mai, zhe xie, deng cao.
			Blood Fen:	Di huang, pu huang, chi ling, zhi zi, dan pi.
		Tonify Deficient Cold	Qi Fen:	Bai zhu, lei wan, hui xiang, sha ken, shen qu, bian dou.
			Blood Fen:	Gui xin, yuan hu suo.
	External Root	Cool Root Heat (Reduce Fire):		Huang bai, huang qin, huang lian, lian qiao, zhi zi.
		Spread External Heat (From Muscles):		Gao ben, qiang huo, fang feng, man jing.
6. Urinary Bladder	Deficiency Excess	Sedate Excess Heat (Drain Fire):		Hua shi, zhu ling, zhe xie, fu ling.
		Tonify Lower Deficiency	Nourish Yin Clean out Heat:	Zhi mu, huang bai.
			Unblock Qi Spread Cold:	Jie geng, sheng ma, yi zhi ren, wu yao, yu rou.
	External Root	Unblock Root Heat (Reduce Fire):		Di huang, zhi zi, yin chen, huang bai, dan pi, di gu pi.
		Remove External Cold (Remove External):		Ma huang, gui zhi, qiang huo, fang ji, huang qi, mu zei cao, cang zhu

	Sedate Water Strong	Sedate The Son:	Qiu niu, da ji.
		Sedate The Bowels:	Zhe xie, zhu ling, che qian zi, fang ji, fu ling.
	Tonify Weak Water	Tonify Mother:	Ren shen, shan yao.
		Qi Fen:	Zhi mu, xuan shen, pu gu zhi, sha ren, ku shen.
		Xue Fen:	Huang bai, gou qi, shou di, suo yang, cong rong, yu rou, e jiao, wu wei zi.
Deficiency Excess	Fire Strong (Sedate Mutual Fire):		Huang bai, zhi mu, dan pi, di gu pi, sheng di, fu ling, xuan shen, han shui shi.
	Tonify Fire Weak (Increase Yang):		Fu zi, rou gui, yi zhi ren, pu gu zhi, chen xiang, chuan wu, liu huang, tian xiong, wu yao, yang qi shi, hui xiang, Hu tao, ba ji, dan sha, dang gui, ge ke, fu pen zi.
	Jing Collapse (Astringe Slippery):		Mu li, qian shi, jin ying zi, wu wei zi, yuan shi, yu rou, ge fen.
	Conquer Root Heat (Down):		Same as Cheng Qi Variations Technique
External Root	Cool External Heat (Clean Out):		Xuan shen, lian qiao, gan cao, zhu fu.
	Warm Root Cold (Warm Interior):		Fu zi, gan jiang, gong gui, bai zhu, chuan jiao.
	Remove Cold Exterior (Remove Exterior)		Ma huang, xi xin, du huo, gui zhi

7. Kidneys

		Sedate The Son:	Huang lian, dai huang.
	Sedate Excess Fire	Qi Fen:	Gan cao, ren shen, chi ling, mu tong, huang bai.
		Xue Fen:	Dan shen, dan pi, sheng di, xuan shen.
Deficiency Excess		Calm Fright:	Zhu sha, niu huang, zi shi ying.
	Tonify Spirit Deficiency	Tonify the Mother:	Xi xin, wu mei, zao ren, sheng jiang, chen pi.
		Qi Fen:	Gui xin, zhe xie, bai fu ling, yuan zhi, fu shen, shi chang pu.
		Blood Fen:	Dang gui, shou di, ru xiang, mo yao.
	Cool Root Heat	Sedate Fire:	Huang qin, zhu zhi, mai dong, mang xiao, chao yan.
External Root		Cool Blood:	Sheng di, zhi zi, tian zhu huang.
	Remove External Heat (Spread Fire):		Gan cao, du huo, ma huang, chai hu, long nao.

8. Heart

9. Triple Heater	Deficiency Excess	Sedate Excess Fire	Sweating:	Ma huang, chai hu, ge gen, jing jie, sheng ma, bo he, qiang huo, shi gao.
			Vomiting:	Gua di, cang yan, ji zhi.
			Lower:	Dai huang, mang xiao.
		Tonify Deficiency Fire	Upper Heater:	Ren shen, tian xiong, gui xin.
			Middle Heater:	Ren shen, huang qi, ding xiang, mu xiang, cao guo.
			Lower Heater:	Hei fu zi, rou gui, liu hang, ren shen, chen xiang, wu yao, pu gu zhi.
	External Root	Cool Root Heat	Upper Heater:	Huang qin, lian chao, zhi zi, zhi mu, xuan shen, shi gao, sheng di.
			Middle Heater:	Huang lian, lian qiao, sheng di, shi gao.
			Lower Heater:	Huang bai, zhi mu, sheng di, shi gao, dan pi, di gu pi.
		Spread External Heat (Remove Surface):		Chai hu, xi xin, jing jie, qiang huo, ge gen, shi gao.
10. Gall Bladder	Deficiency Excess	Sedate Excess Fire (Sedate Gall Bladder):		Long dan cao, niu chi, zhu dan, sheng wei ren, sheng suan zao ren, huang lian, ku cha.
		Tonify Xu Huo (Fire):		Ren shen, ban xia, xi xin, dang gui, chao wei ren, chao zao ren, di huang.
	External Root	Balance Root Heat	Remove Fire:	Huang qin, huang han, shao yao, lian qiao, gan cao.
			Calm Fright:	Hei qian, shui yin.
		Harmonise External Heat (Remove Surface):		Chai hu, shao yao, huang qin, ban xia, gan cao.

11. Liver				
	Deficiency Excess	Sedate Excess	Sedate Son:	Gan Cao.
			Circulate Qi:	Xiang fu, chuan chiong, qu mai, qian niu, qing pi.
			Circulate Blood:	Hong hua, bie jia, tao ren, e zhu, san leng, chuan shang jin, dai huang, shui zhi, mang chong, su mu, dan pi.
			Calm Fright:	Xiong huang, jin bo, tie luo, zhen zhu, dai zhe shi, ye ming sha, hu fen, yin bo, qian dan, long gu, shi jue ming.
			Resolves Wind:	Qiang huo, jing jie, bo he, huai zi, man jing zi, bai hua she, du huo, zao jia, wu tou, fang feng, bai fu zi, jiang can, chan tui.
		Tonify Not Enough	Tonify The Mother:	Gou qi, du zhong, gou ji, shou di, ku shen, bi xie, e jiao, tu su zi.
			Tonify Blood:	Dang gui, niu xi, xu duan, bai shao, xue ji, mo yao, chuan chiong.
			Tonify Qi:	Tian ma, bai zi ren, bai zhu, ju hua, xi xin, mi meng hua, jue ming, gu jing zi, sheng jiang.
	External Root	Cool Root Heat	Sedate Wood:	Shao yao, wu mei, zhe xie.
			Sedate Fire:	Huang lian, long dan che, huang qin, ku cha, zhu dan.
			Conquer Internal:	Dai huang.
		Remove External Heat	Balance Remove:	Chai hu, ban xia.
			Remove From Muscle:	Gui zhi, ma huang.

Section 2
The relationship between the five tastes and channel and collateral theory

The five tastes (wu wei) are the types of tastes: suan (sour), xin (pungent), tian (sweet), ku (bitter), yan (salty) of the medicines. So differentiation of the five tastes mainly depends on the tastes and the five organs and direct differentiation's, and can therefore also be according to the relation effect in practice book.

The using of the five tastes, is according to the medicine tastes differentiation and conclusion of the treatment effect of medicine. For instance, pungent taste medicine can permeate (fa xie), and eliminate from the surface (jie biao), mainly re the qi, and circulating blood (sun qi huo xue). Gui zhi (cinnamon), su ye (perilla leaves), sheng jiang (ginger) taste pungent so usually cure for (jie biao) the surface well; chen pi (orange skin), xiang fu (cyperus root), sha ren (amomum) taste pungent and are used for running the qi and spreading blockage (sen he), sour tasting medicines and should suo (astringe) and gu se (consolidate).

That's why wu mei (black mumes), shi liu pi (pomegranate skin) treat long time diarrhoea condition, shan yu rou, wu wei zi treat sweating, and stop emission. Sweet tending medicines can normalise, tonify, strengthen and balance (moderate). So to use dang shen (codonopsis) for tonifying the qi, shou di for increasing the blood, da zao for sweet moderating and balancing the centre. The bitter tasting medicine can clean out heat and remove fire, pump out the lower (tong bian), remove the poisons / detoxify, strengthen the yin. So to use huang qin (scutellaria), for cleaning out heat and removing the fire, using huang lian (coptis) for cleaning out heat and drying dampness; using dai huang (rhubarb) for cleaning out heat and unblocking the stools; use di ding (rhododendri) to clean out heat and remove poisons. Use huang bai (phellodendron) for conserving the kidney (qu shen) the yin (shen yin). Salty tasting medicines can soften hardness and moisten remove (run xia), so use hai zao (sargassum) for softening hardness and removing phlegm with ruan xia for moisture and unblocking and removing stools (xia tong bian).

Another meaning of the five tastes (wu wei) is in the directing of the medicine with different tastes and having the differing choices re the effects of treatment of the five organs. *Su wen zhi zhen yao da lun* said: "Five tastes into the stomach, each having its own preferable way of attacking, the sour part goes into the liver, bitter first goes into the heart, sweetness first goes into the spleen, pungent first goes into the lungs, salty first goes into the kidneys. Long time then increase the qi, increase for a long time, which is where health comes from." This indicates that the medicine and the organ and bowels having the internal relationship of five tastes, return to five zang. Therefore in practice, best to employ a medicine and intended organ performance, ie. to choose suitable medicines to treat several diseases.

So, five tastes returning to the five organs is not simply using the five elements theory. It is ancient doctors, under the instruction of channel collateral organ or bowels theory, via the practice of summarising the medicine treatment rule. Someone's enumeration of 72 tastes recorded in the *zhong zan yao xue gai lun* results indicate that the five tastes returning to five zang reflect most conditions of the medicines. For example, the salty enters into the kidney occupies 57.1%, sour enters into the liver occupies 56.25%, pungent enters into the lungs and large intestines occupies 50%. Sweet enters into the spleen and stomach occupies 45.61%. See example *zhong yi za zhi* 1961 volume 5, page 40. This illustrates that the five tastes returning to five zang match with the standard law of medicine. It has a practical meaning so that it confirms that the theory of the five tastes has close relations with channel collateral theory.

Section 3
The relationship between rising, lowering, floating, sinking laws and channel and collateral theory

After medicines go into human body, they can produce a recovering raising, lowering down, dispersing (fa san), draining etc. actions. So the summary of these kinds of trends of the medicine is called sheng jiang fou chen. Sheng jiang fou chen mainly depends on the medicines as together and whether the medicines are heavy or light. The *Su wen-yin yang ying nang da lun* said: "taste thick therefore then promotes diarrhoea, thin (bo) promotes unblocking. Qi thin promotes removal from surface (fa xie), thick then expels fever. Sheng jiang fou chen in practice means qi thin has fa san (removing from the surface action) controls raising like ma huang, chai hu, sheng ma, ge gen category. Qi thick has warming internal action, controls floating, like fu zi, gan jiang, rou gui, wu yu category. Taste thick also has promoting diarrhoea, cleaning out fire action, controls sinking (chen); like dai huang, mang xiao, huang lian, huang bai etc medicines. Taste thin has unblocking sinking constantly lowering action, controls (zhu) going down, like fu ling, tong cao, zhe xie, chuan shan jia, shi jue ming etc medicines.

Sheng jiang fou chen dictates the medicine and because of the difference of qi wei (taste) and zhi di can produce different trends of treatment action on the body, this actually reflects the channels and collaterals re the medicine's property having a transmission centre and function classification. If without a cycle transfer of channels and collaterals, then without channels and collaterals as transfer of ying wei, qi and blood pass through, without the channels and collaterals combining the body doesn't become a unit integrating things, then of course there would not be sheng jiang fou chen, ie. this type of treatment trend. Therefore, sheng jiang fou chen is completed, depending on the channel and collaterals. That's why channel and collaterals theory is the main source/reason to form medicine's sheng jiang fou chen theory.

Section 4
Medicines return to the channel, and it's relationship with channel and collateral theory

In accordance to the function of medicine and the study and suggestions that medicines' specific actions and connections to the human body's organs and bowels (zang fu) via the channels and collaterals. This is called "yao wu gui jing".

Ancient people, through long time practice, discovered that the medicine in treatment of yao wu, and jing luo have selectivity. This means there is a special connection between medicine and zang-fu jing luo. However this connection is not only limited to five tastes matching the 5 zang. So, its range is broader, therefore during the study of treatment, relations between medicine and organs and bowels produced the theory of yao wu gui jing. You can see from the literature how Han dynasty Ben cao books, there is not a mention of gui jing. In the book of Wang Hao gu *Tang ye ben cao* started using gui jing statements due to the place. Yi yen's Zhang school of thought (ru pai) progressed/theory promotion, also the "gui jing" theory, itself having practical value. After the Jin Yuan dynasty, a collective of doctors use channels and collaterals with "gui jing" theory. This illustrates that "yao wu gui jing" is in the production of Chinese medicine development. This indicates/emphasises that the ancient people led a non shallow realisation of the classics and their reasons, ie. the medicine's characteristics. So in practice, use only 4 qi and 5 tastes, really raising, lowering, floating, sinking medicine theories cannot illustrate the medicine's specific spread action during treatment such as, for example, some with local condition/syndrome have local coldness, but stomach coldness is different; same with hot condition, there are differences in being hot and stomach hot. So depending on conditions, again have spleen deficiency and kidney deficiency difference. So the medicines that can remove coldness, may not remove the stomach coldness. The medicine can clear being hot, but may not clear the stomach heat; the medicines can tonify the spleen, may not tonify the kidney. This indicates that various zang fu, and in the form two diseases, re medicines, have specific requirements and situations. This is the result produced by medicines "return to channels" (yao wu gui jing) theory, and having the gui jing theory we can closely analyse the specific affects appearing in the practice treatment using different medicines, so as to correctly guide the application of medicine to be suitable for the complex various disease conditions. In practice, treatment such as the "remove heart fire" medicines, like huang lian (coptis) which serves best, huang qin (scutelaria) for removing lung fire (zhi zi assists it), again removing large intestine fire; chai hu (buplerium) serves best in liver and gall-bladder fire (haung lian assists it), again, removes triple heat or fire (huang qin assists it); ba shao removes spleen fire; zhi mu removes kidney fire; mu tong removes small intestine fire; shi gao removes stomach fire; huang bai removes urinary bladder fire. In practice, it helps to choose the most suitable, most effective medicines for the treatment of disease conditions. This not only can handle or reasonably use medicines but also can closely combine the application of medicines and differentiation.

The practical use of 'gui jing' theory and also the treatment principle of the yao wu in disease differentiate treatment, ie. different disease same treatment (tong bing yi zhi, yi bing tong zhi), and the rule of practical application of medicine, such as qi tuo (qi deficiency collapse) ie. prolapse of anus long time diarrhoea; spleen cannot control blood, long term dampness affecting the spleen, in the practical syndrome can be seen as several kinds of total deficiency diseases, however the reasons are spleen deficiency. This can use the principal of different disease, same treatment. All "belong to spleen channel" tonify the spleen medicines like ren shen, bai zhu, huang qi, sheng ma, chen pi, da zao etc. according to the prescriptive components principal in combination becomes the prescription ruling the treatment. Also, an example is oedema. Classic chinese medicine thinks the disease reason is mainly related to the lung, spleen, kidney and urinary bladder. The *Nei jing* says "drinks enters the stomach, increases jing goes up to the spleen qi, spreads jing, goes up to the lungs unblocks and balances the water passages". Also says "shen zhi shui zang, zhu jin ye. Pang guang zhe, zhou du zhe guan, jin ye zeng yi, qi hua za neng chu yi" "the kidney is a water organ, controls the liquids. Urinary bladder is captain of the province/city, those friends (jing yi) are hidden there, qi transform then can go out." Wang Hao gu said, "water, spleen, lungs, kidney, three channels control it". Indicates the lungs re physiology function have the ability to adjust the body's water liquid and pass through action/strategy. The spleen has the action of transport and transfer water liquids. The kidney also has a close relation with water liquids management and adjustment, that's why the lungs, spleen, kidney 3 channels having disease change, all can produce edema. However, the reason for edema type, the medicine selection should also be different. Bai zhu, zhu ling, tong cao, all have move/transport water action. In practice, this tells us bai zhu, zhu ling, tong cao can be used but to treat the edema caused by the spleen: use bai zhu, if lost transporting of water; zhu ling is suitable for those edemas produced by the kidney and urinary bladder disease change; tong cao removes the edema by entering the lung channel and kidney and down, passing it out with the urine. Again the records from Chinese medicine gui jing "return to the channels". bal zhu returns to stomach channel, zhu ling returns to kidney and urinary bladder channels, tong cao returns to lung channel. "Return to the channel" clearly indicates using the medicine techniques for different disease reasons if the same disease.

Yin jing (constricting channels) also belongs to "return to the channel" theory and its specific application. Yin jing means some medicines can guide or conduct the other medicines to treat selectively particular zang fu disease conditions. For example, Zhang yuan su *Zhen shu gao* recorded: "Hand shao yin heart and huang lian, xi xin, hand tai yang xiao chang; gao ben, huang bai, foot shao yin kidney: du huo, zhi mu, gui, xi xin; foot tai yang urinary bladder: qiang huo, hand tai yin lung: jie geng, cong bai, sheng ma, bai zhi; hand yang ming large intestines; bai zhi, sheng ma, shi gao; foot tai yin spleen; sheng ma, ge gen, cang zhu, bai shao; foot yang ming stomach: bai zhi, sheng ma, shi gao, ge gen; hand jue yin; pericardium, chai hu, dan pi; foot shao yang gall bladder: chai hu, qing pi; foot jue yin liver: qing pi, wu yu, chuan chong, chai hu". The guiding channel medicines combines the medicine characteristics, directly reaching the disease portion and have the specific forces and effect. In the practical and the theory, all have certain value.

For example, we have the Dong yuan record of the arm pains, and the Dan xi treatment of headache, using the systemary channel and collaterals and added the guiding channel medicine and treatment have a good effect.

Bao shi: The effect is slightly similar to the medicine guidance. According to the different prescriptions and the distinguished selection to the effect of the main herbs. It's just like Jing zhen said, "the army without a general/guide, then cannot reach the enemies position, so if the medicine's without the guide/general cannot reach the disease location" *Yi xue du shu ji*. So usually use the medicine guidance like "hence as the guide, take to circulate the blood guide the channel; so using jiang as the guide take its function (to spread/remove from surface) ability, da zao can be guide/general to tonify the blood and make the spleen healthy; long yan as a guide/general to settle (ding) the heart; deng xin as the guide/general to help the sleeping system and the spirit, cong bai as the guide/general to take its fa san (spread/disperse evil); lian shi as a guide/general take to clean out the heart, nourish the stomach, harmonise the spleen *(Zhang jie shi zi rong yi jing)*. So if the general medicine application is good/appropriate, it can strengthen the treatment effect of the prescriptive medicine.

Re the above, 'returning to the channel' theory, not only makes the application of medicines more flexible, but also uses some of the specific rules practical. This medicine enlarges the range of medicine application and also is the summary technique of the medicine projection. Of course, we should want very much to follow it blindly. However at best, the 'return to the channel' theory, with its protective value, has confirmed and indicated the channel collateral theory meaning in medicine application.

Section 5
The relationship between the prescription and channel and collateral theory

A prescription consists of medicines in the specific application of the treatment technique. Using research of the contribution of medicine's integral laws must (in a combined prescription), along with medicine theory and practical application theory, be correct in prescription study.

The prescription composition principle is jun (ie. the head/emperor), zhu (the general/leader), fu (assistant), zuo (captain), shi (ambassador); ie. they can be divided as major (zhu), fu (assistant), captain (zuo), shi (ambassador) four parts. The *Su wen zhi zhen yao da lun* said: "The major disease is called the king, the captain helps the king is called the zhu (general), fu is assistant, and the aid to the general is called the shi (ambassador)".

The emperor (king) is the major action medicine for the disease conditions in the prescription; so the general in the prescription otherwise assists or strengthens the king's medicine effects; fu assists; zuo (the captain) is also the assistant (including two meanings), one is the choosing the medicine which is the effect similar to the king medicine so that it can assist the king medicine to treat some secondary important condition; this is called the practical assistant.

Another is to reduce the medicine's side properties as well as weaken the poison properties of some medicines, prevent its side effects and take its opposite however its effect is the same and is called as 'negative assistant'. Using guiding channel medicines, it shapes medicines. In practice, according to the emperor, general, assistant, captain, ambassador grouping method, it makes-up the medicines to become a prescription.

Hence, the prescription is one of the major treatments practiced to treat the disease. Because the prescription is designed to treat the medicine condition, so the components principal of making the prescription have a close connection with channel and collateral theory. "Shi" (using/making) the medicine's action include the meaning of guiding channel, leading the medicine's effect and the whole prescription directing/reading the disease position, performing on the channel and collaterals, and organs and bowels, and producing the treatment effect.

So channel and collateral theory is one of the major theories in the instruction of the prescription forming/formatting. For example, *jiao tai wan* consists of huang lian and rou gui. If one analyses only from the medicine's properties, huang lian is bitter and cold, and belongs to remove heat and remove fire medicines. The major function is remove fire, remove poisons, clear out heat, and "dig out" the dampness; rou gui tastes pungent and sweet, greatly hot, and belongs to removing cold medicines. The major function is warm the kidneys, strengthen the yang, warm the centre and remove cold. However, huang lian and rou gui used together can balance the communication between the heart and kidney, so can treat insomnia. This is due to huang lian entering the heart, spleen, stomach channels, can clear the heart so as to remove the fire; rou gui enters the kidney, liver, spleen channels combine with constricting fire and returning to the source, so it can communicate with the heart and kidney at the same time, in a short space of time, so treating insomnia with a good effect.

Such a type of prescription condition, without instruction of channel and collateral theory, will be very difficult to understand, including the prescription meaning and its suitable application.

Channel and collateral theory is also one of the major theories in instruction of the prescription practical application. For example, *bai hu tang* consists of shi gao, zhi mu, gan cao, geng mi, ie. a yang ming prescription. Shi gao clears the lungs and removes the stomach fire, zhi mu clears the lungs and removes the kidney fire, gan cao balances the centre and removes heart and spleen fire, and geng mi, its son, sedates its mother, ie. doesn't specifically treat the yang ming qi for heat. Lung fire, stomach fire, kidney fire; all these diseases remove fire of the channels and collaterals and the organs and bowels. Shi gao clears out lung and removes the stomach fire, zhi mu clears out the lungs and removes the kidney fire, gan cao balances the centre and removes heart and lung fire. This is the action of the medicines on the channel and collaterals and organs and bowels. The practical application of all such types of prescriptions can be suitably utilised under the instruction of the channels and collaterals theory.

The adding and subtracting change of prescription, according to the conditions, is also under the instruction of channel and collateral theory. For example, *qing shang juan tong tang* (Ming dynasty prescription *shou ao bao yuang* headache gate/chapter. Prescription is mai dong, du hou, qiang hou, fang feng, chuan chiong, dang gui, cang zhu, bai zhi, man jing zi, ju hua, huang qin xi xin, gan jiang, gan cao) is the usual prescription for treating headache. Under the differentiation of disease, removes wind and dampness disease, removes the wind to make the treatment, and one can also add and subtract according to the channel and collateral differentiation/disease position and according to the condition.

For example, "tai yang then qaing huo; shao yang then xi xin; yang ming then bai zhi jue yin then chuan qiong, wu yu; shao yang then chai hu". (See *Ta ye ben cao* xi xin is guidance *(zhen zhu nang)*, this prescription can have a rapid early effect, so the Japanese doctors using this prescription add and subtract, treat wan gu (difficult to treat) headache, chronic headache, trigeminal nerve pain, migraine, period time headache, upper jaw tumour headache and headache caused by brain tumour, all have a very good effect (Japan *Han fang lin chuan* volume 20 no 9 p. 19-25).

Prescription components; no wonder the old prescription and today's prescriptions all have certain principles and suitable ranges. However, they must be used according to the disease change and different disease conditions, the change of the conditions of the medicines or the adding and subtracting change of the medicine, and medicines amount. All need to be added and subtracted according to the disease conditions. In practice, it must be under the instruction of channel and collateral theory so that the changes used can be made suitably, in the treatment of complicated disease conditions. We can skilfully use this method to make any changes to the medicines to treat different diseases.

CHAPTER 4
Case Studies

Case 1 Ding xx, male 40 years old, actor. On the 8ᵗʰ October 1969 ulcer of stomach. Diagnosis as "stomach pain", for 3 weeks, came to hospital to have treatment. The pain is obvious between 1am and 3pm combined with acid reflux. After eating moderately it modified the pain. In any event, three days after had supper by several hours, the pain becomes more serious, combined with vomiting, then vomiting some blood. Body examination shows that zhong wan (CV12), zu san li (ST36) (right hand side), ulcer back point and ulcer sacrum point, there are pressing pain points appearing positive. By the examination of barium meal x-ray, confirms/certifies it is a duodenal ulcer. Taking procain etc. remedies for treatment for 3 days without obviously overcoming the vomiting and bleeding but affecting the sleeping then using 1% procain on the points as block therapy, the back points and zu san li (ST36), each inject 1ml. That night stomach pain and vomiting stopped and can sleep. Afterwards using this treatment for 2 weeks. So the condition totally disappeared and the patient left the hospital. After 5 years the doctor visited him, so the ulcer condition never reappeared. Examination of the above 4 points, proved pain points all are negative (comes from *Chi li jun yi sheng za zha* 1977 volume 7 page 13, Lu Zeng wu).

Note: (1) Ulcer back point: 5ᵗʰ vertebra 3 cun out, (left). Ulcer sacrum point: sacrum upper 3cun sideways 1.5 cun (right).

(2) This case uses 12 skin parts, pressing "pain as shu" as taking the points principle: treatment has an effect.

Case 2: Deng xx, male, 56 years, worker. Case Study 08619, 1975 mid August first diagnosis.

Patient relating his condition.

Left face muscle shaking 2 years. Limited stage, the patient was treated at the local clinic and some hospitals using acupuncture and medicine, the disease condition was not overcome. August 1975 local doctor transferred the patient to our hospital for acupuncture treatment. The condition shows the muscle around the left eye and the left face muscle shaking, happens every day, the pulse bowstring slippery.

Treatment: intensive diagnosis followed by traditional method of select-at-local part face muscle such as tai yang, xia guan, can zhu, jia che etc. Treatment continued until the 4th December. Total remedy 30 times. The condition had some improvement, the effect is not very obvious. This disease re point treatment is normally not going to provide a cure.

Because it has been 30 times without obvious effects, the treatment treatment was changed. Refer to the *Ling shu* and *Zhen jiu da cheng* record of "ju ci's evil guest at the channels, left strong then right disease, reject right strong then left disease", ju ci means left, then take right, right then take left. That is, left disease take right, right disease then left. This is a treatment technique. Then decided to choose and add needles to bai hui (GV 20) and take it as a yang meeting place.

From 5th December using the "ju ci" treatment technique, taking point: bai hui, xia gua (right) quan liao (right), jia che (right) add 6.26 electric needles retain the needles 20 min.

After treating, the face muscles became obviously better. Needling 1 x each day so the condition was gradually overcome or dropped off. 17th December because another doctor didn't know that we changed to new "ju ci" technique, the doctor again used left hand side tai yang, si bai and the lower zu san li point. So the face muscle got worse then 20th of December continue to use "ju ci" technique ie. bai hui, xia guan (right), qian liao (right), jia che (right) add 6.26 electric needle. Retain the needle for 20 min after insert. The face muscle spasm condition was overcome again.

After this using the "ju ci" technique, using the right hand side face muscle as the correct part of taking the points and using bai hui 1 x each 1 – 2 days till 11th March 1976, the face muscle spasms were completely overcome

Lao zhong yi yi su yi huo sun Guang zhou xiong yi xue wan *Xin zhong yi* *page 269*

Note: this cure follows the channels and collaterals, following the afflicted and taking the part, "ju ci" needle technique, in combination with the points, uses extraordinary points to unblock and adjust the face jing qi, the needles change the qi points so it can move freely, resulting in a good effect.

Case 3   Mo, xx, female 38 years old doctor, 1970 both normal initial diagnoses.

Patient had dizziness, combined with tinnitus, hearing ability reduced (especially the right hand side), vomiting, respectively for over 4 years. At the happening of each time, it occurred for 5 – 10 minutes, so the level is relatively high. Following this, the episodes became more frequent, with extended time, so the condition became heavier. Recent years, after episodes, can't get off the bed for several days, going to the hospital for treatment 2 x. In the recent half year used zhen jing (calming) medicine; have a very weak effort, xx hospital suggested an operation (but the frontal nerves could be injured), and the patient didn't agree, but left that hospital and came here for treatment.

According to the disease history, 4 years ago, after giving birth, lost regularity/adjusting and after this the periods were not regular, and found blood colour is pale, additionally, after her period had abdominal pain, at night couldn't sleep, upset combined with palpitations, poor appetite etc. conditions.

The four diagnostic shapes: pale colour, walking unstable even when assisted, tongue red, had little coating, pulse bowstring thin (and excess during the laboratory examinations).

Touch diagnosis examinations:

Gan shu (right) having flat round shaped block sections, hun men (left) having round shape block section, shen shu (right) having thin white stick objects, both feng chi upper appears round shaped block section (right hand side more obvious)

Analysis of disease:

(1)   "zhu feng diao xuan, li shu yu gan" ("all wind changes into dizziness, all this belongs to liver") (gan shu, hun men have positive reactions).

Liver stores blood, blood deficiency, then yin deficiency, yin deficiency so fire is strong (tongue red, coating less, pulse bowstring thin)

(2) "shen kai qiao yu er" (kidneys open onto the ears), kidney deficiency so tinnitus, listening comprehension decreases. Kidney mainly stores semen (jing) and produces marrow, and goes through to the brain; kidney deficiency also may cause marrow to be not enough and dizziness.

(3) Kidney yin deficiency then water cannot submerge wood, wood attacks and flares up (so attacks earth, so vomiting, eats less), liver attacks then heart fire moves, so palpitations and anxiety, and heart can't calm down and cannot sleep.

Differentiation:

Dizziness condition (liver and kidney yin deficiency type), western medicine diagnosis: ear stores water disease ie. Meniere's disease.

Treatment method:

Channels and collaterals treatment technique: choose the medicines vitamin B1, vitamin B12.

Main points:

1. Gan shu, right ding hun pt (1cm above feng chi (GB20) point) moxa: bu hui (GV20)
2. Shen shu, left ding hun pt. moxa: bai hui

Combined point:

tai chong (Liv3), zu san li, tai xi, yi feng, shi shen cong nei guan, all needles.

Needle feeling:

Line sensation (feeling) heavy repeat as combination; use yang type needling medicine as injection as the main method, combined with point needling.

Treatment effect:

> After treatment one time, the patient instantly feels better from the dizziness, and the symptoms obviously better, after four times treatments, symptoms may formally disappear, totally twelve times, then use Chinese medicine to adjust and improve general health. It (the dizziness) doesn't appear again now three years later and the body had no sickness, period was normal, strength increased gradually (adapted from Yunnan Chinese Medicine College, printed by acupuncture treating and research group (Lecture notes on channels and collateral treatment techniques) p. 7-3 Guan Zun Hui).

Note: This example adapts channel and collateral treatment method, identifies symptoms and gives treatment, follows the channel to the point, quickly gets effect, then medicine to improve general health, then the sickness is totally gone.

Case 4:   Mr Zhang xx, male, 44 years old, hospital file number 00627.

Patient diagnosis:

> Right jaw joint sore, beginning half a month ago. This was a self-caused bruised jaw joint pain, effecting the action of opening the mouth. In recent weeks, the jaw joint had become a little swollen and distended. The soreness increased, it affected the jaw area and near tai yang point. After treatment in a non-Chinese medicine hospital, diagnosis is jaw joint inflammation. After taking some anti-biotics, it reduced inflammation and took some pain killers, and jaw joint block therapy with pu lu kai yin (procain) but no beneficial effect happened. Then on the 24th May 1975 came to our hospital to see our doctor.

Check:

> On the surface, looks a painful bitter illness, right jaw joint a little bit swollen, has pressing pain, moving action is not free. Lip is quite red, tongue body is red, tongue surface is a bit yellow, both pulses are a little bit reduced (floating rapid).

Diagnosis:

> jaw joint inflammation. Chinese doctors think this is yang ming and shao yang two channel fire attack on the luo with damage. The treatment has

a better effect and it is felt better to sedate further: si gua lou 12g, chi shao 9g, sheng shi gao 12g, sang ye 9g, xia ku cao 9g, zhu ru 9g, gan cao 3g, gan ju 9g, gou teng 12g.

(Note: the original prescription is using the imperial system, now change to the metric system, percentage of medicine is not changed. Below is the same).

After we are done, jaw joint pain reduced, after, continue 3 doses, jaw joint and nearby pain disappeared, the movement of mouth opening became should now be: smooth and the jaw joint swelling disappeared and totally went (adapted from *New Chinese Medicine* 1977 (2) added volume p32-33, Qu Shao zhang)

Notes:

This example follows channel and collaterals to identify the symptoms, clear out the yang ming shao yang 2 channels fire, helps the channel and collaterals so the pain disappears.

Case 5   The patient Zuo xx, female 34 years old, working as a primary school teacher, first time see the doctor is 1974 July 20th.

Patient began from first 10 days of May, self – feeling the throat is dry and sore and feels like wanting to vomit. After took some bo he hou pian etc. to treat, but no effect, then the voice is not clear and palpitations, early fright, upset, insomnia and continual dizziness. In the early stages of her period, xx hospital concluded: she had ma bi (voice paralysis). In the same hospital used western medicine or later used various antibiotics, which showed improvement, throat part better for more than 1 month. The effect was quite good. Then Chinese medicine was used more than 10 doses, the disease is not reduced. On the contrary, the dry lips, sore throat and head dizziness were increased, coughing but no phlegm. Then came to this hospital to seek treatment.

Initial diagnosis symptoms:

The language is low and weak, the speech is not clear, the throat part is a little bit bleeding, back wall of the throat lymph nodes increase. The side of the tongue and the tip is red, the coating is thin and pale, pulse is thin rapid.

Analysis of the symptoms:

(1)   The throat is dry and the sides of the tongue and the tip are red, pulse thin rapid, which belongs to kidney yin deficiency symptoms.

(2)   Kidney yin deficiency, cannot consolidate, ie. water cannot go up to the heart, water and fire don't cross, then yin deficiency in the lower, yang strong in the upper, so we also can see palpitations and easy to be terrified/frightened, and heart upset, with insomnia and dizziness etc.

(3)   Foot shao yin channel "there is a branch, from the body up to the back diaphragm and circles the lungs, and to the throat, controls the tongue root". Kidney yin deficiency so the channel qi is not enough, cannot go up to the throat to moisten it; yin deficiency produces heat deficiency, fire follows the channels up to the hui yin, to cause the throat to be unclear.

(4)   The throat belongs to the lungs, the lungs are the source of the voice. Checking the patient's history, we found she recently took Chinese medicine. Most of the doses belonged to pungent, cool and jie biao (remove the exterior), and they had no benefit on treating the illness. On the contrary, they adversely changed the lung qi. The channels transported to hui yin, so the illness is increased and not decreased.

Identified pattern:

Lung dryness causes hoarseness.

Treatment:

Nourish the yin and tonify the body, nourish the yin to reduce fire, lubricate the lungs to open the sounds.

Prescription:

nan bei sha shen each 15g, yuan shen 10g, mai dong 12g, sheng di 15g, jie geng 9g, yu zhu 15g, gui ban 15g, shi jue ming 25g, gan cao 5g. Take with 1 raw egg each day, combined with acupuncture zhao hai (K6), tai xi (K3), shenmen (K7), tai yuan (Lu9), yan liang (Ex) etc acupuncture points.

Instant effectiveness:

> The above formula added and subtracted 15 doses, take treatment 21 days, all the patterns disappeared, the voice is normal.

Notes:

(1) This example analyses the illness according to the channel circulation route (ben) combined with the identification pattern of the organs, acupuncture and medicine is used to treat simultaneously, they obtained an effective result.

(2) Acupuncture following the channels to the points and has used extraordinary channel theory: tai xi (K3) for zu shao yin body channel yuan (source) part, shenmen (H7) is for hand shao yin heart channel yuan point; tai yuan (Lu9) is for hand tai yin lung channel yuan point. Kidney channel, heart channel follow internal circulation route to the throat, collects at the throat (yan); by channel jing bie and with hand yang ming together to the throat (hou yan), so all have benefit to opening the sounds of the throat. Tai xi (K3) can tonify the kidney, shen men (H7) can also calm down the spirit, tai yuan (Lu9) can also tonify the lung qi. Zhao hai (K6) is the meeting point of the kidney channel and yin qiao channel, regulating its yin qiao channel qi, and improving its function to treat the blood.

(3) Yan liang point (Ex) is the experimental effective point to treat throat illness. Body position is approximately at the mid-point of Ren channels lian quan (CV23) and tian tu (CV22) points; it is a bit under the thyroid gland between the thyroid and the crickoid cartilage bone ie. the edge and the soft bone bow like upper edge. It has the effect of regulating the nearby channel and to clear the throat (see *Xin zhang yi* 1975 volume 4, p45). Acupuncture needling yan liang point 36 cases (yi bing) type loss of voice condition summary of the 36 cases, Guan Zun hui.

Case 6   Zhang x lan, female 25 years old, married, address: Shanghai xx road x street x no. On the 25th October 1959, the file number is 27348.

The patient has been married 6 years, abortion 1 time, she has no children, her periods often last longer, dizziness, lack of strength in the four limbs, chest stuffy, breast distended, inside sexual organs sometimes have pain (sometimes have spasm feeling when she gets the pain strongly), the tongue body is red, the coating is yellow, the pulse thin bowstring. The pattern belongs to blood deficiency liver dry jue yin and yin wei have illness, treatment should nourish the blood and unblock the liver. *Si wu tang* add jin ling zi, xiang fu, wu yao, ba ji rou initially 10 doses, but still stuffy, breasts were distended, inside sexual organs had spasmed pain, all recovered sooner or later with further treatment. (Adapted from Shen hai medium college extract *Scientific research paper symposium* 1963 (6) page 28 *Yang wei yin wei discussion workshop* Zhu Xiao nan.

Note:

Liver qi stagnancy then blood stagnancy, yin ying weak, so inside the sexual organs get pain. Inside the sexual organs uterus is connected to the kidneys, so also have relationship with foot shao yin. Wang Shu he said "if we check the pulse and get sunken big and forceful, then has bitter chest inside pain, under the ribs full, heart pain. His pulse is like a moving ball, male both ribs excess, waist inside is painful, female inside have sexual organ pain, like a chuang (ulcer)".

This example is foot jue yin, foot shao yin and yin wei combined illness. Treatment mainly uses *si wu tang* add balance the period and unblock the liver and tonify the kidneys, the effective rate is quite good. *Si wu tang* not only regulates periods it tonifies the blood; inside it, the dang gui, bai shao, chuan chiong also enter the yin wei and have the function of stopping pain. The purpose of this example is to demonstrate the use of the yin wei channel in the clinical situation.

Case 7   Ma xx, female, 20 years old, first saw the doctor on May 5th 1975. The patient in May 1975, during the menstrual period she had a lot of menstruation. Several days she was in the rain because of her long work hours. After that, the period lasted longer every month, before the period the abdomen would become very painful, the period blood was dark, the colour becoming black and dark. In the more recent half year, the lips became numb, at night the lower legs and the big toes often become sore like a "cramp", affecting her sleep, appetite was poor, diarrhoea. It was concluded by xx hospital, "Secondary type period pain". Treatment was for several months, but the result was not obvious.

Four diagnostic shapes and the face was pale, felt cold and limbs are cold, the spirit is tired and is too lazy to talk, the tongue body is bland white, coating is white and a little sticky, pulse is sunken tight.

Analysis of illness:

(1) First she got into the rain during the period, and the rain attacked along with evil cold and damp, carrying the uterus blood sea with stagnant blood, and with cold, evil fights with the blood, so less period becoming a dim colour, and abdomen pain felt like stabbing.

(2) *Ling shu wu yan wu wei* says: "if closure of the ren and chong channels, both which come from inside the uterus (bao), upper goes inside the back (bei), it is the sea of channels and collaterals, some floating, (flow) and go out, follow the abdomen and go up, and meet at the throat, and the two (collected together) go to the mouth and lips". The channels are cold and then the collaterals clot. Qi and blood cannot go up fu bu (abdomen part) to moisten it, so the lips are numb. The Chong channel and its branches "from inside of the limbs" and bones obligingly go inside to outside, and then inters the heels of the feet, then to the fu upper, distributed at the feet and toe", the channels and collaterals get cold, cold controls (gets connection), the yin is strong between nights, monthly cause intestinal muscle and toe connection (stabbing) and pain.

(3) The patient's face is pale, and the limbs are cold, the spirit is tired (juan), too lazy to speak, pulse is shen jin (sunken tense) and tongue coating is white and a little bit sticky, all this belongs to cold phenomenon. Cold qi produces turbidity, so the period blood is dim and dark (black ie. hei). The evil of cold-damp goes up to interfere/ interrupt the spleen and stomach, so poor appetite; and goes down to attack large intestines leads to diarrhoea.

Identified pattern:

Chong ren imbalance, cold-damp condensed/accentuated and stagnant/ blocks (ning dai) the sea of blood and uterus (bao gong).

Treatment:

Adjust and tonify the chong ren, remove the cold and transform the dampness, warm the channels and warm the uterus.

Prescription:

Bai zhu 30 g, fu ling 12 g, huai shan yao 18g, ba ji 15g, chao bian dou 10g, jian lian zi 30g, ai ye 6g, rou gu powder mix 3g (take with water and drink), bai guo 15g (approximately).

In the prescription: use bai zhu as jun (gentleman/king), warms and transforms the cold-damp between the waist and the umbilicus; ba ji, bai guo as zhu (minister) warm and unblock the ren channel; bian dou, shan yao, lian zi as zuo (captains), so as to guard and protect the chong channel; fu ling as shi (ambassador); and helps make the spleen healthy; add ai ye to warm the uterus, warm the channels, spreads/disguises the cold and enters the dai channel, rou gui warms the channels and stops pain, tonifies the ning men (life gate) fire and strengthens the kidney yang. Blood gets warm and then dispersed, channels get warm and then unblock; take the medicine 1 dose will have an effect, after 2 doses the period blood will go down smoothly, the abdomen pain will disappear. After more than 3 months treatment more or less, taking 26 doses, the period blood becomes normal. All the illness phenomena/symptoms disappear. He (the doctor) visited the patient 2 years later, the patient was in good health.

Note:

This case used extraordinary channel theory to identify patterns to treat and demonstrates the channel application of the chong ren channels.

Case 8   Fan xx, 28 years old, married, temper. Hospital file is number is 27498 The patient went to her work regularly since 1960, period blood comes only one time and hasn't come for 7 months now and has dizziness and tired spirit/fatigue, sexual desire decreased, two breasts drooped downwards, leucarrhoea and sore waist, impatient etc. symptoms. The gynecology department examination: uterus small (about 5.5 x 3 x 2 cm). The pap smear (and yellow body ie corpeus luteum) examination showed uterus fluid and extent/amount water level, performed 1 time every 3 days, continue to do five times, uterus less and thick, every day observe the pap smear; there was only a little upper cells bacteria showing and there are no crystals shape. The diagnosis is chong ren deficiency weak (xu ruo).

The medicines as follows:

> Dang gui wan 6 pills (swallow), dan shen 10g, ba ji tian 10g, lu jiao shuang 6g, xian ling pi 10g, zi shi ying 10g, yi mu cao 10g, zi he che 3g (taken with water).

The other prescription add and subtract, continuing take 9 doses, within the period of taking medicines. The course examination found that the crystals of the "lambs teeth" shape gradually disappeared, this illness case then used the faster treatment of combining Chinese and western medicine, then the period is recovered (adapted from *Zhang yi za zhi* 1962 volume 8 pages 1-3 *chong ren discussion* Zhu Ren ran)

Note:

> This clinical application of medicine demonstrates the medicines for the chong ren have the effect to remove and improve the sex hormones, so that they verify the theory of the chong ren controlling the sea of blood and uterus (bao tai) in the extraordinary Chinese channel theory as its basis.

Case 9   Tai wu, zhong wu shi gong (official military business leader), 68 years old, early October zhi year (this dynasty), service to the nation teacher; in his official room/office, in the left side of his office is a coal fire oven, gradually feels the face is hot, and the left cheek is a little bit sweaty, all the teachers and the servants go outside because then the left cheek lose warmth and attacked/invaded by wind-cold. The right cheek is tense. The mouth is (slanted) to the right, pulse gets floating and tight, pressing it is surging and moderate, dismissed using *shang ma tang* (sheng ma, shao yao, ge gen, gan cao) add fang feng, qin jiao, bai zhi, gui zhi to spread and disperse the wind and cold, several doses to recover. Somebody asked, doctors if helpful couldn't they normally use *xu ming tang* etc. to treat.

Now you can see *sheng ma tang* add four tastes. What's the reason? The answer is "foot yang ming channel begins from bi jiao (Ex) follows out from the external, enters the upper teeth hand yang ming, also goes to the lower teeth. Also because both cheeks belong to yang ming, *sheng ma tang* is a yang ming channel medicine, xiang bai zhi follows to the hand yang ming channel as well, qin jiao treats loss of sound/voice, fang feng disperses wind evil, gui zhi, fortifies the external, conditions ie. the ying wei (protection qi), makes it so evil cannot attack again, this is the reason." So the illness has differences of external and internal, the channels and collaterals, medicines have differences of thick and thin; check the source of the illness and then choose the medicines, its effects are like the response of drum to a stick. If we don't know the channels and the collaterals and don't know the nature of medicines or only know one side, it will not only be ineffective but also have many cases where the illness is worse. Scholars should think about it carefully (in *wei sheng shi jia reng zhong xue mai zhe yan* volume 8, Luo Tan yi).

Note: Given is an accurate illness case to document the importance of medicines following the channel and collateral theory, and channel and collateral theory guidance significance to the channel prescriptions use.

Case 10 Channels and collaterals re people phenomena (true cases).

According to the very important significant running of the channels and collaterals have phenomena to discuss the channels and collaterals real cases. Now all parts of the whole country, if under investigation, give concern to health proper and all kinds of illness for the channels and collaterals. Re concerns, channels and collaterals have good consensus. Happy results have been obtained through this system of observation and investigation.

Here given are the basic conclusions to demonstrate or explain the basic application of channels and collaterals and their phenomena:

Test case – Huang xx female 49 years old, hospital no 11436, claimed to have a slow gall bladder, xx country so can obtain a staff number, is a sensitive person according to the unified national standards, (?) grew-up and spirit was normal, has no knowledge of channels and collaterals; is cooperative with medical staff, her treatments were uneventful.

(i) Method of stimulation

There are 3 kinds of methods of stimulation

1. Needle prick method (zhen ci fa) use 1.5cun number 32, hao zhen quick needling resulted, prick the 12 jing well points, after the needle is inserted for a better stimulation; after obtain the qi, retain the needle inside.

2. Channel electric stimulation use G6805 low output channel treatment equipment, without off switch, is 3 x 3cm² gian ba (plate), set up and apply the cloth worked in salty water, put on the san yin jiao point (Sp6), stimulation which is measured per the channels and collaterals movement electrical equipment, touch 12 channel jing points, the frequency is 300 times per minute, the strength is considered according to the patients treatment.

3. Match – test rod pressure method: use a moxa-stick and press the 12 true jing points. Its pressure should be as much as possible, the strength should produce numb and sensitive feeling.

Because the jing points are mostly at positions at the ends of fingers or toes, the needle positions are very sensitive to pain, the patient is not easy about it. It is not enough to rotate the needle position point choose 12 turns of the channel yuan points. When the feeling cannot reach all the roots, then another stimulation at the end points of the fingers called jie ti (telegraphic), is used to find the maximum distress and record its route.

(ii) Channel and collateral sensitivity speed movement

After three times of different kinds of stimulation methods, the patient has the feeling transferred from the stimulation point along the channel one direction or two directions. According to the electricity and time to collect its speed.

(iii) The analysis of observation results:

1. Fully transfer route: observe the 12 true channels, its channels and collaterals free transfer route is almost identical to the channel direction, but part of, the channel and collaterals sensation transfer route over or under reasons with the finest points of the channels. Some of them enter the other channels in the middle of the route and go in between two channels. In summary, the feeling and route

in the limbs is quite in agreement with the route as described. Re the main body, it is less in agreement. The feeling transfer route in the head is quite unclear. The 12 true channels feeling transfer route is such a case compared with the four limbs routes and recorded in ancient books. The rate of complete agreement is 33.3%, second to agreement rate is 41.16%, the rate of over-exaggeration is 25%, the under-recorded rate is 0.5%.

The channel and collateral feeling transfer has some kind of stimulation with feeling. Generally speaking, strengthening the stimulation strength, when the needle feeling is obvious, feeling transfer is better; best (over) stimulation, the local part procedure strong pulse feeling as if fully in electrical shock, then the feeling transfer is not good. This demonstrates that only in proper stimulation, strength can produce better needle feeling and feeling transfer.

2.   Feeling transfer proper: it is numb, jumping, hot, distended, sorer etc. feeling as new feelings. These are also the feelings like cramping or jumping. This can be seen when that part/location of feeling transfer passes through a white line (run), if we use G6805 low frequency pulse electrical stimulation on a small channel (SI1) point, when the feeling transfer reaches the elbow joint, on the person's external side appears a fine white line about 8cm long 2 cm width during 2 mins and it disappears by itself.

Needle feeling strength has relationship with stimulation strength, increase the stimulation strength ie. sour, numb, hot, and distended etc. feelings will improve. After the needle is withdrawn, the sour feelings may remain for a period of time even up till several hours.

3.   Feeling transfer directions: stimulate jing points. Feeling transfer shows single direction transfer/conduct. Stimulate yuan points, feeling transferral mostly instantaneously shows double/dual condition ie. opposite directions.

4.   Feeling transfer depth and width. The feeling transfer with it is about 1 – 3 cm strong, where there are differences in the central limb and sides region. The central line is quite thin/fine like the size of a pencil inside, strength and feeling is quite clear, the margin region is not quite so clear, the width of all the feeling transfer lines is about the same but in the different parts of the body the width is quite different,

generally, in the further most location, is found to be narrow, while in the nearest location, the centre is quite broad.

Feeling transfer depth shows between 0.5 - 1 cm, very few channel records can reach the middle inside part, generally in the low limbs it goes deeper and deeper. To the body parts it's not so clear or is fuzzy.

5. Feeling transfer speed. The speed of the channels and collaterals feeling transfer is very slow, the minimal value is 0.047 cm per second, maximum value is 0.180 cm per second; by x^2 measurement p value <0.01 has a very obvious difference.

6. Fully transfer insulated/blocked. Channels and collaterals feeling transfer has its insulation characteristics. Therefore there is a need to stimulate lower kidney and spleen 3 yin channels jing well parts or original points. At the same time, the person's feeling transfer has the feeling of numbness heat, where we can still distinguish the three fine lines, following its own channels going forward; between the three lines there is some distance. They don't interfere with each other, and are not confused with each other and each line channel feeling transfer speed is fixed, with the end part different from each other.

7. Channel and collateral feeling transfer and organs have upper and lower relationship, ie. the relationship of channels and collaterals and organs have been demonstrated under observation, ie. point insertion may cause relative internal organs response. For example, insertion at pericardium channel, when feeling transfer re chart, the patients feel clear pressure, palpitations; needle insertion at stomach channel feeling transfer goes through abdomen parts, the patient said the upper abdomen parts were feeling not comfortable and have pressure feeling; needle insertion at the gall bladder channel, feeling transfer to jing men (GB25), feeling immediately shows ribs side distention and tired/tense feeling. Additionally, re some local and whole body points there may appear, dizziness, fever (fa re), hands and feet centres sweating, local muscle contracted, and vibrating/shaking etc.

This case has extraordinary phenomenon: when the feeling reached the head parts each time, then the patient goes into deep sleep states; call him and has no response. At this time, his heart-beat feeling (xin bo) and pressure are all normal. After strong stimulation 5 – 10 minutes, feeling transfer returns to points or body parts then he became awake (woken up by himself). This case was in 1973 re needle numbness and did the operation on the gall-bladder; also extended to deep sleep states, the needle numbness effect was first-class (ie. very good).

8. Feeling transfer return phenomenon: when feel the transfer reach the end points. If the stimulation does not recur, feeling transfer state stays at the end point and forms a heat feeling region, which emerges slowly, reaching some square distance, then stays unusually, cannot return. Stop stimulation, feeling transfer can follow the original route to return, feeling transfer conducts to the centre, return current go from heat and returns, feeling transfer conducts dual direction return current, however goes to the stimulation points from two ends.

    The return current speed is faster than feeling transfer speed, for example, in one case, a needle was inserted in urinary bladder jing gu (UB64) point. The feeling transfer followed this original channel to conduct in an inverse direction, showing jing gu (UB64) to can zhu (UB2) is about 27 minutes 3 seconds, while returning time needs only 5 minutes 31 seconds.

9. Some "tired" (fa gan) feeling problem in some people is reported in the channels and collaterals, re sensitive people's bodies feeling transfer process: has the phenomena of non-repair period, similar to non-conducting, called tired feeling period. But these cases obstruction results have a not suitable feeling transfer period phenomena (adapted/extracted/taken from *Hu nan yi yan za zhi* 1977 number 3 page 56, (Two cases channels and collaterals sensitive peoples early stage observation). Hu nan zhong yi xue yuan, needles numbness channels and collaterals research development.

Note:

1. This case has demonstrated the objective proof of channels and collaterals.

2. It is very difficult to explain the feeling transfer of channels and collaterals using modern records – physiology. For example, feeling transfer route is obviously the channels and collaterals, not following the normal network, and is quite different from the normal nerves (parts) distribution. The speed of feeling transfer of the channels and collaterals is generally about 0.101 cm per second. However, the speed

of normal conduction of mammals, taking the slowest C normal fibre as an example is about $0.7 - 2$ cm per second. The latter is a usual hundred times faster as the previous.

3. About the basic point input/fundamentals (shu zhi) of channels and collaterals, by a series of clinical practice and basic treatment research in this country and abroad, great progress and good results have now been made. We can predict the basic points of channels and collaterals and these are sure to be recognised in the near future. The theory of channels and collaterals will make a greater contribution to promote the development of world medicine.

Appendix

CHAPTER 1
....
On Ling gui ba fa Theory and Clinical application

Section 1
Ling gui ba fa's origin and significance

Ling gui ba fa is a kind of time combined with points (an shi pei xue fa), using the ba mai jaio hui xue (8 extraordinary channels meeting points) as the main points. "Ling gui's" meaning is according to ancient legend when a race of people, the Da you, conquered Luo (a place), the god/spirit turtle took one Wen ke on his back, which had 9 numbers on it ie. nine on the hand, one is under the shoes, left is three, right is seven, two and four are the shoulders, six and eight are the feet, and five is in the middle. Ba fa used these numbers combine with eight points and daytime main branches, so called ling gui ba fa. The eight points that the ba fa used have reflective and unblocking relationships with the extraordinary eight vessels, eight vessels combined with the eight points belong to the nine palaces and the eight tri-grams; then deduce the opening points according to the main branches each time each day, so also called "qi jing na gua fa" ("extraordinary channels taking the tri-gram method") or "qi jing na jia fa" ("extraordinary channels taking A ie. ABC method").

The twelve channels and vessels have eight points on the four limbs, and go to extraordinary channels eight vessels, that is the "ba mai jiao hui xue" ("eight vessels meeting points") in the clinical situation and are adapted to the illness and related to the ordinary channels. Except for the general applications in the upper and lower combined points method and re the eight points, this method is another special application method combined with daytime main branch opened and closed eight points all of which have representative numbers. Combined these eight points with nine palace numbers, in application, then can get daytime main branch representative numbers by deducing the determined open points. This open points time is the insertion time relating to the flowing time, when these points go through the extraordinary channels. In clinical practice, we use this time's open points to cure the illness related to the extraordinary channels.

Ling gui ba fa originated a long time ago. Early, in the *Nei jing*, there was the theoretical basis for ling gui ba fa. In the Jin-Yuan dynasty's, the famous point expert Du Hu qin in his book *Biao you fu*, pointed out in simple words but with deep meaning, that; "only use eight methods (ba fa) and five gates (wu men), divided into main and not main points and then use needles, no cases were ineffective". Up to and including the Ming dynasty, the application of Ling gui ba fa has been quite general and popularist, eg Xue feng in his book *Zhen jiu da quan* (*Acupuncture and moxibustion complete book*), and Yang Ji zhuo in his book *Zhen jiu da cheng*) (*Compendium of Acupuncture Moxibustion*) etc both have complete and detailed descriptions.

Ling gui ba fa is a kind of acupuncture combined points method, mainly paying attention to the extraordinary channel eight vessels. It has the same meaning as Zi wu liu zhu (midnight to noon flow of energy) circling flow for the twelve channels. The two acupuncture techniques mutually supplement and are mutually different, help each other and quite completely demonstrate the principles of the body's qi and blood circling flow and also maintain the internal change relationship between organs and time. If we can master and use this principle to get the point on time then it's easy to get a quick cure effect. Just as the *Zhen jiu da cheng* said; "like use a rudder on a boat and like an arrow out of a crossbow, through the qi connection and the time dispersion the body's pain can be quickly removed",

Ling gui ba fa's theory is produced by the idea of man and nature in the one whole body. it's a spirit essence, is used to highlight the unity and completeness of the human body and the natural environment's deep relationship. Ling gui ba fa also deduces the change principles of channel and collateral transfer points. Qi and blood open and close, using the mathematical calculations according to yin and yang, ba gua, wu xing, sheng (tonification) cheng (process, sedation), tian gan di zhi, and wu yun hua he (five movements divide and combine). It is a broadly and easily used ancient philosophy and Chinese medicine theory, with the verification of thousands of years of clinical practice and modern science, all of which demonstrate that ling gui ba fa not only contained a deep philosophy, but also has a quite high clinical effect and a certain scientific value. Ling gui ba fa is a precious pearl in Chinese medicine. It will emit a bright light as Chinese medicine develops.

Section 2
Ling gui ba fa's organising context and theoretical fundamental basis

Ling gui ba fa uses the extraordinary channels eight methods, eight vessels eight points, nine palaces eight tri-grams, and tian gan di zhi as the main contents, combined with the body's extraordinary channels qi and blood's meeting points. According to the deducing change of the daytime main branches, and using the principle of mutual adding and mutual dividing, determine the on-time method. Now, we will conduct a comment and discussion on the theory relating to Ling gui ba fa's organising content.

(i)   Qi jing ba mai (extraordinary channels eight vessels)

Qi jing ba mai is a bie dao (another/special route) strange circulating channel and vessels branch, "qi" has a qi ling (extraordinary qi zuo's) meaning, also has a deep relationship with qi han's (qi forever) house, so called "qi jing" (extraordinary channels). Qi jing includes ren, du, chong, dai, yin qiao, yang qiao,, yin wei, yang wei, eight channels; so called "qi jing ba mai" (eight extraordinary channels). Qi jing bai mai physiologically has an adjustment effect on the channels' qi and blood flow and storage, and makes the relationship closer to the twelve channels; qi jing bai mai's functional charachteristics are the classification, combination, conduction and controlling/managing (conquering) effect on the twelve channels. Described individually, the du channel controls all the yang, it has the function of controlling the whole body's yang qi and contains (or conserves) the body's yuan qi; the ren channel manages all the yin and the function of adjusting all of the body's yin qi, absorbs (or gets) the blood, fertility, and nutrition (ren yang); the chong channel is the sea of the zang fu (ie organs and bowels) has the function of closely connecting the organs and bowels with the channels it conserves the xian tian (before birth) and hou tian (after birth) true qi, and controls and absorbs all the yuan qi; the dai channel generally controls all the channels contains/keeps all the qi and blood so it won't go in the wrong direction; the ying and yang qiao control the body's left and right yin and yang; the yin and yang wei control the external and internal of ones body. The qi jing ba mai is an important organising part of the jing luo theory, so ling gui ba fa takes the qi jing ba mai as its main organsing content.

(ii)   Ba mai ba xue (eight channels eight points)

The qi jing bai mai has the effect of controlling and adjusting the twelve channels, qi and blood and the twelve channels themselves, having an upper and down, cycling and intersecting characteristics. So the twelve channels at the four limbs have eight points, which are connected to eight channels:

(1) Hou xi (SI 3): is the hand tai yang small intestine channel, and is external or internal with respect to the hand shao yin heart channel, and is connected with/to the du channel.

(2) Lie que (Lu 7): is the hand tai yin lung channel, and is external or internal with respect to the hand yang ming large intestine channel, and is connected with/to the ren channel.

(3) Gong sun (SP 4): is the foot tai yin channel, and is external or internal with respect to the foot yang ming stomach channel, and is connected to the chong channel.

(4) Lin qi (GB 41): .is the foot shao yang gall bladder channel, and is external or internal with respect to the foot jue yin liver channel, and is connected to the dai channel.

(5) Zhao hai (K 6): is the foot shao yin kidney channel, and is external or internal with respect to the foot tai yang urinary bladder channel, and is connected to the yin qiao channel.

(6) Shen mai (UB62): is the foot tai yang urinary bladder channel, is external or internal with respect to the foot shao yin kidney channel, and is connected to the yang qiao channel.

(7) Nei guan (P6): is the hand jue yin pericardium channel, is external or internal with respect to the hand shao yang triple heater channel, and is connected to the yin wei channel.

(8) Wai guan (TH5): is the hand shao yang triple heater channel, is external or internal with respect to the hand jue yin pericardium channel, and is connected to the yang wei channel

The above eight points are connected with the qi jing ba mai, their channels have a circling and intersecting relationship as follows: the du channel is originally from the lower extremities shu (regular points), then parallel to the spine, goes up to feng fu (GV16), passes through the brain, follows the forehead, reaches the nose, enters the teeth at yin jiao (GV28), follows down to the hand tai yang small intestine channel's "hou xi" (SI3). The Ren channel originates from under the mid-extremities, goes to (tong) the abdomen, goes to the throat, follows the hand tai yin lung channel's "lie que" (Lu7). The Chong channel originates from qi chong (ST30), follows the foot shao yin's channel along next to the umbilicus and goes up the middle of the chest and then disperses, goes to (tong) the foot tai yin spleen channel's "gong sun" (SP4); the Dai channel originates from the 3rd rib, circling around the body once, goes to the foot shao yang gall-bladder channel's lin qi (GB41). The Yin qiao channel originates from the heel (gen) centre (zhao hai point K6), follows the the internal ankle upwards to the throat, intersects the chong channel, goes to the foot shao yin kidney channel's "zhao hai" (K6). The Yang qiao channel originates from the foot ankle centre (shen mai point UB62), follows the external ankle upwards to enter at feng chi (GB20), goes to the foot tai yang urinary bladder channel's "shen mai" (UB62). The Yin wei channel is the controller of all the yin, goes to the hand jue yin pericardium channel's "nei guan" (P6). The Yang wei channel is the controller of all the yang, goes to the hand shao yang's triple heater channel's "wai guan" (TH5).

The eight points which combine with the qi jing ba mai, are selected from the twelve channels, four organs and four bowels, while the ren, du, chong, and dai four extraordinary channels combined points are selected points at the external or internal channels of the liver, heart, spleen, and lungs; only the kidneys and urinary bladder, pericardium, and triple heater have two points ie. more (ie. these four regular channels give one point each). This is because they have special functions. The kidney is the basis or root of before birth (xian tian) (energy). The urinary bladder is the official of the provinces, and the pericardium is the mother of yin blood, while the triple heater is the father of all the yang, at the same time, becomes yin and yang qiao's, and yin and yang wei's. While these last four are connected with the four channels of left and right, internal and external, they systematically circle and distribute. So, each channel is given a point.

The eight points which are intersecting points of the eight channels are also divided into four groups, and have the same intersecting parts and treatment ranges; these are called "fu mu" ("father mother"), "fu qi" ("husband wife"), "nan nu" ("man woman"), "zhu ke" ("host guest") see Table 12 as follows:

Table 12 Eight Techniques Combined With The Eight Channels

8 Points Name	Unblocks 8 Channels	Relations System	Combines At Parts (Controls Cures)
Gong Sun (SP4)	Chong Channel	Father	Heart, chest, stomach
Nei Guan (P6)	Yin Wei	Mother	
Hou Xi (SI3)	Du Channel	Husband	Eye inside canthus, throat, ear, shoulder blade, small intestines, urinary bladder
Shen Mai (UB62)	Yang Qiao	Wife	
Lin Qi (GB41)	Dai Channel	Man	Eye canthus, behind ear, neck, cheek, shoulder
Wai Guan (TH5)	Yang Wei	Woman	
Lie Que (LU7)	Ren Channel	Host	Lung system, larynx and pharynx, chest diaphragm
Zhao Hai (K6)	Yin Qiao	Guest	

The eight points meet eight channels, the relationships names are according to the ba gua and yin yang etc. theories: chong channel and yin wei channel meet each other, both channels follow from gong sun (SP4) and nei guan (P6) because gong sun belongs to qian (male) tri-gram, as heaven (tian) called father, nei guan, pericardium channel, is yin blood's mother, called mother, so the two points are called father mother.

Dai channel and yang wei channel meet each other, the two points follow from lin qi (GB41) and wai guan (TH 5). Because zhen tri-gram is yang male, xun trigram is yin female, so the two points are called male female.

Du channel and yang qiao channel meet each other. The two channels follow from hou xi (SI3) and shen mai (UB62). Because the du channel is the body's yang, follows from the du channel's hou xi point, belongs to the small intestine's bing fire; follows from yang qiao's shen mai (UB62) point, belongs to urinary bladder ren water. Fire is yang, water is yin. So, are called husband and wife.

Ren channel and yin qiao channel meet each other, the two channels follow lie que (Lu7) and zhao hai (K6), because lie que mainly controls the lung system, the lungs go up to the one hundred channels to reach the whole body, belongs to li tri-gram located exactly in the south position, so called host; zhao hai (K6) belongs to the kun tri-gram, and is located at the middle/central palace, so called guest.

(iii)   Nine palaces, eight tri-grams

The ba gua is an ancient select yin yang figure combined with nature's heaven (tian), earth (di), water (shui), fire (huo), wind (feng), thunder (lei), mountain (shan), and lake (ze) formulating it. Where qian is heaven and is ☰ shape, kun is earth and is ☷ shape, kan is water and is ☵ shape, li is fire and is ☲ shape, xun is wind and is ☴ shape, zhen is thunder and is ☳, gen is mountain and is ☶ shape, dui is lake and is ☱ shape, this is the ba gua's name and diagram's figures; the ba gua combined with the four directions, then becomes the nine palaces.

1. The ba gua's origin: *Zhou yi-xi che* said: "Heaven produces god products, great philosophers (sheng ren) respect it, heaven and earth change, philosophers simulate this. Heaven shows figures, see luck (ji) xiang (danger/bad luck), philosophers identify it. Rivers produce figures, Luo produce books, philosophers describe it."

    According to god products, changes, heaven figures, Luo books etc. all are heaven king produced, and he (sea) figures Luo books, are only some of them. But later cultures and peoples use the ba gua as a Zhi he (river) figure. As Kong An guo said, "He figure is Fu xi king's time's dragon horse, out of the river, so write each character to draw the ba gua. In Luo books, Yu controlled the floods, the god turtle took Wen lie on his back, which had nine numbers, and Yu used it for its numbers." Liu qian said "Fu xi followed heaven to be king, get the river figure and drew it, it's the ba gua. Yu controlled the flood and gave us the Luo books to descibe it, its nine areas, and the he (the river) figure in the Luo books. It is longitudinal and distinguished from each other. The ba gua has nine sections which are external and internal with each other."

From the Han dynasty to the Song dynasty, the scholars followed the books. All think the ba gua is produced along with Zhi he (river) figure. Ma rong, Wang shu, Yao xin etc. famous scholars all agree with this. Only the he (river) figure is a kind of unknown object. Therefore, simply have the he (river) to follow.

Today, following the he (river) figure comes from the early Song dynasty's Chen bo, who delivered it from Zhou Mao quan, then from Zhu xi and its theory became very popular. Zhu xi quoted bei wei dynasty Guang nang's words saying "He (river) figure's words, 7 front, 6 back, 8 left, 9 right. In Luo's books words 9 front, 1 back, 3 left, 7 right, 4 front left, 2 front right, 8 back left, 6 back right."

Yi zhuan xi che xia said: "Ancient person Bao shi Se's king controlled the country, looked up to observe the heavens, looked down to observe the earth, observed the birds and animals speech, and the earth's property; selected all the beings in neighbouring places, and selected all things in far-off places. Then began to create the ba gua; using the good spirit to connect to God's spirit, and using the feelings of 10,000 things."

2. Luo's book's 9 palace numbers and the He's diagram numbers, the so-called Luo's books 9 palace numbers are also called the Hou tian ba gua (after heaven ba gua). Luo's books selected the total image. Its numbers are: "head 9, foot 1, left 3, right 7, 2, (and 4) are the shoulders, 6, (and 8) are the feet, 5 is placed in the middle/centre." This figure shows as follows (Figure 6, Luo book 9 palaces figure).

The so-called he tu's (river diagram's) numbers ie. the *Zhou yi- xi chi* said/ stated that the 5 elements (wu xing) produce numbers. *Lei jing fu yi-yi yi* said: "Fu xi, the king, controlled the world, his dragon horse (long ma) back showed figures and a river, its numbers 1, 6 were located below; 2, (and 7) were located in the upper; 3, 8 were located in the left; 4 line was located in the right; and 5, 10 were located in the middle/centre. Fu xi used it to draw the ba gua." River diagram numbers are shown in the following (Figure 7, river diagram sketches)..

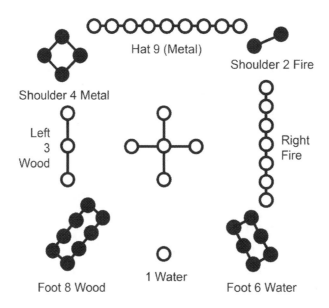

DIAGRAM 6: LUO SHU 9 PALACES DIAGRAM

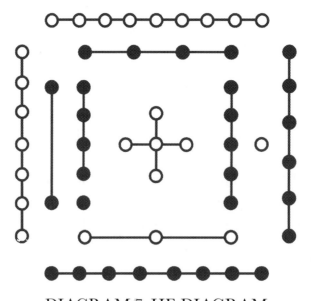

DIAGRAM 7: HE DIAGRAM

3. Before-heaven (xian tian) ba gua and after-heaven (hou tian) ba gua: xian tian ba gua is also called the Fu xi ba gua, divided into yin yang's body use, says 6 combine diagram/figure (xiang); hou tian ba gua is also called Wen Wang ba gua, describes the five elements essence and small details, 'foretelling' the future.

Yi zhuan- xi che said: "Yi has tai ji, is to produce 2 side/aspects (yi), 2 yi produce 4 xiang (diagrams/figures/seasons/directions), 4 xiang produce the ba gua." Lu Xiang shan quoted the Huo people which said: "6, 7, 8, 9 is the four xiang, i.e. old yang ("lao yang"), young yang ("shao yang"), old yin ("lao yin"), young yin ("shao yin"), Old young yin yang, these four as a body, the division of yin and yang starts from internal. 6 and 9 is biao (external), external is normally old, 7 and 8 is internal (li), li is normally young. Shao Kang jia said: "heaven 1, earth 2, heaven 3, earth 4, heaven 5, these are the numbers of heaven and earth. 1, 3, 5 combine to be 9, is heaven's number. Heaven is originally qian so qian is called 9. 2 and 4 combine to be 6, the earth number. The earth is actually kun, so kun is called 6, "The maximum total of the odd numbers is 9, yang attacks forward is taken as the main thing, so is all yang. 7 is shao yang (young yang), yin retreat as the main thing, so 6 is old yin (lao yin), 8 is shao yin (young yin). *Yi zhuan-shuo guan* said: "heaven and earth fixed positions, mountains and rivers unblock qi (tong qi), thunder and wind fight each other, water and fire cannot shoot each other. The ba gua moves in relation to each other. The numbers go, is smooth, not coming is adverse, so easy to adverse/reverse the numbers. Shao Kong jie said: "Qian south, kun north, li east, kan west, zhen north-east, dui south-east, xun south-west, gen north-west. From zhen to qian is smooth (shun), from xun to kun is adverse (ni). After 64 gua's position is similar to this.

Now, before heaven (xian tain) ba gua's order and position diagram is shown below (Table 13, figure 8).

TABLE 13: Fu xi ba gua treatment.

	1.	2.	3.	4.	5.	6.	7.	8.
Ba Gua	Qian	Dui	Li	Zhen	Xun	Kan	Gen	Kun
4 Shapes	9	Tai Yang	Old 8	Shao Yin	7	Shao Yang	6	Tai Yin Old
2 Appearances	Yang					Yin		
				Tai Ji				

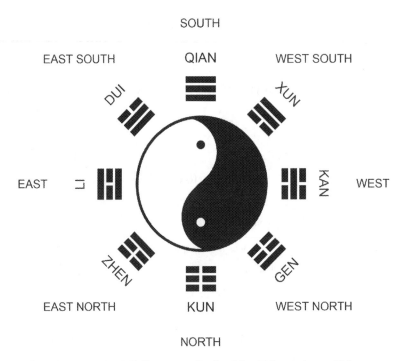

FIGURE 8: Fu Xi Ba gua Suitable Directions Diagram

After birth (hou tian) ba gua, it is said to have been written by Zhou Wen wang (king). Actually, it was summarized by ancient people who through the observation of nature for a long time combined with the season's weather and both characteristics change. After birth (hou tian) ba gua takes south -north as longitude, and east- west as latitude, using xiang's seasons' division classification. Use four times (si zheng) combined with four seasons, east is chun fen, south is xia zhi, west is qiu fen, north is dong zhi. Then use the si you (four corners) combined with the four seasons, north-east becomes li chun, south-east becomes li xia, south-west becomes li qiu, north-west becomes li dong. If use 5 elements (wu xing) creates and processes (or sedates) (Cheng): beginning from zhen gua (tri-gram), then the house (you) has mu (wood); zhen zhun produces li huo (fire); li fire produces earth (tu) (kun), earth (kun) produces gold/metal (gui-qian); gold/metal produces water (kan); water produces wood (combined with gen tu earth), demonstrates five elements produce each other principle. If take west east as the boundary (zhen dui gua or tri-gram). From zhen to li tri-gram is wood fire's place, from dui to kan tri-gram to kan tri-gram is gold/metal water's home. These two also have gen mountain and kun earth, use earth boundary. It demonstrates that true wood and fire produce (metal) and were born of earth, gold/metal and spring water hide under the earth. If use relative divisions then gold/metal attacks wood, water attacks fire.

Now, the after birth ba gua's order and position figure is shown below (Figure 9 and figure 10).

FIGURE 9: Wen Wang Ba Gua Directions Diagram

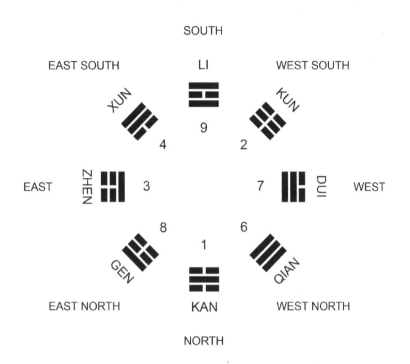

SOUTH

EAST SOUTH   LI   WEST SOUTH

XUN 4   9   2 KUN

EAST   ZHEN 3   7 DUI   WEST

8 GEN   1   6 QIAN

EAST NORTH   KAN   WEST NORTH

NORTH

FIGURE 10: Wen Wang Ba Gua Diagram

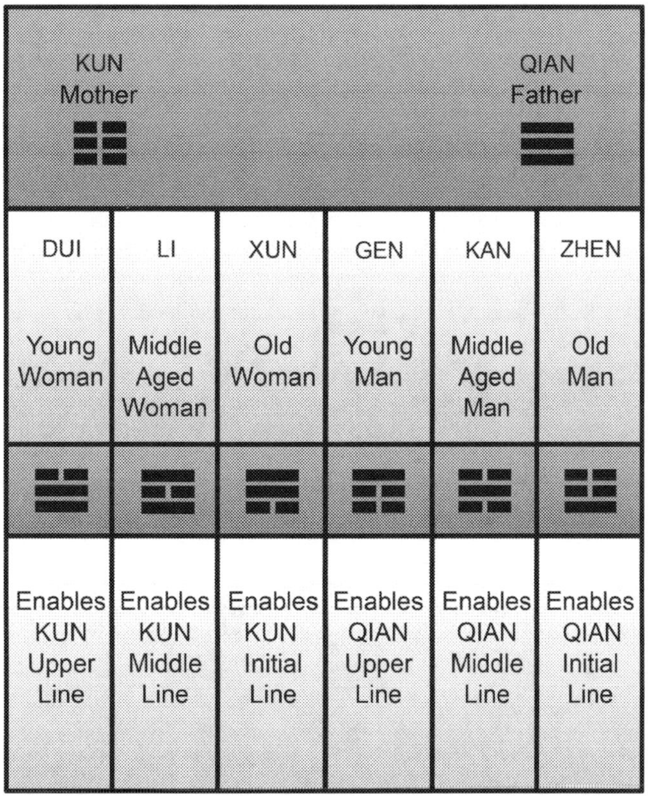

KUN Mother				QIAN Father	
DUI	LI	XUN	GEN	KAN	ZHEN
Young Woman	Middle Aged Woman	Old Woman	Young Man	Middle Aged Man	Old Man
Enables KUN Upper Line	Enables KUN Middle Line	Enables KUN Initial Line	Enables QIAN Upper Line	Enables QIAN Middle Line	Enables QIAN Initial Line

(i)   Eight channels eight points and the nine palaces ba gua's relationship

Ba gua combines with each of the positions, called the nine palaces; each palace combines with a meeting point and an extraordinary channel. Ling gui ba fa open points is derived and calculated according to the combined nine palaces' numbers.

Now, I will list the eight points combined with the nine palaces relationship in the following table:

TABLE 14: 8 Points Combined with the 9 Palaces Table

Ba Gua	Qian	Gen	Dui	Kan	Xun	Zhen	Li	Kun
Direction Position	West North	East North	West	North	East South	East	South	West South Centre
Nine Palaces Number	6	8	7	1	4	3	9	2, 5
Eight Points	SP 4	P 6	SI 3	UB 62	GB 41	TH 5	Lu 7	K 6
Eight Channels	Chong Mai	Yin Wei	Du Mai	Yang Qiao	Dai Mai	Yang Wei	Ren Mai	Yin Wei

Use 8 points and nine palaces ba gua's distribution and belonging relationship, according to the Wen Wang ba gua draw-figure. It is called the *qi jing na gua tu* (Figure 11).

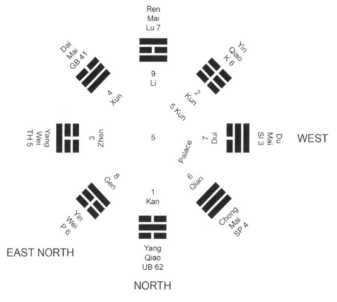

DIAGRAM 11: Extraordinary Channels Na Gua

In the figure, each position's representative number is according to the ba gua's yin yang's evolution/development and production: east position (left) is the number 3. 3 by 3 is nine. So, south position has the number 9. 3 multiplied by 9 is 27, so west position is 7. 3 multiplied 7 is 21, so north is 1. 1 multiplied by 3 is 3, so east is still 3. Heaven belongs to yang, heaven rotates left, so yang counts from 3 to 9, then from 7 to 1, shows heaven's left rotation. The sun comes from the east and down at the west. Yin belongs to earth, earth rotates (turns) right so yin number is from right to left developing circling, from south-west position number 2 starts. 2 multiplied by 2 equals 4, so south. East position is 4. 2 multiplied by 4 equals 8, so north- east position is 8. 2 multiplied by 8 is 16 so, north-west position is 6. 2 multiplied by 6 equals 12, return to the south-east's position number 2. As for the centre's number 5, it is taken as the source of the numbers' derivative. Just like the *Su wen-tian yuan ji da lun* said: "The reason to want to know heaven and earth's yin yang follows heaven's qi moving and not stopping, so 5 years and right movement." And said: "Heaven uses 6 as central, earth takes 5 to manage", it is therefore everything's number, cannot be without 5 and 6. For example, use west east north south etc. each relative direction added together, all is 15. In summary, the ba gua's numbers are also distributed at the four face and eight corners (si mian ba fang), and therefore have unity here as well. These numbers, more or less, represent the four seasons' weather and a day's temperature strong or weak; and shows yin yang's movement forward or backward, whether progressing or static, strong or weak, up or down, shrinking or extended/ stretched, or life or death etc. changes, because of the yin yang changes principle.

Ancient people used these principles and extrapolated and applied them to all aspects of medicine such as the *Ling shu-jiu gong ba feng*, which described the 8 directions' winds effects on the human body's health accordingly. Another example, the *Ling shu- jiu zhen lun* pointed out: left foot should be li chun (spring begins) (gen palace north-east), left rib should be chun fen (vernal equinox) (zhen palace exactly east direction), left hand should be li xia (summer begins) (xun palace south-east), breast throat head (shou tou) should be xia zhi (summer solstice) (li palace exactly south direction), right hand should be li qiu (autumn begins) (kan palace south-west), right rib should be qiu fen (autumn equinox) (dui palace exactly west direction), right foot should be li dong (winter begins) (qian palace north-west), waist, buttocks, lower orifices should be dong zhi (winter solstice) (kan palace exactly north direction), 6 fu (bowels) diagram san chang (three stories - triple heater) should be zheng Zhou (ie. middle palace etc.). This uses the body's upper and lower, and left and right to calculate along with climatic periods and the ba gua, the same meaning as ba gua represents yin yang's, and upper and lower. In addition, there are the "wu lun ba kuo" ("5 wheels and eight corridors") theory, used in the eye disease dept.; and "yun ba gua" etc. which is used in infantile tui na (Chinese massage) etc. Moreover, in the application of ba mai (8 channels) and ba fa (8 techniques), it uses these ba gua numbers which may repeatedly change to represent the name of the channel points.

Ba fa ge concisely summarised the relationship of the ba gua with the ba xue (eight points); if you are using ling gui ba fa you must remember this. Now, I will write down as follows:

Ba fa ge

Kan 1 - connects with shen mai (UB62); zhao hai (K6) kun 2, 5; zhen 3 belongs to wai guan (TH5); xun 4 lin qi (GB41) number; qian 6 is gong sun (SP4); dui 7 hou xi (SI3) house; gen 8 is nei guan (P6). Li 9 lie que (Lu 7) governs,

(ii) Heavenly Stems and Earthly Branches

Ling gui ba fa's composition, except the ba mai (eight channels), and the eight points, the ba gua day times' stems and branches' numbers as the basis of the ba fa (eight techniques) to choose points. Stem and branches' numbers are divided into represented day numbers and represented hour numbers. Represented day numbers heavenly stems uses jia ji as 10; yi geng as 9; ding ren as 8; wu gui bing xin as 7; earthly stems uses chen xu chou wei as 10; shen you as 9; yin mao as 8; si wu hai zi as 7. Represented hour numbers heavenly stems use jia ji as 9; yi geng as 8; bing xin as 7; ding ren as 6; wu gui as 5; earthly branches then uses zi wu as 9; chou wei as 8; yin shen as 7; mao you as 6; chen xu as 5; si hai as 4. Now, I will make a table and appendix as follows:

(Table 15) Eight Techniques According to Gan Zhi Table

10		9		8		7		7	
Heavenly Stems	Earthly Branches	Heavenly Stems	Earthly Branches	Heavenly Stems	Earthly Branches	Heavenly Stems	Earthly Branches	Heavenly Stems	Earthly Branches
Jia Ji	Chen, Xu, Chou, Wei	Yi Geng	Shen You	Ding Ren	Yin Mao	Wu Gui	Si Wu	Bing Xin	Hai Zi

Ba fa zhu ri gan zhi ge:

Jia ji chen xu chou wei shi, yi geng shen you jiu wei qi, ding ren yin mao ba cheng shu, wu gui si wu qi xiang yi, bing xin hai zi yi qi shu, zhu ri gan zhi ji de zhi.

(Table 16) 8 Techniques Clinical Time Gan Zhi Table

9		8		7		6		5		4
Heavenly Stems	Earthly Branches	Heavenly Stems	Earthly Branches	Heavenly Stems	Earthly Branches	Heavenly Stems	Earthly Branches	Heavenly Stems	Earthly Branches	Earthly Brances
Jia	Zi	Yi	Chou	Bing	Yin	Ding	Mao	Wu	Chen	Si
Ji	Wu	Geng	Wei	Xin	Shen	Ren	You	Gui	Xu	Hai

Ba fa lin shi gan zhi ge

Jia ji zi wu jiu yi yong, yi geng chou wei ba wu yi, bing xin yin shen qi zuo shu, ding ren mao you liu xu zhi, wu gui chen xu ge you wu, si hai dan jia si gong qi, yang ri chu jiu yin chu liu, bu jin ling yu xue xia tui.

Ba fa (eight techniques) days, hours, stems and branches numbers arrive according to the 5 elements which create and process (or sedate) (cheng) numbers and stem and branch (favourable) order's (shun) yin yang to determine.

1. Eight techniques following day stem and branch number explanation: he tu shu the river diagram numbers ie. the 5 elements create and process numbers. Five elements create and process (or sedate) (cheng) numbers have 10. *Zhou yi-xi* ci said: "heaven (tian) 1 (creates water) di (earth) 6 processes it; di 2 creates fire, tian 7 processes it; tian 3 creates wood, di 8 processes it; di 4 creates metal, tian 9 processes it; tian 5 creates earth, di 10 processes it." So, the five elements created numbers are water 1, fire 2, wood 3, metal 4, earth 5; five elements becoming numbers water 6, fire 7, wood 8, metal 9, earth 10. The eight techniques represents/substitutes the the following days stem and branch numbers, is use-the-five-elements-process-numbers. Heavenly stems uses mutually combining transforming of the five elements. Earthly branches uses its original-arriving-5 elements, so as to mutually combine the arriving and the five-elements-processing numbers. For example, heavenly stems jia ji combine to transform earth. Earthly branches chen, xu, chou, wei, belong to central pillars earth, earth's processing number is 10. Then 10 represents/substitutes Jia, ji, chen, xu, chou, wei 6 words, so the song says: "jia ji chen xu chou wei shi." "Yi geng shen you gui wei qi" 's meaning. Because heavenly stems' yi geng combine to transform metal, earthly branches' shen you belongs to western direction's metal; metal's processing number is 9, so 9 represents/substitutes yi, geng, shen, you four characters. However, heavenly stems ding ren combines to transform wood, earthly branches yin mao belonging to east directions wood,

wood's processing number is 8, so the eight represents/substitutes ding, ren, yin, mao four characters, so the song says: "ding ren yin mao ba chen shu." "Wu gui si wu qi xiang yi" 's meaning, because heavenly stems wu and gui combine to transform fire, earthly branch si and wu belongs to southern directions fire; fire's cheng (sedating/processing) number is 7, 7 represents/substitutes wu, gui, si, wu four characters. So, as to heavenly stems bing and xin combining to transform water, earthly branches' hai and zi belong to northern directions water; water's combining number is 6; bing xin hai zi four words originally use 6 to represent/ substitute but because water and fire are named under the same category as belonging to before heaven (xian tian) produced things, it is not the case. In the ba gua, if belong to fire's li tri-gram (gua), it is also called Li zhong xu (li central deficiency); the "zhong xu" actually means fire is stored/hidden in true water, ie. Inside the sun is moon's essence (jing) meaning. So, as to the exception regarding bing, xin, hai, and zi not using water 6 cheng number but still using fire's 7 cheng number we can see why; use 7 to represent/substitute bing, xin, hai, and zi four characters. Therefore, the song says "bing, xin, hai, zi, yi, qi, shu."

2. Clinically, the eight methods, (ba fa) are according to the hours' stems and branches' numbers explained meanings: eight methods represent/substitute hour stem and branch number according to the heavenly stem order's yin and yang to determine. The *Su wen san bu jiu hou lun* said: Heaven, earth arriving number, begins from one and ends at nine." Heaven's stem uses "jia" as the first number, jia yi bing ding wu ji geng xin ren, ren is the 9th number, earth branch uses zi as the 1st number, zi chou yin mao chen si wu wei shen, shen is earth branch's number 9. So, stem and branch "ren", "shen" two words are used as the basis derivation of forward and coming/arrival.

Representing /substituting times' stem and branch numbers, is to use combined heavenly stems and opposite earthly branches and combine together to represent the changes of stem's and branch's yin and yang.

Heavenly stems uses jia as head (shou), jia ji meets five (5) combined jia, from jia according to heavenly stems' order count to ren is number 9. Earthly branches uses as head (shou), zi and wu meet 6 opposite (xiang chong), from zi according to earth branches' order, therefore re order count to shen, is number 9. So, jia ji and zi wu, four words are all number 9. It is said, "jia ji zi wu jiu yi yong."

Heavenly stems yi and geng are combined, from yi to ren is 8, earthly branches chou and wei are opposite, from chou to shen is also 8. So it is said: "yi geng chou wei ba wu yi."

Heavenly stems bing xin are combined, from bing to ren is 7, earthly branches yin shen xiang chong (in dispute with each other (can't co-operate), from yin to shen is 7, so it is said: "bing xin yin shen 7 as their number."

Heavenly stems ding ren are combined, ding and ren are 6, earthly branches mao you can't co-operate, mao to shen is 6, so it is said: "ding ren mao you liu shun zhi."

Heavenly stems wu gui are combined, wu to ren is 5, earthly branches chen xu don't co-operate, chen to shen is 5 so it is said: "wu gui chen xu ge you wu."

Earthly branches si hai don't co-operate, si to shen is 4, 4 independently represents si hai, so it is said: "si hai dan jia si geng qi" ("si hai singly adds equals to four").

Section 3
ling gui ba fa's open points method

Ling gui ba fa open points method procedure is:

1. Figure out/calculate that day's daily item, and branch.
2. According to "wu hu jian yuan" ("5 tiger help the source") determine that time's shi chen (2 hour time period) stem and branch.
3. According to "shu re gan zhi" ("according to day's stem and branch") and "lin shi gan zhi" ("according to hour"), to obtain these four 'stems and branches' representative numbers, and then calculate the sum of these four stems and branches.
4. Based on the principles of "yang ri chu jiu ("yang day divide by 9") yin ri chu liu ("yin day divide by 6") to divide this sum, then get the remainder which is in the suitable open the points representative number. Use point representative numbers to check the "qi jing na gua tian" ("Extraordinary channels taken the trigram (diagram"). Then we can know 'should open the points'.
5. All that can be divided and have no remaining numbers, yang day is 9, all are lie que (Lu7) point; yin day is 6, all are gong sun point (SP4).

(i) Day's stem branch direction method.

If there are no reference books for checking the day's stems and branches, only know the calendar month and day, then need to use day stem and branch calculations formula to derive that day's daily stem and branch. Now we'll introduce the method to use *Guan shi gan zhi fang chen sha.* (*Guan's stem and branch equations*) determines the day's stems and branches, but only use as a reference:

Day's heavenly stem representative number =

$$\frac{A + X + \Delta}{10}(+1) = \text{Year one (new years written day)}$$

$$\frac{\text{Heavenly stem representation number and the day's date number use with to calculate the month add and subtract constant}}{10}(+1)$$

Formula explanation:

1. A+X+Δ > 10, then the sum should be divided by 10
2. Every time we next have a leap year, calculate the day after March 1st, must add on to obtain the number.

$$\frac{= \text{Written New Year's day earthly branch calculated day number} + \text{month add and subtract constant (ie total)}}{12}(+1)$$

Foundation demonstration

1. a + x + δ > 12, then the sum should be divided by 12;
2. Every time there is a leap year calculate after March 1st each day should add 1.

When use this equation to calculate we must first understand the meaning of each term.

1. "Day stem branch number" is the stem branch order number's number, see figure 17.

(Table 17) Heavenly stem, earthly branch order number table.

Heavenly stem	Jia	Yi	Bing	Ding	Wu	Ji	Geng	Xin	Ren	Gui		
Number	1	2	3	4	5	6	7	8	19	10	11	12
Earthly branch	Zi	Chou	Yin	Mao	Chen	Si	Wu	Wei	Shen	You	Xu	Hai

2. "New Year's day stem and branch number" is that year's New Year's day's stem branch order number's number. Each year's New Year's days stem and branch is subject to change and has principle's/rules. i.e. this year's New Year's day to next year's New Year's day stem and branch number has 5 days difference but the leap year has 6 days difference. For example, given 1980 is leap year, New Year's day stem and branch is gui you. Want to calculate 1981's New Year's day stem and

branch? Only seriously count 6 stems and branches to obtain Heavenly Stem, gui jia yi bing ding wu ji; Earthly Branch, you xu hai zi chou yin mao, therefore know 1981 New Year's day stem and branch is ji mao. Now list 1980 to 2000 year, each year New Year's day's stem and branch as below tabled, (see Table 18)

(Table 18) 1980 - 2000 Each Year's New Year's day stem and branch table.

Leap year (Yin man)		Normal years (ping man)							
Year	New Year's days stem and branch	Year	New Year's day stem and branch	Year	New Year's day stem and branch	Year	New Year's day stem and branch
1980	Gui you	1981	Ji mao	1982	Jia shen	1983	Ji chou
1984	Jia wu	1985	Geng zi	1986	Yi si	1987	Geng xu
1988	Yi mao	1989	Xin you	1990	Bing yin	1991	Xin wei
1992	Bing zi	1993	Ren wu	1994	Ding hai	1995	Ren chen
1996	Ding you	1997	Gui mao	1998	Wu shen	1999	Gui chou

3. "Month add and subtract constant": according to western calendar to derive the Chinese calendar day's stem and branch. When do the calculation, we must, add or subtract a fixed constant according to western calendar's month. *Ge yue jia jian chang shu ge* as follows:

1, 5 both should minus 1; 2, 6 add 0, 6; 3 should subtract 2 add 10; 4 subtract 1 add 5; 7, 0, 9 add 2; 8 add 1, 7 go

On 10 add 2, 8; with 3 winter 3, 9; leap year beginning from March Remaining number, all add 1

(Table 19) Each month should add-and-subtract content table

Month	Jan		Feb		Mar		Apr		May		Jun		Jul		Aug		Sep		Oct		Nov		Dec	
Stem and branch add and subtract number	H.S		E.B		H.S		E.B		H.S		E.B		H.S		E.B		H.S		E.B		H.S		E.B	
Different years																								
Normal year	-1	-1	+0	+6	-2	+10	-1	+5	-1	-1	+0	+6	+0	+0	+1	+7	+2	+2	+2	+8	+3	+3	+3	+9

4. "Stem and branch periodically rotation number": Heavenly stem from jia to gui has 10 numbers, so Heavenly stem periodically rotation number is 10;

Earthly branch, from zi to hai, has 12 numbers, so, earthly branch periodically rotation number is 12.

After mastering the above constants meaning, one can use equations to calculate any one particular day's stem and branch. For example, calculate 1981 August 28's stem and branch: August 28 heavenly stem = (New Year's day's Heavenly stem number (6) and add the wanted day number (28) and month (add and subtract constant (1)) ÷ 10 (Heavenly stem periodically rotation number = 35 ÷ 10 and the remaining number is 5. According to Heavenly stem series numbers number 5 is represented by wu.

August 28's Earthly branch = (New Year's Earthly branch number (4) add wanted day number (28) and month add and subtract constant (7)) ÷ 12 (Earthly Branch periodically rotation number = 39 ÷ 12 remaining number is 3. According to Earthly branch series number, number 3 is represented by yin.

So we know 1981 August 28's stem and branch is wu yin.

If next Leap Year because February has one day more so from number, need to add 1 to the numbers calculated in the equations. That's the wanted stem and branch number. For example, calculate 1984 May 1st stem and branch. 1984 is a leap year. New Year's day stem and branch is jia wu. Jia's number is 1, wu's number is 7, put into equation. May 1st Heavenly stem equals New Year's day Heavenly stem number (1) add wanted day number (1) minus month add and subtract content (1)) and Leap year's should add day number (1) =2. Because in the formula A + X + Δ < 10 so don't need to be divided by Heavenly stem periodically rotation number. X is heavenly stem's yi's number. So, we know May 1st Heavenly Stem is yi.

May 1st Earthly Branch = (New Year's Day Earthly Branch number (7) add wanted day number (1) - month's add and subtract constant (1)) and Leap Year's should add day number (1) = 8. Because in the formula a + δ + d < 12, so don't need to divide by Earthly branch periodically rotation number. 8 is Earthly Branch's wei's representative number. Therefore, the fifth month first day, is known to many as wei.

So 1984 May 1st, this day's stem and branch is yi wei.

(ii) Two hour period (shi chen) stem branch derivation technique

Two hour period stem branch is according to "wu hu jin yuan fa" ("Five Tiger Construct Elements technique"), a day from the beginning to derive. One day 24 hours is divided into 12 shi chen (2 hour periods) .5 days totally hour 60 shi chen. Exactly 60 jia zi's number, so the following days' shi chen's stem and branch, exactly 5 days exactly rotate one period, try to begin from jia day's beginning (ie. zero hour),

5 days 60 shi chen, to wu day's gui (gui hai) time, ji day's zi time again from jia zi beginning, the each other day's shi chen's stem and branch are also of use. So, once one remembers each day's belonging heavenly stem remember day's beginning time story, one can devise that day's each two hours stem and branch. Day's beginning time song has two kinds, one is frame zi time to derive, is called "wu zi jian yuan fa". The other is from the yin time period to derive, because yin at 12 belongs to tiger it is called "wu hu jian yuan fa".

Wu hu jian yuan ri shi ge

Jia ji zhi ri qi bing yin, yi geng zhi chen wu yin tou, bing xin lin cong geng yin qi, ding ren ren yin shun xing lai.

Wu gui jai yin ding shi hou, liu shi shou fa zhu yi liu

The following: "wu hu jian yuan" day beginning time derivative method, list *shi gan zhi zha dui biao* as following: (see Table 20)

(Table 20) Shi gan zhi cha dui biao

Days stems and branches	Shi gan zhi (Hours of stems and branches)											
	1 o'clock	3 o'clock	5 o'clock	7 o'clock	9 o'clock	11 o'clock	13 o'clock	15 o'clock	17 o'clock	19 o'clock	21 o'clock	23 o'clock
Jia ji	Jia zi	Yi chou	Bing yin	Ding mao	Wu chen	Ji si	Geng wu	Xin wei	Ren shen	Gui you	Jia xu	Yi hai
Yi geng	Bing zi	Ding chou	Wu yin	Ji mao	Geng chen	Xin si	Ren wu	Gui wei	Jia shen	Yi you	Bing xu	Ding hai
Bing xin	Wu zi	Ji chou	Gen yin	Xin mao	Ren chen	Gui si	Jia wu	Yi wei	Bing shen	Ding you	Wu xu	Ji hai
Ding ren	Geng zi	Xin chou	Ren yin	Gui mao	Jia chen	Yi si	Bing wu	Ding wei	Wu shen	Ji you	Geng xu	Xin hai
Wu gui	Ren zi	Gui chou	Jia yin	Yi mao	Bing chen	Ding si	Wu wu	Ji wei	Geng shen	Xin you	Ren xu	Gui hai

(iii)   Ling gui ba fa open points method example

Example 1: Calculate 1981 August 27 afternoon 3:15 according to Ling gui ba fa should open which points?
Solution:

1. Calculate day's stem and branch, check *zhu nian yuan dan gan zhi biao* (Table 18), we know 1981 New Year's day's stem and branch is ji mao, heavenly stem number is 6, earthly branch number is 4. Put them into the equation: August 27 heavenly stem = 6 + 27 + 1 = 34; 34 ÷ 10 the remainder is 4, so we know this day's heavenly stem is ding. August 27 Earthly Branch = 4 + 27 + 7 = 38; 38 ÷ 12 remainder is 2, so we know this day's earthly branch is chou.

2. Calculate hour stems and branch: check *shi gan zhi cha dui biao* (Table 20), we know deng day afternoon 3 - 5 o'clock, hour stem and branch is ou shen.

3. Check *ba fa zhu ri gan zhi biao* (table 15), we know ding is 8, chou is 10 - check *ba fa lin shi gan zhi biao*, we know lou is 5, shen is 7. Day stem and branch, hour stem and branch, together equals 30.

4. According to jia, bing, wu, geng, ren odd numbers are yang days; yi, ding, ji, xin, gui even numbers are yin days. Ding days are yin days, should be divided by 6, 30 ÷ 6 = 5, it is totally divided and has no remaining numbers. Yin day is 6, 6 represents chong mai and gong sun point (SP4). Then know August 27th 1981 afternoon 3:15. According to Ling gua ba fa open points should be gong sun (SP4).

Example 2: Calculate March 16 1982 morning 10:00 should open which point?

Solution:

1. Calculate day, stem and branch: put into *guan shi gan zhi fang chen she*: calculate day, stem, and branch is wu xu

2. Calculate hour, stem and branch: check *shi gan zhi cha dui biao,* know hour, stem, and branch is ding ji.

3. Calculate day, hour, stem, and branches' number sum as 7 + 10 + 6 + 4 =27.

According to "yang days are divided by 9, yin days are divided by 6" this law, 27 ÷ 9 = 3, exactly divided without remaining number. Wu day belongs to yang, yang day is 9, all open lie qie point (Lu7). So we know March 16th 1982 10:00am should open unblock ren mai's bi lie qie point.

Section 4
Ling gui ba fa's clinical examples.

Example 1, Hong XX female 47 years old clothing worker.

This patient, without care, fell and slipped down and rotated, or damaged the foot and waist. This all happened when she went down a slope, with a rod across her shoulders for carrying vegetables in a bucket at 8:00am October 16th 1976. During the same day after a long time the pain increased badly. She was sent to hospital but the waist and back bone were firm and the right lower limb x-ray check didn't discover any bone or any other body damage. She intently took Chinese herbal medicine yun nan bai yao quality pain (pain tablets), and at the waist back bone and sacrum add pu lu kai yin (profane), using block technique, and externally used medical wires etc. treatment for 5 days. The effect is not obvious.

At 8:00pm October 21st 1976, she consented for acupuncture treatment. Check right ankle - seemed blue swollen, locally has pressing pain, cannot walk; waist pain cannot abduct or adduct or rotate to the sides, from lumbar vertebrae to sacrum backbone all have pressing pain. Firstly, vertibrae 4-5 waist backbone pressing pain is obvious, waist vertebrae generally had pressing pain; especially right side waist he la ji (iliocostalis vertibrae) and waist longismis muscle and li zhong muscle (?) and posterior upper illness area etc quarter pressing pain obvious; and herself a comer said recent 3 days has abdomen qi distended gastric cavity full and stuffy, qi adverse (qi ni). Pulse looks chen jin (sunken tense), tongue coating is thin yellow.

Use Ling gui ba fa to select points. 1976 October 21st day, stem, and branch is bing wu. 8:00am according to hour, stem, and branch is ren chen. Day's stem branch number by is 7, wu is 7. Hour's stem branch number ren is 6, chen is 5. These four numbers add to make 25, because bing wu is a yang day, should be divided by 9, remaining number is 7. So open dui tri-gram, goes to/unblocks du channel's hou xi (SI3) point, operating solution technique, then wu semi-conductor treatment machine, switch on for 20 minutes. After remove the needle, the patient's waist has already become movable (can move then add needle to cheng qiang) (Gv1) point, use hand technique (long hu jiao zhan shou fa), retain needle for 20 minutes. After remove the needle, patient's waist pain is reduced greatly, she can extend and flex her back. The next day, the right ankle which was swollen and distended, totally disappeared. She went to see the doctor by herself. Waist pain part moved but needling once again, the illness pain completely disappeared.

Note: du channel originated from lower most points' ji joint, parallel with the spine's upward movement, there was du channel's qi blockage, so there was upper waist pain and cannot extend and flex – yang qiao patient, foot tai yang's bie channel. Its channel qi originates from inside the heel, and exits at the external ankle going down to foot tai yang's shen mai (UB62) point.

Following the thigh external side, goes upwards, yang qiao channel's qi blockage blood stagnancy, so external ankle swollen and distended, waist and back stiff and straight. According to channel's and collateral's intensifying pattern, this is caused by du channel, yang qiao channel's qi blockage. So open hou xi (SI3), combined with shen mau (UB62) together. This is belonging to ba hui xi (fa mu meeting points) "husband and wife" points combined use method. Select left shen mai (UB62) point, because right ankle was blue swollen, is not suitable for needle insertion, the other main reason is according to the words of the *Zhen jiu da cheng*: "left needle, right illness, is to know high or low (gao and xia), use this idea to unblock channels, is the general message".

Example 2, Wan XX, male 38 years old, worker.

Patient got a cold because allergic to western medicine and this type of medicine, self-took *yin qiao jie du pian* to treat for 2 days. The illness become more serious; the patient complained of headache, along with arrival of cold-heat. He came to ask for acupuncture treatment at 2pm September 10th 1980. Upon checking his pulse, it was floating tense (fou jin), tongue coating white, tongue sides coating bland yellow. According to *Ling gui ba fa* to derive, that day is bing xu day, yi wei hour, should give gong sun (SP4) point. Is not in agreement with this pattern, so silent select point he gu (LI4), lie que (Lu7), feng chi (GB20), and tai yang (EX2) are selected.

After needle insertion as treatment, I made an appointment with the patient to come for acupuncture next day at 10:00am. The next day, the patient came on time and said the treatment was effective. Because of yesterday's acupuncture, he had pains a little less however today there was two tai yang points part pain which are quite strong, while the cold-heat was not yet removed.

Then, according to Ling gui ba fa to select points. 10:00am September 11th 1980 is ding hai day yi shi hour, day heavenly stem is ding, number is 8, day earthly branch is hai, number is 7. Hour heavenly stem is yi, remainder number is 8. Hour earthly branch is shi, remainder number is 4. These four numbers added together is equal to 27. Ding hai is yin day should divide by 6. The remaining number is 3, so open zhen tri-gram, connect and unblock with yang wei channel's wai guan (TH5) point.

Simultaneously select zu lin qi (GB41), using selection technique. Retain needles for 20 minutes. After pulling out the needles, the headache is obviously lessened. The same day after sweating-out, the heat was removed.

Next day, the illness fully recovered.

Note: yang wei channel protects (qi's) controls all the collaterals and controls the yang channels, especially tai yang channel, and the shao yang channel which depend on it most deeply. The tai yang controls body's external. The shao yang controls half-external, half-internal. When yang wei etc. is under attack, both have cold-heat symptoms, so if the hand yang wei and the hand tai yang are ill many come bitter cold heat". Connect yang wei's wai guan point (TH5). This is hand shou yang's channel zhu point. The hand shao yang channel follows side of head points, illness symptoms also control "eye brow corner pain". So *jing lin te jiao xue ge* said: "Headache and febrile heat, wai guan (TH5) comes." Yang wei and dai mai intersection combine at eyebrow corner of head bone parts". Connects with dai's zu lin qi (GB41). Should be the foot shao yang's shu point, the foot shao yang channel follows the head temples (ie. the parts of skull next to ear). "The illness" shows that now treat GB41. According to Ling giu ba fa zhen, xun two tri grams intersect. So next needle wai guan (TH5), combined with lin qi (GB41).

Section 5
Discussion and understanding

1. Ling gui ba fa is an acupuncture treatment method, according to the hour select the point, combined with ba gua theory. It is one of the ancient philosophical ideas of this country. It belongs to the area of pure experience theory and self-formation of a time honoured principle. It is a genuine principle summarised from ancient observations of natural phenomena and using yin yang to alternatively compose different areas. The ba gua uses nature, heaven, earth, water, fire, wind, thunder, mountain, etc moves as basis, so it divides qian into heaven, kun as earth, kan as water, li as fire, xun as wind, zhen as thunder, gen as mountain, dui as river etc., eight names. Ba gua theories' basic philosophy observation is the idea to describe the form ie. the so called "yi you tai ji, shi sheng liang yi, liang yi sheng si xiang, si xiang sheng ba gua". The *Yi jing* has tri grams, they produce two yi (opposing forms), two yi produce four shapes, four shapes produce the eight trigrams). It (i.e. the *Yi jing*) is like a geometric progression, from one to two, two to four, four to eight, eight to sixteen, and further subdivide into

32, 64, 384 etc.; uses these numbers to demonstrate the natural phenomena and principle. Because – what then is yin and yang, i.e. they represent the sun, moon, day, night, cold, hot etc. then all of these may represent sunlight change and temperature's change and these changes have a great effect on animals, plants, minerals, and all of the natural world. Especially, also have a deep relationship with human beings lives, human body health, illness production and treatment. So, over several thousand years, ba gua philosophical theory has been widely used in medicine theory. Ba mai ba xue (eight channels eight points), according to the four distribution of points treatment method is the guidance idea of "tian ren he yi" ("heaven and man combined as one") and is one of ba gua's theories' applications in the material aspect.

To demonstrate the natural world and the human body's complicated changes, based on ba gua basic numbers, use the wu xing (5 elements) to produce the numbers; heavenly stems and earthly branches etc. numbers change to describe things and change procedure. Those numbers change in principle. A lot of this is proposed, based on ancient observation of a lot of human and some natural objective changes. So, it is to some extent representative of things change objective principle. For example, the "ren ti nei bu de sheng wu shi zhong li lun" ("human body internal biological time clock theory"), is the name given by recent scientists. On this basis, this is an argument for ba gua theory. The other example, "sheng wu jie cou li lun" ("biological rhythm theory") reveals the period change principle of the body's strength, emotions, and intelligence ie. the so-called body strength cause, emotion cause and intelligence cause. These theories have already been widely used in some Western countries. Moreover this so-called biology rhythm collection method has some initiatives with the deconstructive method of Ling gui ba fa. More examples can be seen as ancient people called it li-lai bo and investigated the relationship between the moon and human beings behaviour. They thought, the moon is full or waning, which may cause the human body's "biological high tide" and "biological low tide" and concluded the moon full or waning has a relationship with people's "invasion or attack behaviour". Actually, li-lai bo's ideas have been mentioned at least 2,000 years ago in this country's ancient medicine's literature and many philosophical works. Recently, some German scholars noticed the *Zhou yi's* 64 tri grams has astonishingly similar effects with 3 body genetic code table in combination as well as listing other aspects. This has caused literary attention in American and Japanese etc. world scholars. Genetic codes means how a biological body's number and control of the combination of protein, controls the principle of biological and genetic characteristics. It is a great discovery in recent molecular genetics. Surprisingly, the genetic side for such beautiful relationship is in Chinese ancient book the *Zhou yi ba gua*. This is a thoughtful consideration.

From the above we can see that the ba gua theory contains a lot of scripture essence and is worthy of deeper search and discussion. Even though it has not got its proper place due to it in history.

2. Recent large scientific research demonstrates that the human body's channels and collaterals objectively exist. The pathogens in the channels and collaterals, and, the strong and weak changes happen during the day and the night has been understood and accepted by people. However, the qi jing ba mai as an important part of this channel and collateral system, by their qi and blood factors opening and closing, strong and weak changes etc. principles, has not been studied and investigated till today. However, this is an important condition when we study channels and collaterals basic concepts, and human body life science, etc. large projects: ie Ling gui ba fa medicines and some principles of qi and blood, whether strong and weak and points, open and close. One idea about this meaning is spoken here. Deep study of Ling gui ba fa and its meaning has scientific value.

3. To investigate and verify the clinical practical value of Ling gui ba fa. Under Guan Zheng zai and old doctors guidance, think of the more than 10 years treatment observation and the 38 kinds of illness and more than 400 patient cases, then the first understandings are as follows:

To use Ling gui ba fa, one should use channels and collaterals to identify the pattern as the main method. Especially, one should pay attention to using actual ordinary channel theory. The accuracy of identifying the pattern is the basis of the treatment effect.

(1) Transport (transmute), selecting point properly and combining point is the key to operate Ling gui ba fa.

(2) Correct group: how to use tonify and sedate hand techniques in treatment, is the important part to determine the treatment effect.

(3) Through clinical illness case analysis, we timidly propose using Ling gui ba fa to treat some urgent illnesses and some painful illness conditions. This can have better treatment effects.

(4) The combination use of Ling gui ba fa and Zi wu liu zhu needling techniques makes the treatment effect more obvious.

Chapter 2
....
Briefly on the clinical application of Zi wu liu zhu ben Zhou (circular) tu (diagram)

Zi wu liu zhu is a type of theory in Chinese oriental medicine theories. It is based on the whole body idea of "tian ren he yi" ("heaven and human being combined as one"). They think the human body's qi and blood is according to a certain circulatory order and has rules like the tides, up and down and appears with periodically strong and weak changes. According to Zi wu liu zhu theory, following the channels and collaterals, qi and blood strong and weak and point position open and close principle combines with yin yang, wu xing (5 elements), tian gan (heavenly stems) di zhi (earthly branches). Of course all this is according to time to open point prudent method, is called Zi wu liu zhu making techniques.

Section 1
The composition of Zi wu liu zhu circular diagram.

Twelve channels jing, ying, shu, yuan, jing, he, 66 points one cycle (2 weeks/fortnight). Day by day liu zhu (flowing), according to time open points, periodically and comes back to the beginning again, like a circle without an end. So, it is called zi wu lin zhu circle diagram. This diagram is compound of 5 circles. Now, I will demonstrate according to the diagram example as follows.

1. The 1st circle: 10 stems main day: the first circle with knowledge use the 10 characters, anaylse earthly (branches) five transformations (wu yun), are divided into 5 yin, 5 yang: 5 yin is combined at 5 yang, 5 yang combined at 5 fu, jia day yang work (nu) combines with the gall bladder fu (bowel). Yi day combines with the liver yang (organ). Bing day yang fire combines with the small intestine: ding day yin fire combines with the heart; wu day yang earth combines with the stomach fu, ji day yin earth combines with the spleen zang; geng day yang metal combines with the large intestine; xin day yin metal combines with the lung zang (organ); ren day, yang water

combines at urinary bladder; gui day yin water combines at father's home's zang (organ). There is little representing pericardium collateral and triple heater by itself, a bowel. According to *Zhen jia da quan, Zhen jiu ju ying, and Zhen jiu da cheng* etc books all said "san jiao yi xiang ren zhong qi, bao luo tong gui ru gui fang" ("Triple heater is also positioned at ren inside, the pericardium collateral categorized under the gui position.") My father thought the triple heater and the pericardium collateral as external and internal, both of them belonging to mutual fire (xiang huo), also the heater is "jui du" ("small ditch/creek that bursts its banks") You can say ren, but really is opposite to the heart and centres it, so how can one say it is gui? He agreed with Zhang Jing yue's theory "san jiao yang fu, xu gui bing, bao luo cong yin ding huo pang" (triple heater is a yang bowel, should belong to bing, bao luo follows the yin, ding is a fire site") With regards to the lesser of the two, the triple heater's classifications, this diagram's stem rotation follows Mr Zhang's theory but the zi wu liu zhu tu follows Mr Shu's.

2. The second circle the stem and branch's fixed time: the secong circle is divided so one day is 12 hours, beginning from zi and ending up at hai. Up to now normally the heavenly stem's have the characteristics of 10 days, totalling 120 hours. Earthly branches are used 10 times. Heavenly stems are used 12 times. Jin ji's day, both begin from jia zi: yi geng's days both begin from bing zi; bing xin's day, both begins from wu zi; ding ren's day both begins from geng zi: wu gui's day, both begins from ren zi. From jia day's jia zi time, after 10 days (one go - 120 hours) has passed, the relation to jia zi, circulating repeatedly like this, periodically beginning again.

3. The third circle shu points of Zi wu liu zhu: this circle is arranged according to the contents of Xu Run bo's book *Zi wu liu zhu jia ri an shi ding xue ge*. In its diagram marked" "is the main channel of this day's beginning to open up the jing (well) points, then after follow the other Zi wu liu zhu's points, including "fa ben hai yuan" ("return to the origin") and "mu zi xiang sheng" ("mother and son produce each other") (the triple heater points produce that day's main channel, the points of the five elements produce the channel's five elements and are the mother points, ie. that day's main channel produced 'biao luo points" channels five elements, (channels five elements produced points are son points). No matter if the connecting time is that day or the next day both subscribe with that main channel. For example, at jia day xu time open gall bladder jing-well's qiao yin (GB44), before jia day xu time's you wei, se, mao, chou 5 yin times, the listed/

corresponding are zhong chong (P9), chi zi (Lu 5), shang qiu (SP5), shen men (H 7), xing jian (Liv2) each zangs' yin day, following wood-fire-earth-metal-water produce each other's order. Jia day meets jia at xu hour again, only should open qiao yin (GB44) one point. Jia at yang day open at yang hour; hai at yin hour, so don't open any points, circulate insert on yi day bing zi yang time, open small intestine ying point qian gu (S12) because jia gall-bladder belongs to wood, bing small intestine belongs to fire; gall bladder opens the first point and connects to small intestine's second point, wood produces fire, yang jing well giao yin (GB44) belongs to metal, yang ying (a spring) qian gu (S12) belongs to water, is also the meaning of metal and water produce each other. Then, insert on yi day wu yin time, should open stomach's shu (stream) point xian gu (ST43). Small intestine belongs to fire, stomach belongs to earth, fire produces earth then passes through qiu xu (GB40) one point. Because the six fu liu shu points, each have one more yuan (origin, or source) point, goes outside of 5 elements producing each other, so passes through shu (stream) points, conversely, search for its source (ben). It's committed with qiao yin (GB44's), channel then pours through it, listed at a lower position. Yi day's geng chen time, insert large intestines yang xi point (L15). Ren wu time, insert urinary bladder wei zhong (UB40) point. Say its fu (bowel), the large intestine belongs to metal/gold, urinary bladder belongs to water, metal and water produce each other; say its points then yang channel fire, yang shu earth (tu), fire earth produce (each other). The end is jia shen time, repeat list triple heater ying point ye men (TH2) because the triple heater is only/solely a fu (bowel), the six shu have no position to put it anywhere, so list it at the extreme end of each bowel as a kai xue (opening point); respectively select its ying point. It is because the yang ying (stream) point is a water point, and the gall-bladder is a wood bowel, this has the meaning of water produces wood. Jia day xu time cycling continues and add yi day shen time totalling eleven hours, 6 bowels (fu) open one point each. The gall-bladder is located at a main position. Pass one original point more, totalling 7 points. This jia day (zi wu) liu zhu details are as follows: the remaining 9 days, while periodically liu zhu, zang (organs) have five shu each. The (bowels) have six shu each. The bowels are yang, zang are yin. Yang jing metal, yin jing wood, each following the order of producing each other (zi wu) liu zhu circulating and therefore select bowels pass one yuan (point), zang (organs) use shu (points) to replace yuan (points) and pass it. End one point, yang day qi na (grasp) triple heater select "produce me." Yin day blood returns to bao luo, select one which "produces me", to give a day which loses 10 hours, kidney doesn't open chou hour but moves to hai hour, this is because the kidney controls water, is the root of the human body's life; pay attention to producing wood. If you cannot turn to insert jia day, then flow (liu) (doesn't zhu) but doesn't count, is not in agreement with the rule of yin and yang produce each other. Gui water although is also one of the 10 days stems, is not listed according to the five elements producing numbers, is called heaven (tian) one produces water, since gui water belongs to tian one. Use the beginning yin stem to combine with the end yin branch, heaven (tian) one (1) gives water, combines with the earthly branches ie. The last double hour hai hour. This equals yang stem, begins at jia wood, must combine with the last one (1) yang hour xu time, as beginning to open the jing (well) points time. And moreover, 10 days stem's periodically circle according to the yang forward, yin backwards principle. For example, gui day's hai time begins, then the heavenly stems which enter into jia wood. Earthly branches return to wu time, then the heaveny stems enter into jia wood. Earthly branches returns to xu time. Again, Heavenly stems enter into yi wood, earthly branches returns to you time, then the following bing, ding, wu, ji, etc. days are inside this heavenly stems enters and earthly branches returns rule. This is supportive of the jia day xu hour opens at qiao yin (GB44) idea, that yi day you hour opens at da dun (Liv 1) belief, and that bing day shen hour opens shao zi (SI1) view etc. order, and therefore follows in an orderly and contributively fashion without stopping. Gui water is having the channel's representative name, but the kidney channel's jing (well) point is yong quan (K1), so at the gui day's gui hai hour should open yong quan (K1) point.

4. The fourth circle: same thing with crossing the disorder: heavenly stems 10 characters, earthly branches 12 characters, one day 12 hours, 5 days 60 hours, earthly branches use 5 times, heavenly stems use 6 times. Jia zi xiao zhou (little period), 5 days one time/visit (hour) 6 days also begin another jia zi hour, is the same as one day. Then one six has the same ancestor. This means jia ji have the same ancestor. Jia day ji day, one old one new, one yin one yang, day stem yin yang is different but hour stem branch are all the same. So, jia day liu zhu (flow) all the points. Also, follows (list under) jia day stem. Two (2) seven (7) are yi geng; 3, 8 are bing, xin; 4, 9 are ding, ren; 5, 10 are wu, gui: all are one yin's one yang's same ancestor liu zhu each point, except one pass point that's not crossing the following. Remaining all

cross each other, list it in that circle. So, it is called same ancestor cross (tong zong jiao cuo). Use this circle for the day (i.e. meeting day), select introducing point and yun use. That is, so called "wife needles her husband" ('qi bi zhen qi fu"), "husband can needle his wife" ("fu bi zhen qi qi"); husband and wife point substitutes. Husband represents yang channels and yang days, wife represents yin channels and yin days, yang days and yin days combine and add (these) 2 days points together. It will improve many opportunities for opening points. This is called husband and wife use each other ("fu qi he yong"). For example, jia day jia xu hour, the open point is the gall-bladder channel's jing (well) point qiao yin (GB44), at that day's yi hai hour, originally doesn't open the point but ji day's yi hai hour, the open point is liver channel's jing (channel) point zhong feng (Liv.4), because husband and wife use each other's yuan (source) at jia day yi hai hour, may also insert zhong feng point (Liv.4). Qiao yin fu (GB44) belongs to gall-bladder channel's jing jin (well metal/gold) point, zhong feng (Liv.4) which belongs to the liver channel's jing jin (well metal/gold) point. Liver and gall-bladder are externally and internally related to each other, two points distribute the 5 elements. Yang jing well (metal/gold) and yin channel's metal/gold is also related externally and internally, so jia yi 2 days open points using, each other or yun use, moreover which, if true, has a relative relations unit. The *Zhen jiu da cheng* said, "yang ri yi yin shi, yin ri yi yang shi, ze qian xue ji bi, qu qi he xue zhen zhi. He zhi, jia yu ji he, yi yu geng he …" (Yang day meet in yin hour, yin day meets yang hour, then previous point has been closed, combined points insert. Combined means jia and ji combined, yi and geng combined …"), this circle is according to "its combined point meet" the "five gates" (wu men), and the "10 changes" (shi bian) theory, and is listed according to husband and wife points. However, in clinical conditions, yun is used not to note each channel's original point (yuan xue), originally following that day's main channel return to origin's time to open point. Is only suitable for that day, but cannot use each other. Each yin channel shu (stream) point represents original points return to the origin point (yuan xue). Is the same, cannot use each other. When choosing the open point time, this point must be noted.

5. The fifth circle: mother son fills in (tun chong): according to the Zi wu liu zhu's nia jia method, the day rotates periodically according to the stems and branches, 5 days become a cycle, 10 days is another cycle, 10 days count as 120 double hours (ie. 2 hour periods) (shi chen) and combines with 66 points. Remove 6 points which are the open points to the original points,

same as open points open at the same time with shu points, only has 60 points. On average, open a shu point each double hour (ie. 2 hour period). 10 days has only 60 double hours, which have points can open. Then add some ancestor cross (tong zong jiao cu) - 36 husband and wife points may use each other. Still have remaining 24 double hours "bi xue" ("blocked points"), which have no points to open. Zi wu liu zhu's na zi method (na zi fa) has specially double hours as the main thing, 12 channel liu zhu fa method. It is different to na jia fa, following the day's combined stems branches to open hours rule. However, in the treatments adapted by doctors at the same time (ie. parallel), has become the organisational contents of Zi wu liu zhu needling technique. This circle chooses na zi fa's "mother son point" in "bi xue" ("closed/blocked points), a so-called "mother son fill in". For example, jia day geng wu hour 'closed/blocked point," therefore no point then many choose, mother son points. If the heart channel has excess condition, choose channel point shen men (H7). Is called "welcome and role it" (yin er duo zhi"), the excess then will be settled (or reduced) via the son. If spleen channel deficiency condition, choose spleen channel mother point da dun (SP2), follow and sui/help it ("sui er ji zhi"), deficiency transfer and tonifies its mother. Like this, then the following day, following hour both have points to open, makes Zi wu liu zhu needle technique more perfect.

Section 2
Zi wu liu zhu circle charts use method

Re Zi wu liu zhu needling technique open points first should calculate the patient's diagnosis time for year's, month's, day's, hour's, stems and branches and then for the following day according to the time to open points. This needs grasping – this is the year's stem and branch, month's stem and branch, day's stem and branch, hour's stem and branch derivative method.

Heavenly stems begin at Jia and end at Gui totalling has 10 numbers, earthly branches begin at Zi and end at Hai, totalling has 12 numbers. Heavenly stem and earthly branches combine with each other begin at jia zi, then return to the first stem and branch jai zi hour, you need the heavenly stem to rotate 6 times, Earthly branches rotate 5 times ie. heavenly stem multiplied by 10 multiplied by 6 equals 100. Earthly branches 12 is multiplied by 5 equals 60. This is the 60 circle method. It is the basis of calculating year's, month's, day's, hour's stems and branches.

(1) <u>Year's stem and branch derivation method</u>

The simple and commonly used year's stem and branch derivation method has 2 types:

1. Starting with derivative method, is year stem and branch list following the year, after according to the sixty cycle method. Once we know a certain year's stem and branch, the other year's stem and branch can be derived according to the order, using 60 circle method remember 1960 is geng zi, 1970 is geng wu, 1980 is geng shen, using these three years as a standard we can quickly derive nearly 30 year's any stem and branch. For example, to calculate 1975 year's stem and branch, we use 1970 year's stem and branch according to the order to derive the 5th year, then we know it is yi mao. If we want to know 1983's year's stem and branch, use 1980 year's stem and branch according to the order, shift across 3, know it is gui hai. Now we list 1981 to 2000 year's stem and branch in the following table as reference (see table 21)

Table 21 1981 to 2000 following the year's stem and branch table

Year	Stem Branch	Year	Stem branch	Year	Stem Branch	Year	Stem branch
1981	xin you	1982	ren wu	1983	gui hai	1984	jia zi
1985	yi chou	1986	bing yin	1987	ding mao	1988	wu chen
1989	ji si	1990	geng wu	1991	xin wei	1992	ren shen
1993	gui you	1994	jia wu	1995	yi hai	1996	bing zi
1997	ding chou	1998	xu yin	1999	ji mao	2000	geng chen

2. Year's stem and branch formula calculation method

If you don't know, as previously stated, any year's stem and branch number, and want to transfer the AD calendar to stem and branch ji nian (a way of remembering years in the lunar calendar), may choose the year's stem and branch calculation formula to derive it.

Year's stem and branch calculation formula:

1. $\dfrac{X-3}{60}$ .... remainder (Y)

2. $\dfrac{Y}{10}$ .... remainder (J) is the wanted year's heavenly stem number

3. $\dfrac{Y}{12}$ .... remainder (L) is the wanted year's earthly branch number

Formula note:

i   Formula can be used to for any year after 4 A.D.

ii   In the formula X is representative of the wanted year's A.D. number

For example: to calculate 1982 year's stem and branch.

Solution: $Y = \dfrac{1982 - 3}{60} = \dfrac{1979}{60}$ ...... remainder 59

$J = \dfrac{59}{10}$ remainder 9

According to the Heavenly stem order 9 is Ren's number so we know that the year's heavenly stem is Ren

$L = \dfrac{59}{12}$ remainder 11.

According to the Earthly branch order 11 is xu's representative number. So we know that the year's Earthly branch is xu. By the formula's calculation we know 1982's year's stem and branch is ren xu.

(2)   Monthly stem and branch derivation method

One year has 12 months, calculated according to the lunar calendar, in the monthly stem and branch, earthly branches are fixed and don't vary. Every year's 11th month (ie. November) is "zi", 5th month (ie. May) is "wu", the 1st month (ie. January) is "yin" so to derive the monthly stem and branches, actually only need to derive the monthly heavenly stem, as that year's yearly stem and branch is long. Remember the following song and it can be quickly derived.

Jia ji zhi nian bing zuo shou, yi geng zhi sui wu wu tou
Bing xin zhi sui geng yin shang, ding ren ren shun xing liu
Ruo yan wu gui he feng gi, jia yin zhi shang qu xun qiu.

(Jia ji year big is the head, yi geng year lou is the head,
Bing xin year geng yin is the upper, ding ren ren yin following the flow,
If ask wu gui comes from where, go to jia yin's upper to search)

For example, to derive 1981 March month's stem and branch, 1981 is xin you year. According to "bing xin zhi sui geng yin shang", January is geng yin, stem and branch in order shift two, March stem and branch known to be ren shen. Now list 2000 to 2019, each stem and branch in the following table for reference. (See table 22)

Table 22 Years 2000 to 2019 each month stem and branch

		Jan	Feb	Mar	Apr	May	Jun	Jul	Aug	Sep	Oct	Nov	Dec
2000	Geng chen	Wu yin	Ji mao	Geng chen	Xin si	Ren wu	Gui wei	Jia shen	Yi you	Bing xu	Ding hai	Wu zi	Ji chou
2001	Xin si	Geng yin	Xin mao	Ren chen	Gui si	Jia wu	Yi wei	Bing shen	Ding you	Wu xu	Ji hai	Geng zi	Xin chou
2002	Ren wu	Ren yin	Gui mao	Jia chen	Yi si	Bing wu	Ding wei	We shen	Ji you	Geng xu	Xin hai	Ren zi	Gui chou
2003	Gui wei	Jia yin	Yi mao	Bing chen	Ding si	Wu wu	Ji wei	Geng shen	Xin you	Ren xu	Gui hai	Jia zi	Yi chou
2004	Jia shen	Bing yin	Ding mao	Wu chen	Ji si	Geng wu	Xin wei	Ren shen	Gui you	Jia xu	Yi hai	Bing zi	Ding chou
2005	Yi you	Wu yin	Ji mao	Geng chen	Xin si	Ren wu	Gui wei	Jia shen	Yi you	Bing xu	Ding hai	Wu zi	Ji chou
2006	Bing xu	Geng yin	Xin mao	Ren chen	Gui si	Jia wu	Yi wei	Bing shen	Ding you	Wu xu	Ji hai	Geng zi	Xin chou
2007	Ding hai	Ren yin	Gui mao	Jia chen	Yi si	Bing wu	Ding wei	We shen	Ji you	Geng xu	Xin hai	Ren zi	Gui chou
2008	Wu zi	Jia yin	Yi mao	Bing chen	Ding si	Wu wu	Ji wei	Geng shen	Xin you	Ren xu	Gui hai	Jia zi	Yi chou
2009	Ji chou	Bing yin	Ding mao	Wu chen	Ji si	Geng wu	Xin wei	Ren shen	Gui you	Jia xu	Yi hai	Bing zi	Ding chou
2010	Geng yin	Wu yin	Ji mao	Geng chen	Xin si	Ren wu	Gui wei	Jia shen	Yi you	Bing xu	Ding hai	Wu zi	Ji cjou
2011	Xin mao	Geng yin	Xin mao	Ren chen	Gui si	Jia wu	Yi wei	Bing shen	Ding you	Wu xu	Ji hai	Geng zi	Xin chou
2012	Ren chou	Ren yin	Gui mao	Jia chen	Yi si	Bing wu	Ding wei	We shen	Ji you	Geng xu	Xin hai	Ren zi	Gui chou
2013	Gui si	Jia yin	Yi mao	Bing chen	Ding si	Wu wu	Ji wei	Geng shen	Xin you	Ren xu	Gui hai	Jia zi	Yi chou
2014	Jia wu	Bing yin	Ding mao	Wu chen	Ji si	Geng wu	Xin wei	Ren shen	Gui you	Jia xu	Yi hai	Bing zi	Ding chou
2015	Yi wei	Wu yin	Ji mao	Geng chen	Xin si	Ren wu	Gui wei	Jia shen	Yi you	Bing xu	Ding hai	Wu zi	Ji chou
2016	Bing shen	Geng yin	Xin mao	Ren chen	Gui si	Jia wu	Yi wei	Bing shen	Ding you	Wu xu	Ji hai	Geng zi	Xin chou
2017	Ding you	Ren yin	Gui mao	Jia chen	Yi si	Bing wu	Ding wei	We shen	Ji you	Geng xu	Xin hai	Ren zi	Gui chou
2018	Wu xu	Jia yin	Yi mao	Bing chen	Ding si	Wu wu	Ji wei	Geng shen	Xin you	Ren xu	Gui hai	Jia zi	Yi chou
2019	Ji hai	Bing yin	Ding mao	Wu chen	Ji si	Geng wu	Xin wei	Ren shen	Gui you	Jia xu	Yi hai	Bing zi	Ding chou

(3)   <u>Day stem and branch derivative method</u> To use Zi wu liu zhu weekly technique the most important thing is to derive the day's stem and branch. However the lunar calendar's big small and leap year's month's are not fixed, so it's quite difficult to derive day's stem and branch according to months. On the other hand, the Christian calendar is different. Each year's big and small months are fixed and unchangeable, except for one leap year each four years, so it's much more convenient to use the Christian calendar to derive the lunar calendar's day's stem and branch. For calculation method, please refer *Lun ling gui ba fa de li lun ji lin chuang yun yong's* "day's stem and branch derivation method" section.

(4)   <u>Hour's stem and branch derivative method</u>

Please refer to *Lun ling gui ba fa de li lun ji lin chuang yun yong's* "double hour stem and branch derivation method" section.

(5)   <u>Zi wu liu zhu cheng zhu (circular diagram)'s use example</u>

Example:

1981 December 14th 10:00am, a kidney deficiency patient came for acupuncture treatment. How to open points?

Check (table 21) (table 22), know 1981 December is xin you year geng zi month. Use *Guan shi gan zhi fang chen shi Mr Guan's stems and branches equations,* calculate the fourteenth day's heavenly stem is bing. Then check *Shi gan zhi cha dui bino Hour's stems and branches check table,* know that day 10:00am hour's stem and branch is gui shi.

First find out bing day one segment or section (ge) within the first circle of zi wu lui zhu circular diagram (10 stems govern one day) in that day's beginning hour, at the 2nd circle (stem and branch fixed time) fix gui shi hour; in that hour's open points check the 3rd circle (shu point liu zhu), should kidney channel yin gu (K10) point; according to the fourth circle (same ancester to cross) can or may select ran gu (K2) point at same time. Clinical pattern time, except according to zi wu liu zhu, and according to the hour open points, we can probably choose other combining points (pei xue) in accordance with the identification of pattern requirements.

Section 3
Zi wu liu zhu needling techniques clinical use and understanding

1. <u>Zang-fu (organs and bowels), jing luo theory is the theoretical basis of Zi wu liu zhu needling technique.</u> Zang fu theory is the study of the human body's zang-fu (organs and bowels) physiological functions, illness properties changes, and their relationship theory; jing luo theory is the study of the human body's channels and collaterals systems physiology, illness property change, and their relationship with zang-fu theory. Both have an inseperable relationship, they tightly combine with and compensate for each other. They verify each other, they completely represent Chinese medicine's basic principle re the human body's physiology and illness properties, they form the nucleus of the Chinese medicine system. With regard to Zi wu liu zhu needling technique's clinical use the theoretical basis is zang-fu jing luo theory.

Example 1: Chen XX, male, 18 years old, 1965 April 15th 10:00am first diagnosis.

The patient suffered from acute nephritis in August 1962, then stayed in hospital for treatment for more than one month, the symptoms disappeared and he was firstly finally released from hospital. Recently, in the last 2 years, he had numerous urine tests, all show albumen + - ++, red cells 4 - 6, white cells 2 – 4, then took Chinese medicine more than 100 doses, but in the urine there was still albumen. First diagnosis, the pattern was seen as the face colour pale, tired and weak with regard to strength, food desire is not good, waist and knees sour and soft. In the afternoon, feet and ankles had slight swelling, tongue pale and coating thin and white, pulse sunken and thin. Yi shi year, geng chen month, yi hai day, yi shi hour, open points yin bai (SP1) shang qiu (SP5), combined with pi shu (UB20), moxa ming men (GV4), guan yuan (CV4). April 17th 10:00am, open points ran gu (K2), yin gu (K10) combined with shen shu (UB23), moxa shui fen (CV9), pi shu (UB20). According to the above method, and according to the hour for opening points, properly combined points today treat 36 times (treatments). On July 12th tested urine again, urine is normal or clear. Then test many times, no protein in urine then visit 3 years later, body healthy and no illness.

Note: Urine has a lot of protein, spleen weak and cannot consolidate yin, face pale, tired and without strength is qi weak, central yang is not strong,

255

spleen is not healthy enough to transport, so appetite decreases, waist and knees sour and soft, pulse chen xu (sunken and weak), kidney deficiency pattern, pattern belongs to spleen and kidney yang deficiency. Treatment should nourish both spleen and kidney, so open points should be the spleen and kidney 2 channels as main channel for treatment, combined with moxa ba shun techniques and nourish spleen and kidney, cultivate (or nourish, strengthen) jing and tonify the qi.

Example 2: Gong XX, male 58 years old. September 7th 1974 2:00pm first diagnosis.

Patient has had high blood pressure for 5 years. On September 5th 1974, after some physical work, he drank 2 cups of alcohol, then suddenly felt a headache, with dizziness, and fell down unconscious. With urgent treatment at a hospital, a day later his conscious state gradually became better, blood pressure 190/115 mm Hg, speech was still unclear, right side mouth corner slanted to one side, the philtrum was flat, right side paralysis, tongue red and pulse bowstring. At this time it was jia yin year ren shen month xin hu day yi lou hour, open points diagnosis the open points were tai chong (LIV3), tai yuan (Lu9), lao gong (P8), combined with guang ming (GB37), zu san li (ST36), tai xi (K3). Four days later, blood pressure is 130/90 mm Hg, spirit is clear, right side paralysis, right upper limb muscle strength 0 grade, right lower limbs can strengthen and bend back, muscle power grade 2 Babinsky test positive, tender response to strong, September 12th 8:30am. Bing day chen hour, open points on affected side: qi chi (LI11) combined with he gu (LI4), zu san li (ST36), jie xi (ST41). September 13th 8:00 am ding day chen hour open points on affected side: yang ling quan (GB34), xia xi (GB43), combined with tian jing (TH10), zhi gou (TH6), zheng zhu (TH3). The patient was treated 6 times, and after he could lie down on the bed by himself and move around the room. Then, combined with lou zhen (scalp needling), and point injection treatment for 12 times, he could walk outside with the help of a walking stick. Two months later, limbs and body function greatly recovered. He was visited on October 1976, and his blood pressure was normal, limbs and body movement sensations were normal, only hands and fingers movements were not quite as flexible as they should have been.

Note: Patient is a stroke patient, September 7th was first diagnosis. Blood pressure was still high, liver wind was moving internally, hence the open points for treatment source mainly for balancing the liver, and to extinguish the wind.

On September the 12th, the liver wind gradually became more balanced, then it was possible to concentrate on the paralysis. Following the principal of "zhi wu du qu yeng ming" ("to treat atrophy/flaccidity condition, solely select yang ming."), first open hand yang ming large intestine channel mother point qu chi (LI11) combined with the channel's yuan (source) point chi gu (LI4), and foot yang ming channel bin (original) point zu san li (ST36), mother point ji xi (ST41). On September 13th, the following shu points liu zhu (flow) according hour to open points. Combined with head needling etc. treatment which can improve the unblocking of the channels and the circulating of the collaterals, and adjust qi and blood.

2. <u>Channels and collaterals identification pattern is the main identification pattern method of Zi wu liu zhu needling techniques</u>

The channel points used by zi wu liu zhu needling techniques are from the 12 channels distributed below the elbows and the knees jing (well), ying (spring), shu (stream), yuan (source), jing (river), he (sea) 66 particular points. These particular points on the locations of the channel qi's output and input, qi and blood exchange, yin and yang cross – meet, and are also in the treatment experience confirmed important points. To accurately and affectively use these points, we must become very familiar with each channel's circulation and related illness conditions. After grasping the channels and collaterals identification pattern methods, we will be able to apply the clinical applications of Zi wu liu zhu's needling techniques.

Example 3: Xu xx male 42 years old April 13th 1978 5:00 pm, first diagnosis.

The patient waist vertebrae parts distended, painful, hui yin (CV1) part felt not good, and had the feeling of dripping urination etc. symptoms half a year ago. The effects of the medicine treatment on the problem were not obvious. In recent months, the hui yin parts distended painful became more serious, after urination, there was white fluid like secretion, and couldn't calm down and get to sleep, tongue coating thin white, pulse sunken. Rectal diagnosis: prostate gland showed a little enlargement, pressure pain is obvious, after massaging and squeezing out a little prostate fluid for microscopic examination: phosphatidylcholine small body only has a little, white cells 15-20. Diagnosis: chronic prostatitis. Wu wu year, bing chen month, yi si day, yi you hour first diagnosis open points: da dun (LIV1), combined with tai xi

(K3), zhong ji (CV3), pang guang shu (UB28). April 11ᵗʰ 10:00am bing day si hour, open points: yin gu (K10), ran gu (K2), combined with li gou (LIV5), hui yin (CV1). April 17ᵗʰ 5:15pm ji day you hour, open points: tai xi (K3), tai bai (SP3), combined with fei yang (UB58), chang qiang (GV1). After needling treatment 3 times, hui yin parts distended painful feeling disappeared, urine dripping became smooth, without white fluid-like secretion. After needling treatments totalling 12 times, rectal digital examination: prostate gland showed normal size, pressure pain disappeared, prostate fluid microscope examination phosphatidylcholine small body showed increase, white cells were 2-4. December 1979, visited the patient, who said that all the symptoms became well, body health without illness. Note: Chronic prostatitis main illness mechanism is turbid dampness is stored internally, qi mechanism loses its unblocking and transforming abilities, because illness change mainly shows at the anterior private parts, must pay particular attention to foot three ying channels' points. For liver channels and collateral's reproductive organs, first open liver channel's jing (well) point da dun (LIV1), to smooth the channel qi, and remove liver fire to stop pain; tai xi (K3) is the kidney channel's yuan (source) point, is beneficial for helping kidney water, to clear it's source. At the same time, choosing pang guang shu (UB28) and zhong ji (CV3), shu and mu points combined with each other, to smooth the urinary bladder mechanism. Bing day, si hour open kidney he (sea) point yin gu (K10), according to husband and wife points use each other principal, at the same time select ran gu (K2), zu jue yin collateral "shang gao, jie yu jing" ("testes go up, blockage at the penis") so combine to select liver channel and collateral points li gou (LIV5); ren mai "qi yu zheng ji zhi xin, shao fu zhi xie, hui yin zhi fen ...", ("beginning below zhong ji, inside the lesser abdomen, at the dividing line of the hui yin ..." so select hui yin (CV1). Ji day you hour, open kidney channel shu (stream) point tai xi (K3), according to "fan ben huan yuan" ("return to origin") principal. At the same time open tai bai (SP3) to balance the middle heater, and adjust the qi mechanism; tai bai is the spleen channel's shu point because yin channel has no yuan (source) point, so use shu (stream) point instead of yuan point, combined with fei yang (UB58) is host-guest yuan (source) collateral combined point method. Also because the du channel "qi luo xun yin qi, he cuan jin" ("the collateral follows through the reproductive organs, combines and takes control of that which is in between"), so therefore is combined with the du channel and collateral's chang qiang (GV1).

Example 4 Fu XX female 38 years old, primary school teacher. May 23 1964, 10:00AM, first diagnosis.

Patient caught a "cold", in January 1963 but kept giving lectures, gradually felt throat painful, speech became hoarse. In March 1963, she was diagnosed as having "vocal cord polyps" by X army hospital, who then carried out an operation to cut them out. After the operation, speech at once became better, in the recent half year, sounds of unclearness became stronger, throat dry, and insomnia, tongue body red, coating less, pulse thin and rapid. Though the treatment of Chinese and western medicine and I (iodine) ion conduction insert, effect is not obvious, so ask for acupuncture treatment. Jia chen year, ding mao month, xin wei day, gui si hour. First diagnosis open points: ran gu (K2), yin gu (K10), combined with yin liang (EX pt). March 26th 5 minutes past 5:00PM, bing day, si hour open points: yin gu (K10), ran gu (K2), combined with yin liang (CV23), shen xiang (EX pt), total treatment 24 times. Speech returned to normal, sleep is good as well. May 1966, visit, for 2 years has been no recurrence. Note: patient gave lectures with illness, diagnose and damage lung yin reaches to kidney. Lung – kidney yin deficiency, deficiency fire flares up and causes throat pain and speech dimness. The foot shao yin kidney channel, "qi zhi zhe, cong shen sheng guan gan gi, ru fei zhong, xun hou lung, xi shi bin" ("the branch goes from kidney up, goes up through liver diaphragm and enters the lungs inside, follows the throat, controls the tongue root"); in the xi sheng bing", and also mainly has "hou re, shi gen, yen zhang, shing qi, yi gu, ji tong: ("mouth hot, tongue dry, throat swollen, qi goes up, throat has a dry sensation in the pharynx and painful. So open kidney points to tonify the kidney yin, yin chou points, shu and hui is at the foot shao yin, select zhao hai (K6) to unblock yin qiao channel qi; ren channel zhi yan points follows to the throat", so choose tian tu (CV22), lian quan (CV23) to smooth the lungs, benefit the throat, open sounds up. Yin liang (EX pt), shen xiang (EX pt) are the author's family traditional experienced points, and they have good effects on speech unclear, lose speech, throat dry, hou bi.

3. <u>Choose open points, combined points is the key for using Zi wu liu zhu needling technique.</u> Regarding Zi wu liu zhu, one must choose points according to day and hour, using time as the main consideration, but to open channel points, must be consistent with the identified pattern. To choose the combined points, also must consider the requirements of the illness pattern. If the combined

point prescription is suitable or not, it will directly relate to the clinical affect, therefore accurately choosing the yuan points and combining points becomes the key to using Zi wu liu zhu needling technique.

Example 5. Shang XX. Male 19 years old, September 8th 1965 5:00PM first diagnosis.

The patient suddenly appeared to have dian xian (epilepsy) when he went to sleep in December 1963. Later, it began to happen one time per month approximately. Before it happened, he felt upset and a few minutes later, he shouted loudly, the four limbs shaking and convulsing, the mouth vomiting white foam (ie froth or saliver). Sometimes he wet himself. It took around ten minutes each time to complete an attack. After he woke, he would be tired and want to sleep. He went to X hospital to have a check-up: leucocytes 7000 per cubic millimetre, oxyphilic granular cells were 2%, blood sugar 100 mg%; blood calcium 12.4 mg%, EEG shows shuang er zhong yang qu (double forward central area) has dispersed negative medium spikewave, it appears as a peaked slow wave combination, at temple left central conducting connection degree extraordinary EEG, characteristic of epilepsy condition. After more than 1 year's medicine treatment, the happening time approached something of a pattern. It always happened at dusk or before sleep every time, but the happening times gradually happened more frequently. They happened 1-2 times each week. Tongue coating thin and sticky, pulse bowstring and slippery. Yi si year, yi you month, yi chou day, yi you hour, first diagnosis open points: da dun (LIV1), combined with zhao hai (K6), shen mai (UB62), jiu wei (CV15). September 9th 2:00pm bing day, wei hour, open points: lao gong (P8), tai chong (LIV.3), combined with zhao hai (K6), yao qi (Ex pt). By using the above treatment, 3 weeks didn't have an epileptic episode. September 30th 8:00pm, ding day chen hour open points: yang ling quan (GB34), xia xi (GB43), combined with da zhui (GV14), moxa bai hui (GV20), on the same day epileptic attack happened, the symptoms were serious and time lasting was long, one week later moxa bai hui (GV20) again, 4 hours later the epilepsy attack happened again. Later, according to the treatment method of extinguish the wind and remove the phlegm, calm down the heart and open the orifices, mainly open the liver channel points, one by one choose zhao hai (K6), shen mai (UB62), yao qi (Ex pt), jiu wei (CV15), feng long (St.40) etc. combined points. Didn't use moxa technique. After needling technique treatment 36 times, epilepsy pattern didn't happen again.

Example 6: Bai xx, female, 28 years old, 1968 3rd December first diagnosis. Illness involved being overly sensitive and emotions irregular. Rash, not calm, crazy talk and delusional speech. Stayed in x mental hospital for 2 months, illness not any better. Transferred to acupuncture hospital for treatment. Initial diagnosis here: spirit slow, speech irregular. Often speaking to herself, at times sad at times laughing, doesn't like food or drink, sleeps restless, tongue coating white sticky, pulse bowstring thin. Wu shen year, gui hai month, ding wei day, ding wei hour open points: shao chong (H9) combined with shen men (H7), feng long (St.40). December 4th 10:00am wu day si hour open points: da ling (P7), combined with a selection of feng chi (GB20), bai hui (GV20), shen xing (GV23), tai yang (Ex2), jian shi (P5), tai chong (LIV.3), zu san li (St36), electric needling strong stimulation. After needling, the patient was impatient and not calm. Drinks and food greatly decreased. That night had insomnia. December 10th 6:45am jia day mao hour open points shen men (H7). When have the needle, the patient wanted to sleep. After removing the needles, she went to sleep quietly, then according to the note about liu zhu point selected, shen men (H7) combined with biao li channels and collaterals zhi zheng (SI7), treatment for 2 months. Patient spirit and understanding completely returned to normal. March 1st 1969 go to work. Visited after 11 years, the illness had recovered.

Note: selected points prescription tries hard to be precise and appropriate. If combined points are too much, you will result in extra channels attack or fight each other, affecting channel normal results and recovery slow. It not only means double use but halves the effect. If so, can be difficult to get a good affect. But also may cause the qi and blood to obey adversely and will interrupt the spirit brightness and cause not good results.

Suitable tonifying and sedating hand techniques are important considerations to get good effects from Zi wu liu zhu needling techniques.

The evil gathers, then the patient's qi must be weak, the illness is formed, and there is deficiency and evil in excess. The rong wei (protective qi) also loses balance, qi and blood loses its unblocking ability, and so this is the total principle or rule of chinese medicine, insofar as illness cause and illness mechanism. Therefore deficiency, so tonify, excess then sedate it, this is the big law of chinese medicine identification patterns for diagnosis and treatment. The *Ling shu-jiu zhen shi er yuan* said, "xu *shi* zhi yao, jiu zhen zui miao, bu xie zhi shi, yi zhen wei zhi" ("For deficiency and excess's essence, the nine needles are the best, when tonify and sedate, use these needles to do them." Zi wu liu zhu also has uncovered the principle that if the qi and blood are strong and provided beneficial conditions one can open points according to time ie. to reach the goal of to tonify the deficiency and sedate the excess, support the true and remove the evil, balance the nutritive qi and the defensive qi, and unblock the qi and blood. Therefore, we must accurately use hand techniques.

Example 7: Jing xx, male, 34 years old, March 19ᵗʰ 1980 4:00 pm first diagnosis. The patient at 4:00 pm March 1980, fell down from a balcony 2 metres high and injured his right side waist and back, and the upper leg positive side. Internally, he took medicine alcohol but the waist and back pain re-occurred and became more serious ie. when breathed deeply and coughed, the pain cannot be tolerated and cannot literally rotate, and cannot sleep at night. Geng shen year, yi mao month, xin day, shen hour first diagnosis. Check right side waist and back, muscles straight and cannot move, a little swollen and distended, right side fang muscle, bai kuo muscle, and di ji muscle all have obvious pressing pain. Select points: wei zhong (UB40), "tou tian liang" ("through the heaven cooling") hand technique, right side da chang shu (UB25) needle through to san jiao shu (UB22), right side yi shi (UB45) needle through to po hu (UB42), "long hu jiao zhen" ("dragon tiger fight each other") hand technique, add electric needling.

When the needles were inserted, there was a "cooling and comfortable feeling". After pulled them out, suddenly felt the pain seemed to disappear. Then can bend flex smoothly and rotate laterally. That night, the patient calmly slept, and the next morning the pain completely disappeared.

Note: The patient's injury time uses yi day, shen hour, and the illness pain part belongs to the urinary bladder channel. According to the twelve channels distribution, combined with the twelve hours na zi fa (technique), shen hour is exactly the time the qi and blood flows into the urinary bladder channel. The qi and blood circulation is at the strong time, suddenly is attacked by an illness which causes qi and blood to become condensed and stagnant. The channels and collaterals, once blocked, then are painful. Needling treatment time meets the shen hour again, so choose the urinary bladder points, face and attack them. Except wei zhong (UB40), use sedation technique on the back shu points and also choose adverse the channel through-and-through techniques and electrical stimulation to strengthen the adjusting the channel qi, unblocking the channels, and circulating treatment effects. So, the effects were very good.

Example 8: Hao xx, male, 32 years old, April 14ᵗʰ 1979 8;00 am first diagnosis. The patient half a month ago, his right hand was injured by a wooden board. The right index finger's second joint was blue and swollen, and the x-ray showed no evidence of bone body damage. Externally, he applied chinese herbal medicines then the swelling disappeared, and the pain stopped but there then appeared right upper limbs numbness. A week later he was given he gu (LI4) point treatment but the between the bones back side muscle became numb, the ball muscle group and the hong rau muscle extension and strength decreased and there appeared different degrees of muscular atrophy. The right hand when it came to holding objects, unconsciously dropped them. And when holding a pen to write or when holding a chop-stick to eat, would find them difficult to do. Ji wei year, wu chen month, xin day, chen hour, first diagnosis. Open points, qu chi (LI11) combined with he gu (LI4), "shao shan huo" ("fire on top of the mountain") hand technique, and after needling added moxa. Ask the patient to come for treatment every day at 8;00 am. After acupuncture 3 times, the right limb's numbness disappeared, then was able to treat every other day. In total, acupuncture was given 7 times, and right limb muscle extension and force recovered, while movement function completely became normal.

Note: "Yang ma xu bu, teng tong shi xie" ("itching and numbness are deficiency so tonify, pain is excess should sedate"). This example, takes right limb numbness as the main consideration accompanied by light degree muscular atrophy so should tonify. Illness parts belong to hand yang ming large intestines channel, large intestines channel qi and blood flow time is mao hour. Tonify the large intestines channel deficiency condition, and should at chen hour tonify its mother point. So, we made an appointment with the patient for treatment at 8:00 am. Tonify qu chi (LI11) and then save the patient. He gu (LI4) is the yuan point, shang yang (LI1) is the ben point, and also belongs to and can adjust and tonify the original channel's qi and blood. Although important points, they can be used as combined points alternatively with shou san li (LI10), and yang xi (LI5), to assist the unblocking of the channels and to re-continue the flow of qi. The yang ming is a channel of much qi and much blood. Needling and moxa used together to strengthen the function of tonifying and the qi and blood is strengthened to its fullness so the pattern disappears by itself.

Zi wu liu zhu needling technique's basic characteristics are: "an ri qi shi, xun jing xun xue, shi shang you xue, xue shang you shi" ("according to the day's beginning hour/time, follow the channels to search for points. On time has points, on points has time"). In clinical use, first you need to derive the patient's arrival time and diagnose the day, hour, stem and branch, under the conditions of identification patterns combined with the human body's channels and collaterals and qi and blood circulation. In addition, you will need to consider the jing (well), the ying (spring), the shu (stream), the jing (river), and he (sea) 's 5 elements production of each other's laws, re open points for treatment. Needling open points means using for some illness, should acupuncture some channels and some points at some time of day at some hour open points principle. Also, one hundred illnesses may be needled using one point According to time therapy (an shi zhi liao), should use open channel points as the main thing. First, insert open points, then insert combined points. This is called: "yong xue xian zhu er hou ke" ("use points first the host (zhu) and, then the guest (ke). These are the basic principles which Zi wu liu zhu needling technique should follow in clinical use.

To use Zi wu liu zhu needling technique, we must not simply fix some hour to open some points for treatment. Instead, we should use flexibly on the basis of according to day and hour opening points, in turn, according to illness case conditions. Combined with the shu points main treatment function. If one meets an acute condition, when it is not suitable for liu zhu open points, not only may choose husband and wife points, and mother and son points, but also can choose other points suitable for this condition. As generally as possible to carry out the treatment, this is called "yong shi ze qi zhu er cong bin" ("when we get rid of the host but follow the guest").

The human and nature's whole body idea is the guidance idea forming Zi wu liu zhu theory. In clinical conditions, we must consider the natural environment's effect on the human body's qi and blood, just as the *Biao you fu* said: "cha sui shi yu tian dao, ding xing qi yu yu xin, chun xia shou er ci qian," ("absorb year time by heavenly low, fix forming qi by your heart, Spring and Summer body thin, insert shallowly, Autumn and Winter fat, then insert deeply"). Only by being good at according to time, according to locality, and according to man's flexible treatment, can we get better treatment effect from this technique.

Zi wu liu zhu needling technique is a long term medical practice, by applying special treatment effect – it has shown its advantages and its scientific value. By further research in modern medical science and Zi wu liu zhu theory, this pearl in the chinese medicine treasury room must radiate more glorious colour.

CHAPTER 3
Channel and collateral identification pattern clinical use outline

The heartland's medicine's spirit is in identification pattern treatment. Identificationpattern treatment is the basis of how to guide acupuncture clinical diagnosis and the treatment of illness. Chinese medicine identification pattern method mainly has the channels and collaterals identification pattern, the ba gang (8 conditions) identification pattern, the zang fu identification pattern, the qi, blood and fluids identification pattern, liu jing (6 channels) identification pattern, the wei qi ying xue identification pattern, the triple heater identification pattern, and the illness evil identification pattern etc. Each method has particular characteristics and pays particular attention to or gives considerations to various points when using them. But regarding academic sources and theory content, the channels and collaterals identification pattern is the basis. The zang fu identification pattern is nuclear, while the ba gang identification is the main law.

In the acupuncture clinical situation, one should pay particular attention to the channels and collaterals identification pattern. According to the conditions for treatment, one should use the following channel identification pattern as the main rule. The illness condition identification pattern as a secondary consideration, incorporated with the extraordinary channels identification pattern and pi bu (skin parts), jing jin (tendino-muscular channels) etc. related theory, and must deeply combine the zang fu identification pattern, and the ba gang identification pattern etc., combined together and flexibly used.

Channels and collaterals identification is based on the guidance theory of the channels and collaterals theory and zang fu theory. It takes channels and collaterals as its basis and is a synthesized clinical identification pattern method. Channels and collaterals identification patterns' main characteristic is the use of twelve channels and the qi jing ba mai to analyse and summarize pattern conditions. Combined with zang fu etc. theory, to investigate illness mechanism, judge illness change properties and the state of true evil, whether strong or weak. According to the different hannels', zang fu's physiological functions and illness mechanism change, analyse pattern conditions, identification patterns, and divide into channels. (This is the basic method of channel and collateral identification). Therefore, to get familiar with each channel's circulation, physiological functions, shi dong, suo sheng bing's illness conditions etc. principles are the basic things needed to group channels and collaterals into identification patterns. Just, as the *Ling shu-jing bie* said, "fu shi er jing zhe, ren zhi suo yi sheng, bing zhi suo yi cheng, ren zhi suo yi zhi, bing zhi suo yi qi, xue zhi suo tai, gong zhi suo zhi ye" ("the twelve channels are produced by man, illness comes from them, one's study should begin there, and also stop here.") The *Ling shu-jing mai* said, "Jing mai zhe, suo yi jue shi sheng, qu bai bing, tiao xu shi, bu ke bu tong" ("Channels decide life or death, and can treat the one hundred illnesses, adjust deficiency and excess, this must be grouped.")

Section 1
Follow the jing (channels) conditions as if new.

Follow-the-channel conditions, as if new, in detailed speaking, have the following several aspects:

(1) The channels self-illness adjusts its own channels. According to the channels conditions distribution, illness happens at a channel, then choose this channel's shu point to treat. "Channel go through somewhere, then the main treatment should go there". This is the basic principle of follow the channel investigation to treat, like hand yang mai channel" enter lower teeth come out of xia kou" so lower teeth select he gu (LI4); foot jue yin channel "covers the ribs", liver qi … adverse (heng ni) rib pain, select zhang men (Liv13).

The Ling shu zhang shou said: "So yin yang cannot move each other, xu shi cannot help ie. cannot tend to each other, select its channel." One channel's channel qi imbalanced/ maladjusted and has not returned to other channels. Only select this channels points to adjust.

When following channels to select the point, we can combine with this channel's zi mu (son mother) points application. For example, pain at temple site (nu) "shao yang headache", can select xia xi (mother point) to strengthen water, needle yang pu (son point) to reduce fire one tonifies, one sedates, applies to them both the same channel at the same time, to supply its deficiency and sedate its fire, adjust channels qi imbalance, of course can treat by balancing the other. Also the example is pain in the forehead is yang ming headache, then tonify jie xi

(ST41) (mother point), sedate li dui) (ST45), tonify wei zhong (UB40) (according to this reason), should tonify zhi yin (UB67), but because zhi yin (UB67) is different should manually treat with shou fa (hand needling), according to "tonify jing (UB67) should tonify the he (UB40)" but transformation is noted, so change to tonify wei zhong (UB40) to exercise and benefit the channels). The same theory, if pain at top/apex of head, "jue yin headache," can tonify qu quan (LIV8), sedate xing jian (LIV2).

(2) Some positive channels illness patterns, external and internal channels treatment are at the same time: in the twelve channels, each channel has internal and external relations with each other ie. have 3 yin channels and have 3 yang channels that are external and internal with each other. The foot 3 yin channels and foot 3 yang channels are external and internals with each other; yin channels belong to the zang collaterals' fu, yang channel belong to the fu collaterals' zang. According to the channel's circling order, the twelve channels detailed external and internal relationship is: hand tai yin lung channel (jing), and hand yang ming large intestine channel external and internal relationship with each other; foot yang ming stomach channel and foot tai yin spleen channel is external and internal relationship with each other; and shao yin heart channel and hand tai yang small intestines channel are indicative of channels which have an external and internal relationship with each other. Although the external and internal relationship with very close, there connection ways belong to the collateral's relationships in the body covering; ie. has channel qi exchange relationship at the four limbs; has the channel bie's "exit and enter" combination, for strengthening the deep channels under the body; has "bie luo's" connection for strengthening the external channels qi relationship. So, the channels have illnesses, external and internal treatment at the same time follow-the-channel identify pattern and to treat is one of the important methods. If stomach qi xu han (deficiency and cold) select zu san li (ST36) combined with gong sun (SP4); for spleen deficiency cold select yin ling quan (SP9) and combine with zu san li (ST36) etc.

(3) Ben (original channel) has illness, combine and adjust son and mother channels: according to the illness change position, first determine its illness changes to the belonging channels, best adjust the original ben channel's qi blood. According to the principles of "deficiency (xu) then tonify its mother, excess (shi) then sedate its son", adjusting its son and mother channels is also belonging

to the arm of the following channels to identify the pattern. Now, one illness case is given to demonstrate this

Case 1: Zhong x 4 female, 30 years old, first diagnosis at August 2 1959. Eight days after giving birth, the milk cannot come out, right breast upper part swollen and distended painful, press it its hard like an egg size. That night (temperature is 39.6c). She is impatient (fan zao), face hot and firey bright red. No stools passed for 2 days. The pulse hong jin (surging tense), tongue body red, coating yellow. Follow the channel to identify the pattern, illness is at foot yang ming stomach channel.

It is yang ming hot, milk blocks the collaterals and then comes the illness, illness is ru yong ("breast ulcer"). Select points li dui (ST45) (prick to bleed), nei ting (ST44) (sedate), chi zi (Lu5) (sedate). After needling point 2 times, swollen pain decreases gradually, body heat also disappears. The needle treatment 2 times and give chinese medicine external application, milk begins to flow down, swelling pain gradually disappears, needle treatment 6 time and then recovers.

Note: "deficiency then tonify its mother, excess then sedate its son." So, sedate the stomach channel's son point li dui (ST45) and son channel (lung channel) son point chi zi (Lu5), because the foot yang ming stomach channel has more qi and blood, li dui (ST45) is its jing (well) point. The jing (well) is the channel qi's exit so in this situation by releasing blood, to unblock its flow and help its origin (source) chi zi (Lu5), which is the he (sea) point of the jing. Sedate chi ze (Lu 5) also clears the qi fen (qi part), and sedates the channel's fullness effect. Nei ting (ST44) is the foot yang ming ying (stream) point. The *Nan jing* said: "Yang controls body heat," so sedate the yang ming blockage unblocks the collaterals.

Section 2
Pay attention to the pi bu and jing jin theory

Skin parts (pi bu) are the parts of the channel and the collaterals on the skin. In general understanding, skin parts are the human body's shallow surface parts reflecting externally. It is the body's surface organisation which the channels and the collaterals system, use to directly connect to the external environment. It has the function of defending the body, attacking external evils, and has adjusting and adapting functions on the external environment.

Skin parts in a narrow concept is the distribution are of twelve channels on the body surface. The *Su wen- pi bu lun* said: "pu bu yi jing mai wei ji", ("Skin parts take channels as the rule"). "Fan shi er jing luo mai zhi, pi zhe bu ye" ("The twelve channels and collaterals are the skin parts"). This means this:

(1) Twelve skin parts applications in identification parts: In normal diagnosis procedures, note skin and fou luo (floating collaterals) colour changes according to skin parts and then according to the channels. If qi blockage and blood condensing, then pain and colour is qing (blue/green); long time coldness and long time painful, then bi (blockage/arthritis) and the colour black; if see heat yong zhong (ulcer swelling) then the skin is hot and the colour yellow red; qi deficiency blood less then skin is cold and colour is white, if 5 colours variously seen then it is yin yang imbalanced cold and heat condition. So, note skin parts colour change, also can measure parts of the illness. The *Ling shu- lun yi zhen chi* it said: "zhen xue mai zhi, duo chi duo re, duo qing tong, duo hei wei ru bing, duo chi duo hei, duo qing ci jian zhi han re." (Diagnosis of blood vessels, much red means much hot, colour blue/green means much pain, much black, means long time bi: much red, much black, much glue/green all seen means cold-hot.") The *Ling shu-jing mai* said: "Wei zhong han shou you zhi luo duo qing yi wei zhong you re ziu ji luo chi: qi bai hei zhi liu ru bi yo qi you chi you hei yo qing zhi han re qi ye, qi qing duo zho shao qi ye" ("if stomach internal has cold, hand yu ji collateral have qing, if inside the stomach has heat yu ji's collaterals are chi (red), if very black means long time bi, if has red, has black has qing (blue-green) it means cold hot qi. If qing (blue-green) short means less qi".)

Next, note the skin's formation changes according to skin part's fen jing (disseminated channels). For example, according to different parts, generally produce qiu zhen (popular rash) red patch (hong xian) obviously convex or concave, very thin skin, etc to delegate disseminated channels and collaterals. If calf parts muscle skin weak and reduce demised is foot tai yang channel, but if breast part upper lower tan he (phlegm lump) bao kuai (lump/mass) disease is foot yang ming channel. Or, according to disease changes, the skin parts position and characteristics identify the discussed channels and zang fu. If bin ju (temple have poisonous sore or boil), according to designated position, then the diseased channels is foot yang ming stomach channel etc.

Pulse diagnosis (qie zhen) can be according to the skin parts, divided into channels designated skin sensations extraordinary, such as numb (ma mu), long time cold pain, fa re (fever) etc., based on these to analyse the parts changes belong to one channel or sever qi channels. Next, chu mo (touch rub), under skin formations change such as bumps (jie he), stick-like structures, mai bao (ball like swelling), use as responses for channels and collaterals identification patterns, or follow according to zhen points assistant diagnosis of internals organ's disease. For example liver illness, has press-pain at gan shu (UB 18), and qi men (LIV 14). Intestinal yong (ulcer), beginning stage, pressure painful at large intestine channel lower he point-shang ju shu (ST 37) (or lan wei xue Ex point-appendix point).

In addition, one can ask the patient about any specific feelings on the body surface and other symptoms, these provide more evidence of related channels and collaterals identification patterns.

(2) Twelve skin parts applications in treatment. The *Su wen- pi bu bu* said: "xie ke you pi, ze chou li kai, kai ze xie ru ke you luo mai luo mai man, ze zhu ru jing mao king mai, jing mai man, ze ru she you fu zang ye. Gu pi zhe you fen bu bu you er sheng da bing ye" ("evil guest on skin then the pores are open, its open then evil enters as a guest in to the channels and collaterals, collaterals and channels are full then flow into the channels, the channels are full then they enter into the fu zang (bowels and organs) so the skin has differentiated parts, if not corrected will produce big illness. "Re treatment aspects, can use half insertion (ban ci), high level insertion (mao ci) to strengthen skin parts and excitated skin parts functions to defend against evil qi as a guest on skin surface, against various diseases. For some kinds of skin parts diseases like pi shen jing yan and shen jing xing pi yan (neuro dermatitis), then use a mei hua zhen (plum-blossom needle) to excite the skin parts channels' qi to treat. In addition, for some kinds of skin disease patterns, also can choose suitable treatment method according to skin part theory such as yang chuang (sores, ulcer), use separated-by-garlic moxa, dan du (erysipelas) by using prick-and -bleed techniques treatment, and wind stroke and zhong luo (ie final paralysis) by more through-and-through needling etc. Regarding zang fu or channel and collateral diseases, their corresponding skin parts often have

responses (such as a node (jie jie) or press pain etc.). Also, re node use of fan lai (?) to treat this zang fu disease. For example, "chuan" ("panting) condition, often needle inserts point positions at node areas at kong zui (LU 6), fei shu (UB 13), zhong fu (LU1) etc. points skin parts lower parts and jie jie (nodes) get an extraordinary effect each time.

(3)   The application of jin li (number channel) theory: the twelve jing jin are the channel and collateral system connecting parts on the external surfaces of the limbs. Because of their circulation distribution, disease conditions, and functions etc. all at "jin rou" ("tendons and muscles"), so they are called jing jin. The jing jin have their own particular "jie zhu san luo" ("node accumulation spread collaterals"), distribution form circulating the four limbs, the trunk parts, the chest parts, and the abdominal wall, constricting the channels and collaterals system's "jin rou" system, externally which becomes the "jing jin". The relationship amongst the twelve jing are particularly represented by the "si jie" ("the four nodes") relationship ie. the foot 3 yang jin combined at the qui (ie. zygomatic bone - face cheek bone parts); the foot 3 yin combined at the sexual organs (reproductive organs); the hand 3 yang combined at the horns (ie. the head parts); and the hand 3 yin combined at the ben (ie. the chest /diaphragm parts). The jing jins' physiological functions mainly are to connect the bai gu (the one hundred bones), manage the whole body, and has a protective function on the whole body's various parts organizational zang qi (visceral organs). The jing jin's functional activities are also deprived of the nourishment of the zang fu's channels and collaterals qi and blood, and hence the body's surface function tendon flesh diseases, and the channels and internal organ's physiological and pathological changes, which connect with each other. The jing jin's illness conditions are fundamentally condition groups of channels related tendon flesh systems.

In the clinical situation, for all the jing diseases, you may select from the 8 hui xue, and use the "jing hui" (the tendon meeting or resting point) - ie.. yang ling quan (GB34) and commonly combine the liver channel shu point gan shu (UB18), and the liver channel yuan point - tai chong (Liv.3) - and then according to the illness change position, i.e. "suan tong qu ah shi".

For some illness, change positions, which are quite broad (ie. big or large), the related channels show that there are quite a lot of jing jin illness conditions.

Still, you can use the "si jie" ("the four nodes") relationship, and select point methods to treat. For example:

Case 2. Li xx male, 50 years old, November 1967 because of work relocations he relocated and because he was mostly working in water, ie. the living environment was cold and damp, then his right side gastrocnemius muscle became especially painful, and his right side elbow was sprained, with his thumb contracted inwards, and his other four fingers sprained painfully. One week later his right shoulder and neck were weak sprained ruined and painful, and his arms were unable to lift themselves. He walked with a limp, and his right hand couldn't hold objects. After having at x hospital an examination, it was found that his blood pressure was 140/86 mm Hg. This eliminated the possibility of brain blood vessel abnormalities. After taking medicine, on the basis that this was an external injury-caused problem for 7 days, the illness didn't decrease. Then came here for diagnosis. Diagnosis: no facial paralysis, but head and neck couldn't look backwards, right side feng chi (GB20), tian liao (TH15), bing feng (LI12), tian zong (SI11), gao huang shu (UB43) etc. areas pressing pain was obvious. The right shoulder and arm still couldn't lift up. All external extremities or backward rotations of the right elbow were unable to extend straight. By way of external force, he could only extend approximately to 160 degrees, but the right hand fingers themselves could hold a fist. The right knee joint couldn't extend straight, the knee joints were cold, with no red swelling, and the foot instep was downwardly internally curled a little. The pulse shape on the right side was sunken uneven, left was sunken moderate, tongue bland purple and damp moist, coating white. Appetite and liquid consumption was ok. Stools were loose. This was an attack by cold evil, flowing into the channels and collaterals, the qi and blood transformation and cycling was not well and the cold being a yin evil was causing the tendon channels to contract, and the blocking of the joints. The condition was belonging to cold dampness stagnates and blocks the tendon channels. Therefore, we needed to warm the channels and spread the cold, and circulate and balance the tendon channels. Select points: left tou wei (St.8), left quan liao (SI18), right qu chi (LI11), right yang ling quan (GB34), right tai chong (Liv.3). Tou wei and quan liao used "hui ci fa" ("slow insertion technique"), combined with "long hu jiao zhen" ("dragon and tiger combined diagram") hand techniques. Qu chi, yang ling quan, and tai chong used "long hu sheng jiang" hand techniques. After removing the needles, the hands and feet could move freely, the elbow joint could basically curl up and extend out by itself. Next diagnosis: select points like right side tou wei (St.8), right side quan liao (SI18), right side qu chi (LI11), tai chong, both yang ling quan (GB34), after needle treatment as with the previous two types, the hand techniques used were the opposite, travelling the pathways to the origin. After 5 times, the neck and back pain reduced and went, the upper and lower limbs recovered, and only the knee joint had its sensation of pain, while at nights occasionally he had the spasming pain in the lower limbs. Because of some reason, the patient couldn't continue treatment.

Note: the hand 3 yang jing jin cross at the "horns" (ie. the sides of the head), so select the neighbouring points tou wei (St.8), cross select (ie. counter-lateral select) points to match the idea that "wei jin xiang jiao" ("the head wei and the tendons cross each other"). The foot 3 yang channels tendons cross at the face cheek bones points. So, select the mutually proximal point quan liao (SI18), which also belongs to the technique of "bing zai xia zhe gao qu" ("if the illness is at the lower, select in the upper"). The *Ling shu* said: "shi er jing mai, san bai liu shi wu luo, qi xue qi ci shang yu mian, er zou kong qiao" ("the twelve channels and the three hundred and sixty-five collaterals all their blood and qi goes up to the face and goes to the empty orifices"). The *Zhen jiu da chen* said: "tou wei zhu yang zhi hui, bai mai zhi zong" ("the head is the meeting place of all the yang and the operator of the hundred vessels"). Cold is a yin evil, easily injures the yang qi. If on the head and face select points, on the hand 3 yang channel tendons combined, to help the yang qi, and spread the channel tendons' cold.

"gan zhu jin" ("the liver controls the tendons"), so select the liver channel source point tai chong (Liv.3). Yang ling quan (GB34) is the tendon's meeting point, it can adjust the tendons and also remove the lower limbs sprain painful. Qu chi (LI11) adjusts the yang ming jing jin channel qi, and can smooth the elbows', the arms', and the necks' spasms (contractions).

Section 3
Channels and collaterals identification pattern

Should have whole body view of points.

Using the channels and collaterals to identify patterns, also one should have a whole body view or perspective on points. One must also pay attention to channels, zang fu, and the human body's individual organisation of each organ, and their related connections and related influence principles. Channels and collaterals identification patterns, except for the identification of disease patterns and their related channels and zang fu, should also analyse its pattern belonging to the principles like cold, heat, deficiency and excess, and channels and collaterals, zang fu qi and blood and whether yin yang's more strong or weak. For these, we must simultaneously use the ba gang, and qi and blood etc, identification patterns method. Then one can be more complete and detailed re illness understanding and treatment in the clinic. This can represent the completion and orderliness or identification patterns for treatment. For example:

Case 3: Zhou, xx male 56 years old, case. He felt dizzy, beginning from June 1957, and was found to have high blood pressure when examined and became better after taking medicine. April 8th 1960, first diagnosis, he himself said, in recent years the waist has been sore and the legs soft. Ear sound like tinnitus, hand centres were upset hot, head dizziness and distended painful, found he couldn't concentrate his attention, spirit and body tired, continually took medicine for ½ a year. Illness happened when tired and illness situation then would recover. Examination: blood pressure: 170/110 mm Hg. Face total red, tongue red less coating, pulse bowstring thin. Chest x-ray: both lower lung texture thick and in disorder. Heart left side and heart boundary increase or become large "towers" left side, lower parts. The main artery and the main artery vein bends extremely and has large curves. Eye internal examination: visual web membrane small vessels harness, urine normal check protein (4). Western medicine diagnosis: high blood pressure illness. Identification patterns; liver and kidney yin deficiency, deficient yang flows upwards. Treatment technique: balance the liver, and nourish the kidney, select points; bai hui (GV20), feng chi (GB 20), tai chong (LIV3), tai xi (K3), ran gu (K2). Needling technique, for bai hui (GV 20) use *Nei Jing's* "he gu ci" ("crane needling") combined with man zhang xie fa (needling sedation technique), sedation feng chi (GB 20), tai chong (LIV 3), to soften the liver and hide the yang. For tai xi (K3), ran gu (K2), use tonification technique with fire and tonify the kidney jing (excess), nourish water and therefore wood (bu mu), "conduct the dragon into the sea" introduce the fire to return to the origin. Later diagnose and treated, each time check pulse and tongue. The four diagnoses combine as a reference - select points according to pattern. Needling treatment 18 times, blood pressure went down to 136 over 84 mm Hg. Waist sore, legs soft problem decreased a lot. Head and eyes were clear and comfortable, sleep calm and appetite good. Urine check: normal. Totally treated more than 60 times.

Blood pressure stabilized at about 140/86 mm Hg. He briefly felt body healthy again, etc normal. Visit again in 1967, he was still healthy and had no illness.

Case 4: Wang xx male 41 years old. Worker, April 5th 1957 first diagnosis: reportedly got headaches for more than 1 year. Recently caught cold, then the pain became more serious. Left side was more strong. Face sometimes had hot feeling, accompanied by nausea, mouth bitter, urine red, pulse floating true, tongue body red, less coating. Identification pattern; after catching a cold, it cause the headache to become more serious, the pulse became floating and true, this is wind-cold attacking the collaterals. Tongue body red, less coating, face hot, tinnitus wanted to vomit, mouth bitter and urine red, all are liver fire flaring up information. Following the channels upwards and then interpreting. This belongs to: first heat, later cold. Should use: "yin zhong yin yang" ("heat yang inside hidden yin") hand technique. First above: gall bladder channel, combine points yang ling quan (GB 34). Insert the needle into earth level (di bu), slowly press tensely lift 6 times, return the needle to the heaven level (tian bu), truly press, slowly lift 9 times, then use opposite this technique 3 times. The patient himself said the headaches lessened, then choose feng chi point (GB 20). After this procedure, the headache reduced more than half. April 8th diagnosis again choose yang ling quan (GB 34), tai chong (LIV 3) and use "yin zhong yin yang" hand technique, add, to combine with lie que (LU 7), tou wei (ST 8), after two times totally removed.

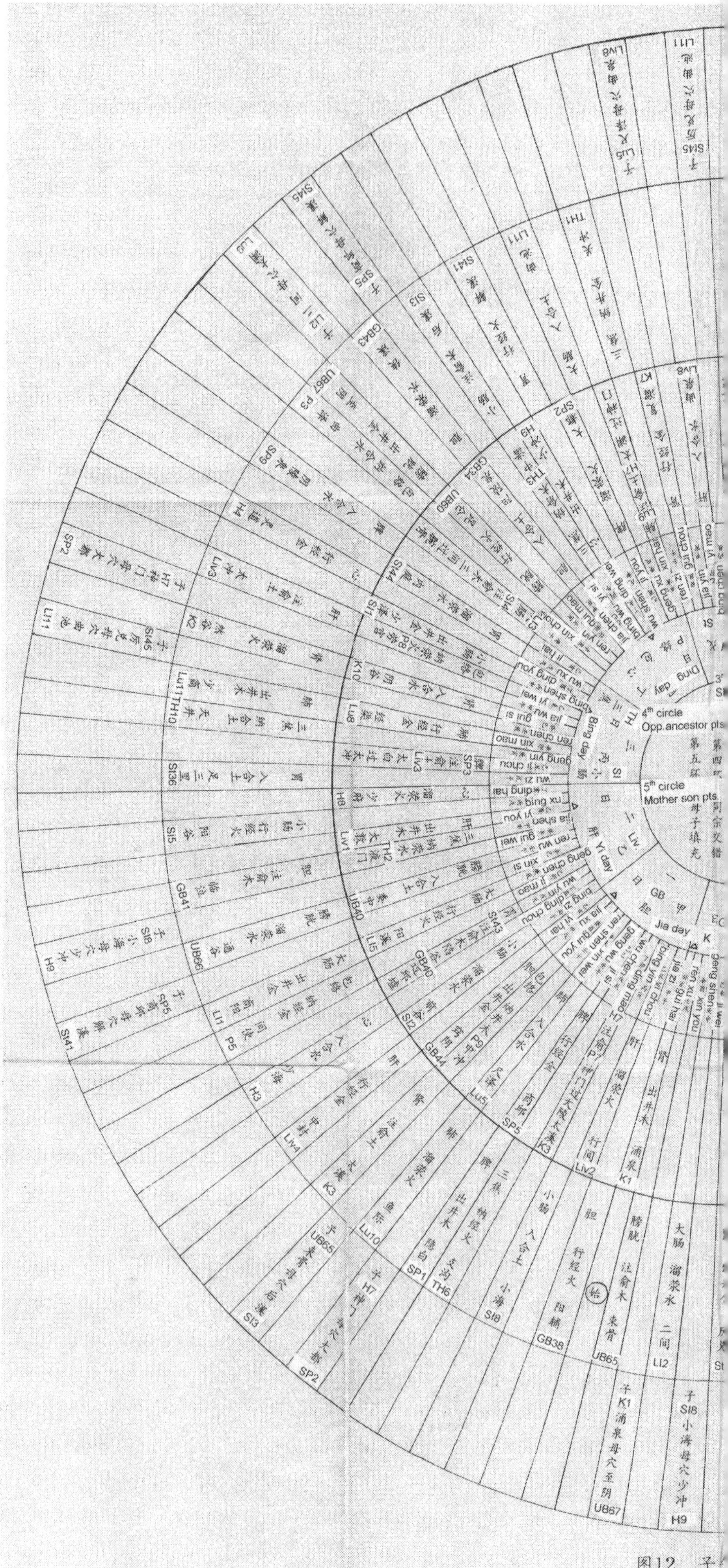

图12 子

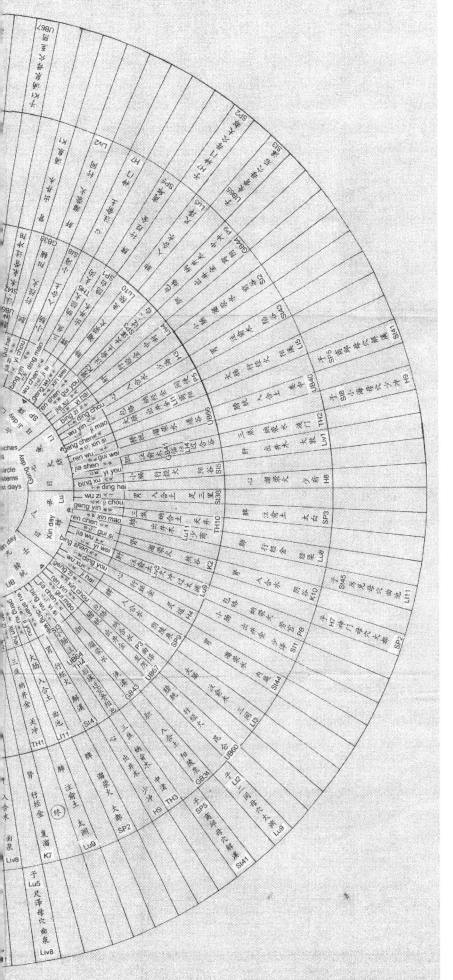

周图

GUAN ZUN HUI

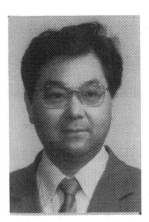

Guan Zun hui is a Director of the Acupuncture Department, China, Kunming City Chinese Medicine Hospital. He is a Professor and also one of the famous Chinese medicine doctors of Yunnan Province, and a member of the standing committee of the Chinese Academia Sinica.

Also, he is a Yunnan Acupuncture Society member, a Canada - Chinese Medicine Acupuncture College (Govt.) Visiting Professor, and a Canada Chinese Medicine Acupuncture Society Honorary Consultant. He has published more than 120 academic papers, published 3 books, and has been awarded a National Invention Patient for G2H heat needle equipment. Soon after, he was awarded 6 awards re national, provincial, and city science technology equipment. He has been awarded special government grants and contracts.

ANDREW MCPHERSON

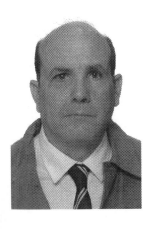

Andrew McPherson has a B.A. (Modern Asian Studies) Degree from Griffith University and is a govt. recognised member of AHPRA. He has been a Doctor of Chinese Medicine for some 30 years or more. He is the president of A.N.A.C.H.A. (the Australian National Acupuncturists and Chinese Herbalists Association) and has written numerous articles for newspapers, magazines, and books. In addition, he has studied in PRC China for extended periods and is a long term student of Professor Guan Zun hui.

d in the United States
er & Taylor Publisher Services

Printed
by Ba